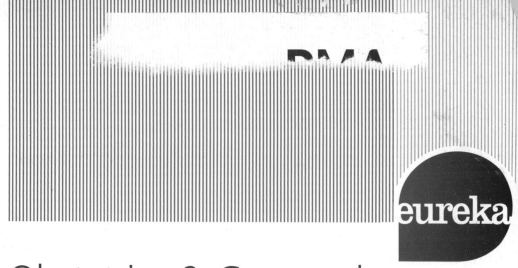

eureka

Obstetrics & Gynaecology

D1427706

0759735

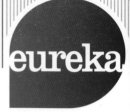

Obstetrics & Gynaecology

Hannah Kither MBChB MRCOG
Clinical Research Fellow in Maternal
Fetal Medicine
Specialty Registrar in Obstetrics and
Gynaecology
University of Manchester
St Mary's Hospital, Central Manchester
University Hospitals NHS Trust
Manchester, UK

Sarah Kitson MB BChir MA MRCOG
Clinical Research Fellow in
Gynaecological Oncology
Specialty Registrar in Obstetrics and
Gynaecology
University of Manchester
St Mary's Hospital, Central Manchester
University Hospitals NHS Trust
Manchester, UK

Y Louise Wan BSc MBBS MSc MRCS
MRCOG
Wellcome Trust Clinical Research Fellow
in Gynaecological Oncology
Specialty Registrar in Obstetrics and
Gynaecology
University of Manchester
St Mary's Hospital, Central Manchester
University Hospitals NHS Trust
Manchester, UK

Emma Crosbie BSc MBChB PhD
MRCOG
Senior Lecturer and Honorary
Consultant Gynaecological Oncologist
University of Manchester
St Mary's Hospital, Central Manchester
University Hospitals NHS Trust
Manchester, UK

Series Editors

Janine Henderson MRCPsych
MClinEd
MB BS Programme Director
Hull York Medical School
York, UK

David Oliveira PhD FRCP
Professor of Renal Medicine
St George's, University of London
London, UK

Stephen Parker BSc MS DipMedEd
FRCS
Consultant Breast and General
Paediatric Surgeon
St Mary's Hospital
Newport, UK

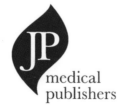

JP
medical
publishers

London • Philadelphia • New Delhi • Panama City

© 2017 JP Medical Ltd.

Published by JP Medical Ltd, 83 Victoria Street, London, SW1H 0HW, UK

Tel: +44 (0)20 3170 8910   Fax: +44 (0)20 3008 6180

Email: info@jpmedpub.com   www.jpmedpub.com, www.eurekamedicine.com

ISBN: 978-1-907816-98-7

British Library Cataloguing in Publication Data
A catalogue record for this book is available from the British Library

Library of Congress Cataloging in Publication Data
A catalog record for this book is available from the Library of Congress

Publisher:	Richard Furn
Development Editors:	Thomas Fletcher, Paul Mayhew, Alison Whitehouse
Editorial Assistants:	Katie Pattullo, Adam Rajah, Sophie Woolven
Copy Editor:	Kim Howell
Graphic narratives:	James Pollitt
Cover design:	Forbes Design
Page design:	Designers Collective Ltd

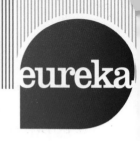

Series Editors' Foreword

Today's medical students need to know a great deal to be effective as tomorrow's doctors. This knowledge includes core science and clinical skills, from understanding biochemical pathways to communicating with patients. Modern medical school curricula integrate this teaching, thereby emphasising how learning in one area can support and reinforce another. At the same time students must acquire sound clinical reasoning skills, working with complex information to understand each individual's unique medical problems.

The *Eureka* series is designed to cover all aspects of today's medical curricula and reinforce this integrated approach. Each book can be used from first year through to qualification. Core biomedical principles are introduced but given relevant clinical context: the authors have always asked themselves, 'why does the aspiring clinician need to know this'?

Each clinical title in the series is grounded in the relevant core science, which is introduced at the start of each book. Each core science title integrates and emphasises clinical relevance throughout. Medical and surgical approaches are included to provide a complete and integrated view of the patient management options available to the clinician. Clinical insights highlight key facts and principles drawn from medical practice. Cases featuring unique graphic narratives are presented with clear explanations that show how experienced clinicians think, enabling students to develop their own clinical reasoning and decision making. Clinical SBAs help with exam revision while Starter questions are a unique learning tool designed to stimulate interest in the subject.

Having biomedical principles and clinical applications together in one book will make their connections more explicit and easier to remember. Alongside repeated exposure to patients and practice of clinical and communication skills, we hope *Eureka* will equip medical students for a lifetime of successful clinical practice.

Janine Henderson, David Oliveira, Stephen Parker

About the Series Editors

Janine Henderson is the MB BS undergraduate Programme Director at Hull York Medical School (HYMS). After medical school at the University of Oxford and clinical training in psychiatry, she combined her work as a consultant with postgraduate teaching roles, moving to the new Hull York Medical School in 2004. She has a particular interest in modern educational methods, curriculum design and clinical reasoning.

David Oliveira is Professor of Renal Medicine at St George's, University of London (SGUL), where he served as the MBBS Course Director between 2007 and 2013. Having trained at Cambridge University and the Westminster Hospital he obtained a PhD in cellular immunology and worked as a renal physician before being appointed as Foundation Chair of Renal Medicine at SGUL.

Stephen Parker is a Consultant Breast & General Paediatric Surgeon at St Mary's Hospital, Isle of Wight. He trained at St George's, University of London, and after service in the Royal Navy was appointed as Consultant Surgeon at University Hospital Coventry. He has a particular interest in e-learning and the use of multimedia platforms in medical education.

About the Authors

Hannah Kither is a Clinical Research Fellow in Maternal Fetal Medicine and a Specialty Registrar in Obstetrics and Gynaecology. She teaches medical students in lectures, tutorials and on the wards, and hopes to inspire new doctors to follow a career in the specialty. She is currently studying the link between stillbirth and systemic lupus erythematosus.

Y Louise Wan is a Wellcome Trust Clinical Research Fellow in Gynaecological Oncology and a Specialty Registrar in Obstetrics and Gynaecology. She has always enjoyed teaching, examining and mentoring medical students. She is investigating the role of targeting the oncofetal antigen 5T4 in ovarian cancer treatment.

Sarah Kitson is a Clinical Research Fellow in Gynaecological Oncology and a Specialty Registrar in Obstetrics and Gynaecology. She enjoys teaching medical students and is an Associate of the Higher Education Academy. She is currently investigating novel treatment strategies for endometrial cancer.

Emma Crosbie is a Senior Lecturer and Honorary Consultant Gynaecological Oncologist at the University of Manchester. She has extensive experience in teaching undergraduates and postgraduates and is a Fellow of the Higher Education Academy. She is currently developing strategies for the prevention of obesity-related endometrial cancer.

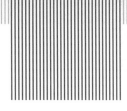

Preface

Obstetrics and gynaecology is a diverse and exciting specialty. Obstetricians are involved in some of the most important moments in a woman's life: her birth, planning her family and the subsequent birth of her own children. Gynaecologists focus on the reproductive and sexual healthcare needs of women outside pregnancy, from the cradle to the grave.

Eureka Obstetrics & Gynaecology equips students with the knowledge needed for exam success and confident clinical practice. It is structured to make it easy to access information and is highly illustrated with images and artworks to aid understanding of key concepts. Cases are included to give an insight into how an experienced clinican would approach a patient and include graphic narratives to illustrate how patients are managed in real life.

Effective clinical care requires an appreciation of the scientific principles and mechanisms that explain how and why things go wrong: these are described in chapter 1. The clinical approach to patients, including relevant signs and symptoms, examination techniques and management options are covered in chapters 2 and 3. Normal and abnormal pregnancy, and specific gynaecological diseases are covered in subsequent chapters, followed by chapters dedicated to emergency situations and integrated clinical care. Finals-style SBA questions are included for effective revision and exam preparation.

We hope *Eureka Obstetrics & Gynaecology* stimulates your learning and inspires your interest in this fascinating specialty.

Hannah Kither, Y Louise Wan, Sarah Kitson, Emma Crosbie
August 2016

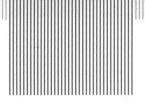

Contents

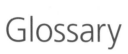

Glossary

AFP	α-fetoprotein
AMH	antimüllerian hormone
APTT	activated partial thromboplastin time
BA	bile acids
BMI	body mass index
BRCA	breast cancer susceptibility gene
CA	cancer antigen
CEA	carcinoembryonic antigen
CN	cranial nerve
COCP	combined oral contraceptive pill
CRP	C-reactive protein
DHEA	dehydroepiandrosterone
DHEA-S	dehydroepiandrosterone sulphate
DNAR	do not attempt resuscitation
DVT	deep vein thrombosis
ECV	external cephalic version
FBC	full blood count
FGM	female genital mutilation
FIGO	International Federation of Gynecology and Obstetrics
FSH	follicle-stimulating hormone
G	gravidity
G+S	group and save
GnRH	gonadotrophin-releasing hormone
GP	general practitioner
β-hCG	β-human chorionic gonadotrophin
HELLP	haemolysis, elevated liver enzymes and low platelets
hMG	human menopausal gonadotrophin
HPO	hypothalamic–pituitary–ovarian
HPV	human papillomavirus
HRT	hormone replacement therapy
HSV	herpes simplex virus
ICSI	intracytoplasmic sperm injection

Ig	immunoglobulin
INR	international normalised ratio
IVF	in vitro fertilisation
LDH	lactate dehydrogenase
LFT	liver function test
LH	luteinising hormone
LLETZ	large loop excision of the transformation zone
LSD	lysergic acid diethylamide
MRSA	methicillin-resistant *Staphylococcus aureus*
NSAID	non-steroidal anti-inflammatory drug
P	parity
PCOS	polycystic ovary syndrome
PID	pelvic inflammatory disease
PMDD	premenstrual dysphoric disorder
PMS	premenstrual syndrome
PT	prothrombin time
Q	perfusion
Rh	Rhesus
SRY	sex-determining region Y gene
STI	sexually transmitted infection
TENS	transcutaneous electrical nerve stimulation
U+E	urea and electrolytes
V	ventilation
WHO	World Health Organization

Acknowledgements

We would like to thank those friends, family and students whose infectious curiosity about what makes us all tick inspired us to put pen to paper.

We are indebted to Chris, Mike, Richard and Phil, for their never-ending love, support and cups of tea.

And finally, to Susanna, Thomas and Louisa: may this book stimulate your love of learning and inspire you to achieve great things.

HK, YLW, SK, EC

Chapter 1
First principles

Overview of the female reproductive system

Starter questions

Answers to the following questions are on page 74

1. What makes us male or female?
2. Can eating foods high in plant oestrogens affect the reproductive system?

The female reproductive system is a collection of organs that enable women to conceive and bear children. Together, these organs:

■ develop female gametes (reproductive cells that contain half the number of chromosomes of a somatic cell)
■ create the ideal environment for their fertilisation (the fusion with a male gamete to form a zygote)
■ support a developing fetus
■ give birth

The endocrine system governs the ways in which the reproductive system develops and changes throughout a woman's life.

The reproductive organs start to develop during gestation, but the system remains immature and non-functional until after puberty. At puberty, increasing levels of sex hormones stimulate the reproductive system to mature (see page 11). During the reproductive years, the cyclical changes of the menstrual cycle cause the maturation and release of

oocytes (female gametes) that enable fertilisation and prepare the uterus for pregnancy
(see page 44).

The quantity and quality of a woman's
oocytes decline over time, so as she ages the
reserve of oocytes capable of fertilisation is
depleted. When the reserve is exhausted,
menopause occurs, marking the end of her
fertility (see page 72).

Structure

The female reproductive system comprises
both internal and external structures with
specific functions (**Table 1.1**).

- The internal structures are the ovaries,
  fallopian tubes, uterus, cervix and vagina
  (**Figure 1.1**)
- The external structures are the vulva, clitoris,
  and labia minora and majora (**Figure 1.2**)

The internal reproductive organs are located
in the pelvis (**Figure 1.3**). The external reproductive organs are situated in the urogenital triangle of the perineum (Figure 1.22).
Innervation and blood supply to these areas
reflect their embryological origin.

Hormonal regulation

The function of the reproductive system is
tightly regulated by the endocrine system,
which ensures that the body maintains a
state in which it is working as efficiently as
possible, i.e. homeostasis. Reproductive

Functions of the female reproductive organs	
Organ	Function(s)
Ovaries	Develop and release oocytes, and secrete female sex hormones
Uterus	Hosts the fetus during pregnancy
Fallopian tubes	Site of fertilisation
	Transport the ovum to the uterus
Cervix	Forms a seal between the internal and external environments
	Facilitates the passage of sperm into the uterus
Vagina	Receives the penis during sexual intercourse
	Provides a passage for the loss of menstrual blood
	Acts as a birth canal
Breasts	Produce milk to feed the infant

Table 1.1 Organs of the female reproductive system and their functions

hormones are chemical messengers that co-
ordinate changes in multiple sites around
the body (e.g. the breasts, the female reproductive tract, the brain) to facilitate sexual
reproduction. Reproductive hormones are
secreted directly into the bloodstream by
endocrine glands, specifically the pituitary
gland and ovaries, where they are transported
to their target organs.

Internal structures of the female reproductive system

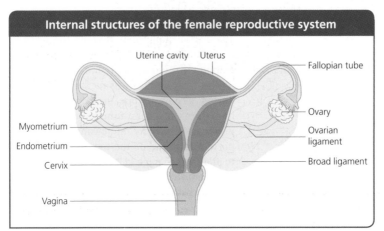

Uterine cavity   Uterus
Fallopian tube
Ovary
Myometrium
Ovarian ligament
Endometrium
Broad ligament
Cervix
Vagina

Figure 1.1 The internal structures of the female reproductive system: the ovaries, fallopian tubes, uterus, cervix and vagina.

External structures of the female reproductive system

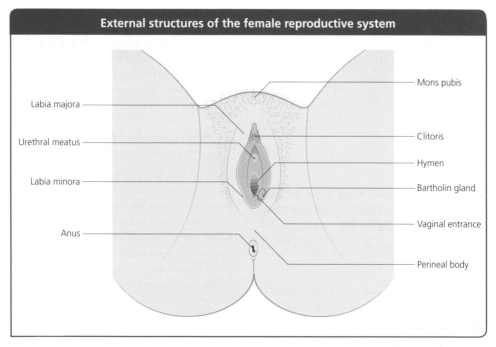

Figure 1.2 The external structures of the female reproductive system. The labia minora and majora protect the clitoris, urethral meatus and vaginal entrance. The vulva includes all these structures as well as the mons pubis. The Bartholin gland opens into the vagina.

Anatomy of the female pelvis

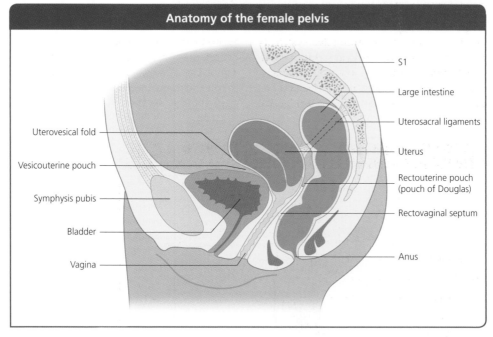

Figure 1.3 Anatomy of the female pelvis (sagittal section). In this view, the ovaries lie lateral to the uterus and are not visible.

Feedback loops

Levels of reproductive hormones are regulated by both internal and external factors. For example, high levels of circulating oestrogen and progesterone inhibit further production of oestrogen and progesterone from the ovary (**Figure 1.4a**). This is known as a feedback loop. Feedback loops can be either negative or positive.

Negative feedback

In a negative feedback loop, as in the previous example, the effects of the hormone include inhibition of further secretion; this ensures controlled release. Most hormones are regulated by this type of feedback.

Positive feedback

In a positive feedback loop, a hormone's effects potentiate further release of hormone. This amplifies the hormone's signal and continues until its level reaches a threshold at which an event occurs that returns the system to basal levels. The control of ovulation is an example of positive feedback. The release of luteinising hormone (LH) causes an increase in oestrogen production by the ovaries, which in turn stimulates the anterior pituitary gland to release more LH (**Figure 1.4b**). This results in the LH surge that triggers ovulation.

Hypothalamic hormones

Production of reproductive hormones is inhibited by external factors such as stress and malnutrition; in this way, the body prioritises energy for survival over reproduction. The hypothalamus acts as a control hub to integrate feedback from the pituitary gland and the ovaries with other factors from the environment.

The hypothalamus is a small gland in the brain that controls the release of hormones from the pituitary gland. Release of hormones from the anterior pituitary gland is controlled by releasing and inhibiting hormones secreted by the hypothalamus. Hormone release from the posterior pituitary gland is controlled by

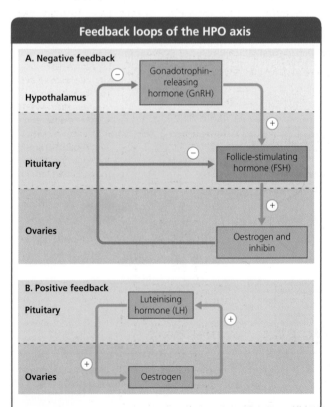

Figure 1.4 Feedback loops of the hypothalamic–pituitary–ovarian (HPO) axis. (a) Negative feedback. Stimulation of the ovaries by follicle-stimulating hormone (FSH) leads to follicular maturation and an increase in oestrogen. The increased levels of oestrogen inhibit further secretion of the stimulating hormones FSH and gonadotrophin-releasing hormone (GnRH). (b) Positive feedback. Luteinising hormone (LH) stimulates the production of oestrogen, which in turn potentiates further secretion of LH. Once LH levels reach a threshold, ovulation occurs and oestrogen levels fall.

neural signals from the hypothalamus. Anatomically, the hypothalamus sits between the thalamus and the pituitary gland.

The hypothalamus synthesises various hormones (**Table 1.2**). These enter:

- the circulatory system via the posterior pituitary gland
- the hypophyseal portal system (blood vessels connecting the hypothalamus with the anterior pituitary) to exclusively stimulate the anterior pituitary

The hypothalamic–pituitary–ovarian axis comprises negative and positive feedback loops thats act via the hypothalamus, pituitary and ovaries to control the female reproductive system (**Figure 1.5**).

Oxytocin

This peptide hormone (a short chain of amino acids), is synthesised in the cell bodies of magnocellar cells found within the hypothalamus. The axons of these neuroendocrine cells (neural cells which secrete hormones) project into the posterior pituitary. Oxytocin is stored in membrane-bound vesicles at the tips of these axons in the posterior

Pituitary hormones and female reproductive function		
Hormone	Site of production and/or secretion	Action(s)
Oxytocin	Produced by the hypothalamus and secreted by the posterior pituitary	Stimulates uterine contraction
		Stimulates milk ejection ('let-down')
		Promotes bonding and sexual arousal
Luteinising hormone	Gonadotrophic cells in the anterior pituitary	Stimulates sex hormone production
		Triggers ovulation
Follicle-stimulating hormone	Gonadotrophic cells in the anterior pituitary	Stimulates development of ovarian follicles
Prolactin	Lactotrophic cells in the anterior pituitary	Stimulates milk production

Table 1.2 Hormones secreted by the pituitary gland with roles in female reproductive function

pituitary and is released into the circulatory system in response to electrical activity from the hypothalamus. Peptide hormones, like oxytocin, cannot pass through cell

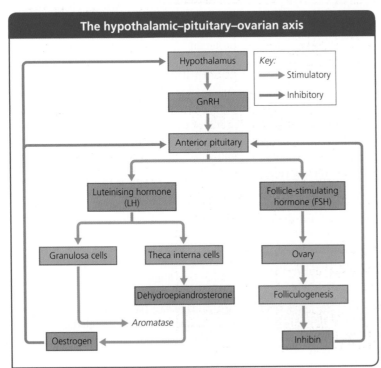

Figure 1.5 The hypothalamic–pituitary–ovarian axis. The hypothalamus, pituitary and ovaries secrete hormones that regulate their own production and secretion. Together, they control the function of the female reproductive system.

membranes and must bind to cell surface receptors to trigger changes within target cells.

The main functions of oxytocin are to:

- stimulate uterine contractions during labour (see page 65)
- stimulate milk ejection ('let-down') during lactation (see page 71)

Oxytocin is also thought to have a role in social behaviour, for example enhancing the development of the bond between mother and baby and strengthening the emotional bond between sexual partners. The mechanisms through which these effects occur are not well understood.

> **Oxytocin has a mild antidiuretic effect.** This is because its chemical structure differs from antidiuretic hormone by only 2 amino acids. In large doses, such as when used to augment labour for a prolonged period, this can cause hyponatraemia.

Gonadotrophin-releasing hormone

This is a peptide hormone produced by the hypothalamus. It stimulates the anterior pituitary to produce gonadotrophins. These hormones, namely LH and follicle-stimulating hormone (FSH), stimulate the activity of the gonads.

Gonadotrophin-releasing hormone (GnRH) is secreted in bursts known as pulses, causing circulating levels to rise and fall in short periods of time. The frequency and amplitude of these pulses are more important than the presence or absence of GnRH in determining the body's response. For example, in childhood GnRH secretion is low. GnRH pulses increase in frequency and amplitude to trigger sexual maturation at puberty. During the reproductive years, the characteristics of GnRH pulses vary throughout the menstrual cycle.

- High-frequency GnRH release during the first 14 days of the menstrual cycle favours secretion of LH
- Low-frequency GnRH pulses after ovulation favour secretion of FSH

Thus, changes in the frequency of GnRH pulses control not only the amount of gonadotrophins released but also the ratio of LH to FSH.

> **Continuous release of GnRH leads to a rapid decrease in the production of LH and FSH.** As a result, oestrogen production is blocked. Slow-release GnRH analogues are used therapeutically to treat oestrogen-dependent conditions such as endometriosis.

Negative feedback controls GnRH release. Increasing levels of oestrogen down-regulate both the release of GnRH by the hypothalamus and the release of LH and FSH by the anterior pituitary.

Pituitary hormones

LH and FSH are synthesised in the anterior pituitary and released in response to GnRH secreted from the hypothalamus. These hormones are known as gonadotrophins, because they act on the ovaries to regulate the production of ovarian hormones (see page 7) and stimulate oocyte maturation during folliculogenesis (see page 36).

Gonadotrophin production is stimulated by GnRH but inhibited by inhibin (a by-product of folliculogenesis), oestrogen and prolactin.

Luteinising hormone

This is a glycoprotein secreted by gonadotrophic cells in the anterior pituitary in response to high-frequency GnRH pulses. It stimulates production of sex hormones (see page 7) in both males and females and in females triggers ovulation.

In women, sex hormone secretion begins with the stimulation of thecal cells (secretory cells that form a shell around the maturing follicle) to produce dehydroepiandrosterone (DHEA). DHEA is converted to oestrogen by granulosa cells, which make up the ovarian follicles (see **Figure 1.5**). Positive feedback by the increasing levels of oestrogen stimulate further LH release (see **Figure 1.4**). This results in an LH surge, midway through the menstrual cycle, that triggers ovulation (see page 37).

After ovulation, LH causes granulosa and thecal cells to differentiate to form a temporary sex hormone-secreting structure known as the corpus luteum, which secretes oestrogen and progesterone. High oestrogen and progesterone levels cause negative feedback, inhibiting the release of FSH and LH, and preventing further follicle development and ovulation. Once LH falls below a certain level, the corpus luteum degenerates and oestrogen and progesterone levels fall. This releases the negative feedback inhibition and a new menstrual cycle starts.

Follicle-stimulating hormone

This hormone is secreted by the anterior pituitary in response to low-frequency GnRH pulses. FSH stimulates the recruitment and growth of ovarian follicles (see page 37). These follicles secrete oestrogen, which in turn inhibits the release of FSH (see **Figure 1.4**). Because of this negative feedback, FSH levels decrease rapidly during the follicular phase of the menstrual cycle (see page 37).

Larger, more developed follicles are less dependent on FSH for their continued development. As FSH levels fall, it is only the largest follicles that continue to mature. The oestrogen produced by these follicles suppresses FSH release further. This process selects for a single follicle, known as the dominant follicle, that matures to the point of ovulation each cycle.

Prolactin

This peptide hormone is synthesised primarily by lactotroph cells in the anterior pituitary. It is also secreted by the uterus, placenta and mammary glands during pregnancy and lactation.

Prolactin promotes milk production (lactation) and maternal bonding. Unlike the secretion of other anterior pituitary hormones, prolactin is secreted continuously and only inhibited by the release of dopamine from the hypothalamus. When dopamine levels fall, its inhibition is released and prolactin is secreted again.

> **Drugs that block the effects of dopamine**, such as the atypical antipsychotics risperidone and quetiapine, may cause excess prolactin secretion (hyperprolactinaemia). A drug history should always be taken in women presenting with symptoms of hyperprolactinaemia, such as amenorrhoea or galactorrhoea.

Ovarian hormones

Oestrogen and progesterone are commonly referred to as sex hormones. These steroid hormones are produced by the ovaries and are responsible for preparing the reproductive system for possible pregnancy. As steroid hormones, they diffuse through the cell membranes and bind to receptors in the nucleus to modulate the expression of genes.

Their secretion is stimulated by the pituitary hormones LH and FSH as part of the hypothalamic–pituitary–ovarian axis. Oestrogen and progesterone levels rise and fall cyclically in response to LH and FSH after puberty; this continues until a woman reaches the menopause. The release of LH and FSH is stimulated by the hypothalamic hormone GnRH. Oestrogen inhibits the production of LH, FSH and GnRH through negative feedback.

Oestrogen

This hormone prepares the body for pregnancy. Specifically, oestrogen enables the development of female secondary sexual characteristics, thickens the endometrium and triggers ovulation (**Table 1.3**).

Once secreted into the circulation, 95–98% of oestrogen molecules bind to transport proteins such as albumin and sex hormone-binding globulin. This prolongs the life of steroid hormones and makes them more soluble in the blood. Only 1–2% of oestrogen is unbound: this fraction is free to diffuse into target cells where it modulates expression of target genes. The level of sex hormone-binding globulin, therefore, controls the amount of biologically-active oestrogen available to act on cells.

Ovarian hormones: sites of production and actions		
Hormone	Site of production	Action(s)
Oestrogen	Thecal and granulosa cells	Promotes development of female sex organs at puberty
		Prepares body for pregnancy
		Promotes fat distribution in female pattern
Progesterone	Corpus luteum	Prepares and maintains the endometrium
		Prepares the breasts for lactation
		Thickens cervical mucus
		Inhibits uterine contractility in pregnancy
Androgens	Thecal cells	Promotes bone mineralisation
		Increases sexual desire

Table 1.3 Sites of production and actions of ovarian hormones

Girls who are obese are more likely to have early menarche (onset of menstruation). Obesity leads to lower levels of sex hormone–binding globulin and increases levels of biologically active oestrogen. Prolonged action of biologically active oestrogens predisposes obese girls to hormonally driven cancers, such as endometrial cancer, in adulthood.

Progesterone

This hormone opposes the proliferative effect of oestrogen on the endometrium, and helps to mature the endometrium by promoting the differentiation of glandular structures. Progesterone maintains the body in a suitable state to support pregnancy. It dampens the maternal immune response to placental and fetal tissues, and decreases the contractility of uterine smooth muscle.

Development of the female reproductive system

Starter questions

Answers to the following questions are on page 74.

3. Why are some babies born with ambiguous genitalia?
4. Why is the average age of puberty falling?

The female reproductive system develops in stages: the organs are formed during fetal life, but mature and become functional during puberty. The onset of menstruation (menarche) occurs in response to increased activity of the hypothalamic–pituitary–ovarian axis. It takes 3–4 years for regular menstrual cycles to become established; the onset of which is a sign that an individual's reproductive system has reached maturity.

Fetal development

Sexual differentiation occurs during the first trimester of pregnancy (weeks 1–13). The female reproductive organs develop in three main stages:

- differentiation of the gonads
- differentiation of internal reproductive organs
- differentiation of external genitalia

Differentiation of the gonads

Male and female embryos are indistinguishable until the 7th week of pregnancy. The first reproductive organs to differentiate are the gonads.

Differentiation of the gonads into either testes or ovaries depends on whether or not the embryo has a Y chromosome. In males, expression of the sex-determining region Y gene (SRY), located on the Y chromosome, activates a series of further genes that induce the primordial gonads to develop into testes.

Because females lack a Y chromosome, SRY is absent, so ovaries develop instead.

Sex is usually considered an objective biological category – male or female – based on distinct physical characteristics determined by an individual's sex chromosomes. However, intersex conditions challenge this binary classification. For example, an individual with androgen insensitivity syndrome, who has a Y chromosome and is therefore genetically male, may develop female external genitalia and identify as female.

Gender is generally regarded as a construct based on what a particular society considers 'masculine' and 'feminine'. As such, it is subjective and may not match an individual's sex. For example, a transgender person has a gender identity that differs from the sex they were assigned at birth.

Differentiation of the internal reproductive organs

The internal reproductive tracts in men and women develop from embryonic structures known as the mesonephric and paramesonephric ducts. If the gonads develop into ovaries, no testosterone or antimullerian hormone are produced; these hormones usually suppress the differentiation of the

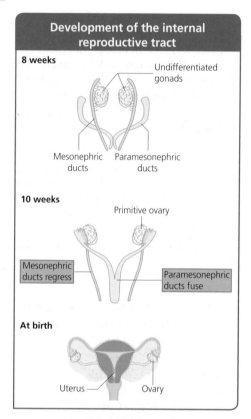

Development of the internal reproductive tract

8 weeks

Undifferentiated gonads

Mesonephric ducts   Paramesonephric ducts

10 weeks

Primitive ovary

Mesonephric ducts regress

Paramesonephric ducts fuse

At birth

Uterus   Ovary

Figure 1.6 Development of the internal reproductive tract. The paramesonephric ducts fuse to form the fallopian tubes, uterus, cervix and upper part of the vagina. The mesonephric ducts regress. The vaginal plate grows and canalises to form the lower part of the vagina.

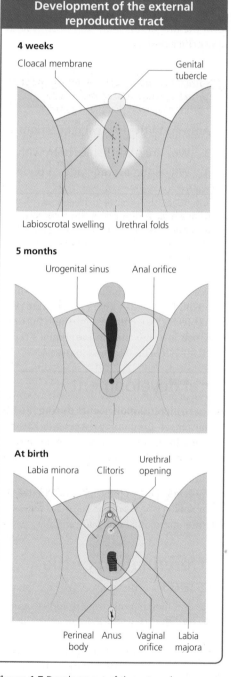

Development of the external reproductive tract

4 weeks

Cloacal membrane   Genital tubercle

Labioscrotal swelling   Urethral folds

5 months

Urogenital sinus   Anal orifice

At birth

Labia minora   Clitoris   Urethral opening

Perineal body   Anus   Vaginal orifice   Labia majora

Figure 1.7 Development of the external reproductive tract. Without the influence of androgens, the fetus develops female external genitalia. The labioscrotal swellings form the labia majora. The urethral folds develop into the labia minora, urethral opening and vaginal opening. The genital tubercle forms the glans of the clitoris.

paramesonephric duct. In the absence of these hormones the uterus, fallopian tubes, cervix and upper third of the vagina develop from the paramesonephric ducts while the mesonephric ducts, which in males become the epididymis, regress (**Figure 1.6**). This process is completed by the 4th month of pregnancy.

Differentiation of the external genitalia

The external female genital tract forms during the first trimester. As with the differentiation of female internal organs, differentiation of the female external genitalia occurs by default in the absence of testosterone (**Figure 1.7**). In both sexes, the urethral folds elongate and fuse to form the cloacal membrane. This membrane separates to form the urogenital sinus anteriorly and the anal orifice posteriorly.

> **Normal ovarian function is not essential for the development of the female reproductive tract.** People who have complete gonadal dysgenesis (Swyer's syndrome) develop a female reproductive tract despite having an Y chromosome. Their gonads fail to differentiate into testes, and therefore they are unable to produce the testosterone and antimüllerian hormone necessary to form a male reproductive tract. Because they have no functioning ovaries, they do not develop female secondary sexual characteristics at puberty.

The upper third of the vagina is formed by the paramesonephric ducts. The lower two thirds derive from the vaginal plate, a thickened area of endoderm lining the urogenital sinus. The cells at the centre of this thickened tissue break down to form a lumen by the 5th month of pregnancy. A thin membrane known as the hymen remains, which separates the lumen from the urogenital sinus. A small opening forms in this membrane around the time of birth. The urethral orifice is located anteriorly and the vagina posteriorly within the vestibule of this sinus. The urogenital folds lying lateral to these openings also remain unfused and develop into the labia minora. The labioscrotal folds form the labia majora, and the genital tubercle forms the clitoris.

Puberty

Puberty is the process by which physical changes make the body capable of sexual reproduction. In both girls and boys, the onset of puberty is triggered by an increase in the frequency and amount of GnRH released by the hypothalamus.

In girls, the first signs of puberty usually appear between the ages of 8 and 14 years (**Table 1.4**). It is usually completed within 3–5 years of onset.

Puberty is a period of accelerated growth, redistribution of body fat and development of secondary sexual characteristics:

- development of breasts
- development of axillary hair
- redistribution of body fat
- development of pubic hair
- accelerated growth and fusion of epiphyses

These changes occur in a set order and can be classified into the distinct stages of the Tanner

Stages of puberty			
Stage	Defining feature(s)	Average age at onset (years)	Requirements
Growth spurt	Accelerated growth, fusion of growth plates	8–10	Functional hypothalamic–pituitary–ovarian axis, increasing oestrogen levels, growth hormone
Thelarche	Breast bud development	8–10	Functional hypothalamic–pituitary–ovarian axis, increasing oestrogen levels
Pubarche	Growth of pubic and axillary hair	10–13	Increasing androgen levels as a result of adrenal maturation
Adrenarche	Increased secretion of androgens from the adrenal cortex, resulting in oily skin, acne, pubic hair and body odour	10–11	Adrenal function and maturation May occur independently of gonadal maturity
Menarche	Menstruation	12–13	Functional hypothalamic–pituitary–ovarian axis, increasing oestrogen levels

Table 1.4 Stages of puberty

scale; those for girls are shown in Table 8.3. The appearance of each characteristic marks the maturation of different components of the reproductive system, and the absence of certain features is useful in determining the cause of any abnormalities in puberty.

■ The first sign of puberty in girls is the development of breast buds (thelarche)
■ This is followed a few months later by the development of pubic hair
■ Menarche occurs about 2 years after thelarche

> **In the first few years after menarche, 90% of menstrual cycles are anovulatory. Girls experience heavy and irregular bleeding during this time.** Within 3–4 years, their periods become more regular as ovulatory cycles become established.

Menarche

At puberty, increased hypothalamic secretion of GnRH stimulates secretion of FSH by the pituitary. FSH, in turn, stimulates the development of ovarian follicles, which secrete oestrogen as they mature. During puberty, increasing oestrogen levels increase the frequency and amplitude of GnRH secretion by positive feedback; this results in an LH surge, ovulation and the onset of menstruation.

The average age of menarche is 12–15 years. The timing of menarche is affected by factors such as diet, genetics and overall health. For example, girls with higher dietary energy intake have earlier menarche, while girls with chronic illnesses, such as Crohn's disease or kidney diseases, have delayed menarche.

The ovaries

Starter questions

Answers to the following questions are on page 74.

5. Why is ovarian torsion an emergency?
6. Does removing one ovary affect the length of the menstrual cycle?

The ovaries are two almond-shaped organs about 2 cm wide, 5 cm long and 1 cm thick. They lie within small depressions in the pelvic side wall, known as the ovarian fossae, and are held in place by the infundibulopelvic (suspensory) ligament, the ovarian ligament and the broad ligament (**Figure 1.8**).

Arterial supply and venous drainage

The blood vessels supplying and draining the ovaries reflect their embryological origin in the abdomen. The right and left ovarian arteries arise directly from the descending abdominal aorta and pass over the pelvic brim as they enter the pelvis to reach the ovaries via the infundibulopelvic ligaments (**Figure 1.9**). Venous drainage is via the two ovarian veins, which travel, along with their corresponding arteries, within the infundibulopelvic ligament.

- The right ovarian vein drains directly into the inferior vena cava
- The left ovarian vein drains into the left renal vein

Nerve supply

The ovaries receive sympathetic and parasympathetic innervation arising from abdominal and pelvic plexuses. Visceral pain travels via sensory afferent fibres that accompany the sympathetic fibres to the level of T10-T12.

Lymphatic drainage

The ovaries drain to the para-aortic lymph nodes (**Table 1.5**).

Histology

Each ovary is covered by a single layer of flat cuboidal epithelial cells (ovarian surface

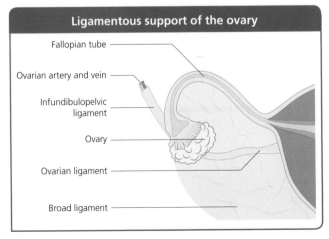

Ligamentous support of the ovary

- Fallopian tube
- Ovarian artery and vein
- Infundibulopelvic ligament
- Ovary
- Ovarian ligament
- Broad ligament

Figure 1.8 Ligamentous support of the ovary. The ovary is held in position by the infundibulopelvic ligament, the ovarian ligament and the broad ligament.

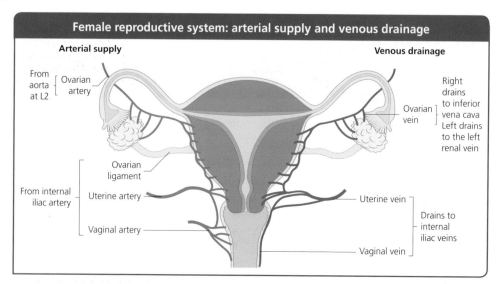

Female reproductive system: arterial supply and venous drainage

Arterial supply

Venous drainage

From aorta at L2 — Ovarian artery

Right drains to inferior vena cava — Ovarian vein

Left drains to the left renal vein

Ovarian ligament

From internal iliac artery — Uterine artery

Vaginal artery

Uterine vein

Drains to internal iliac veins

Vaginal vein

Figure 1.9 Arterial supply and venous drainage of the female reproductive system.

Lymphatic drainage of female reproductive organs	
Organ(s)	Lymph node drainage
Ovaries and fallopian tubes	Para-aortic lymph nodes
Uterine fundus	Para-aortic lymph nodes
Uterine body and isthmus	External iliac lymph nodes
Cervix	Internal and external iliac lymph nodes
Vagina	Iliac and superficial inguinal lymph nodes
Vulva	Superficial inguinal nodes

Table 1.5 Lymphatic drainage of the female reproductive system

epithelium) and a thick layer of connective tissue called the tunica albuginea. The ovary has two histological compartments (**Figure 1.10**):

- the cortex, which contains the developing ovarian follicles
- the medulla, its vascular central core

Function

The ovaries have two main functions:

- production and release of female gametes (secondary oocytes) capable of being fertilised
- production of oestrogen and progesterone to control the development and function of the female reproductive system (see page 7)

The development of secondary oocytes from precursor egg cells (primordial germ cells) occurs by a process called oogenesis. This requires the development of a surrounding support structure known as a follicle; this process is folliculogenesis. Each oocyte develops within a single follicle, meaning oogenesis and folliculogenesis occur in conjunction (**Table 1.6**). They start during embryonic development, pause during childhood, restart with the onset of puberty and continue until the menopause.

By the time she is born, a female infant has all the primordial follicles (dormant follicles) she will ever develop. Thus, women are born

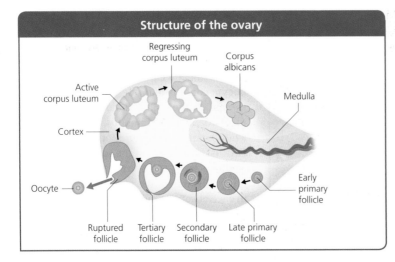

Structure of the ovary

Regressing corpus luteum
Corpus albicans
Active corpus luteum
Medulla
Cortex
Oocyte
Early primary follicle
Ruptured follicle
Tertiary follicle
Secondary follicle
Late primary follicle

Figure 1.10 Structure of the ovary. The ovary consists of the cortex, which contains developing follicles, and a vascular central core, the medulla.

Stages of folliculogenesis and oogenesis

Stage of folliculogenesis	Appearance of follicle	Stage of oogenesis	Stage of cell division within oocyte
Primordial follicle	Single layer of granulosa cells (follicle is dormant and awaiting recruitment)	Oogonia become primary oocytes	Meiosis until prophase I
Primary follicle	Granulosa cell layer thickens, zona pellucida forms, thecal cells start to grow	Primary oocyte	Meiosis halted
Secondary follicle	Thecal cells separate into theca externa and interna	Primary oocyte	Meiosis halted
Tertiary follicle (graafian follicle)	Follicular fluid is produced, resulting in a fluid-filled antrum. Oocyte projects into antrum of follicle surrounded by a thickened mound of granulosa cells (cumulus oophorus; see **Figure 1.12**)	Secondary oocyte	Meiosis restarts and continues until metaphase II

Table 1.6 Stages of folliculogenesis and corresponding stages of oogenesis

with a finite number of both eggs and follicles. Over the course of her life, the follicle count gradually declines: each day around 30 primordial follicles start the 13-month long process of folliculogenesis. Less than 1% of follicles mature to the stage where ovulation occurs, instead undergoing atresia (cell death). Menopause occurs when there are no follicles left. In contrast, men continue to produce new gametes throughout adulthood.

Oogenesis

Oogenesis is the production of a mature egg (ovum) with a single set of 23 unpaired chromosomes, i.e. a haploid cell (n), from a primordial germ cell with two sets of paired chromosomes, i.e. a diploid cell (2n) (**Figure 1.11**). The process begins in utero and is not fully completed until after fertilisation.

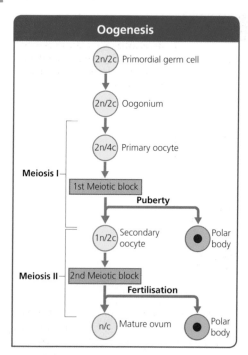

Figure 1.11 Oogenesis. Oocytes are held in meiosis I until puberty. Meiosis is completed only after fertilisation. c, chromatid number (numbers of copies of DNA); n, haploid number (23 chromosomes); 2n, diploid number (23 pairs of chromosomes, i.e. 46 chromosomes).

Before birth

In the third week of development primordial germ cells migrate into the gonads and differentiate into oogonia. These cells then divide by mitosis to produce millions of oogonia. By the 5th month of pregnancy, there are up to 7 million oogonia. These cells enter into meiosis and become primary oocytes. Primary oocytes contain two sets of chromosomes: a maternal and a paternal set. During the first meiotic division, each set duplicates to form two daughter chromosomes (4c chromatids). Meiosis pauses here until puberty (1st meiotic block). Many of the oogonia that start differentiating do not survive this process: by birth, approximately 2 million oogonia have differentiated to become oocytes, the rest degenerate.

After puberty

From puberty, a single primary oocyte is triggered to undergo maturation by the cyclical peak in LH each month. One to two days prior to ovulation, the primary oocyte completes its first meiotic division to form two haploid cells: a secondary oocyte, containing most of the cytoplasm, and a polar body. Each secondary oocyte contains half the number of chromosomes (23), but each chromosome is still made up of 2 daughter chromatids. Meiosis is halted again until fertilisation (2nd meiotic block). Fertilisation triggers the oocyte to divide again to form a mature ovum and a polar body. This halves the number of chromatids in each chromosome, leaving a cell with a single set of chromosomes, each made up of one chromatid. The polar bodies degenerate and never become mature oocytes.

Folliculogenesis

Follicles comprise a shell of somatic cells that develop in stages over about 13 months by a process called folliculogenesis (**Figure 1.12**).

During fetal development, each primary oocyte becomes enveloped by an outer layer of support cells to form a primordial follicle. These follicles remain dormant until puberty when 20–30 primordial follicles begin to develop each day. As the follicle develops, granulosa cells form multiple flattened layers around the oocyte. Follicular cells and the oocyte secrete glycoproteins that establish a coat around the oocyte called the zona pellucida. When this process is complete, the follicle is called a secondary follicle.

As the follicle develops into a tertiary (graafian) follicle, it recruits further layers of thecal cells and develops a large fluid-filled cavity called the antrum. The follicular fluid in the antrum nourishes the oocyte.

The thecal cells form two layers: the theca externa and the theca interna.

- The theca interna secretes androgens in response to stimulation by LH; these are converted into oestrogen by aromatases produced by the granulosa cells
- The theca externa contains smooth muscle cells that facilitate rupture of the follicle at ovulation

This process can take up to 300 days, during which the developing follicles are not gonadotropin-dependent. All but 0.01% of

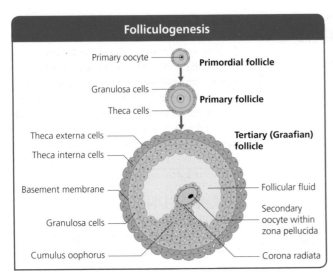

Folliculogenesis

Primary oocyte — **Primordial follicle**

Granulosa cells —
Primary follicle
Theca cells —

Theca externa cells —
Tertiary (Graafian) follicle
Theca interna cells —

Basement membrane — — Follicular fluid

Granulosa cells — — Secondary oocyte within zona pellucida

Cumulus oophorus — — Corona radiata

Figure 1.12 Folliculogenesis. After menarche, a dominant follicle develops each month. Increasing numbers of granulosa and thecal cells surround the oocyte during this process.

the developing primordial follicles die before reaching the tertiary follicle stage. If a follicle reaches this stage, it becomes responsive to FSH, which causes it to grow rapidly. As the follicle grows, it secretes increasing amounts of oestrogen and inhibin. Oestrogen and inhibin reduce FSH production by negative feedback. The follicle best able to continue maturing despite decreasing levels of FSH becomes the dominant follicle during that cycle. The other follicles degenerate; this is known as follicular atresia.

The fallopian tubes

Starter questions

The answer to the following question is on page 74.

7. Why are fallopian tubes often the site of ectopic pregnancies?

The fallopian tubes, also known as the salpinges, are ciliated seromuscular ducts that convey the fertilised ovum to the uterine body. They are situated within the upper edge of the broad ligament. At the distal end are the fimbriae. These are finger-like projections closely applied to the ovarian surface. From distal to medial, the rest of the fallopian tube is divided into the infundibulum, ampulla, isthmus and interstitium (**Figure 1.13**).

Arterial supply

Their blood supply is via the uterine and ovarian arteries located within the mesosalpinx (see **Figure 1.9**). They are drained by the corresponding venous plexuses.

Nerve supply

The fallopian tubes are innervated by both sympathetic and parasympathetic fibres. Sensory signals travel via fibres from T11 to L1.

Lymphatic drainage

The fallopian tubes drain to the iliac and para-aortic lymph nodes (see **Table 1.5**).

Histology

The tubal wall consists of three layers (**Figure 1.14**):

- the internal mucosa
- the intermediate muscular layer
- the outer serosa

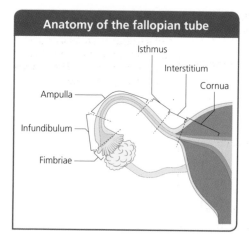

Anatomy of the fallopian tube

Isthmus

Interstitium

Cornua

Ampulla

Infundibulum

Fimbriae

Figure 1.13 Anatomy of the fallopian tube. The fallopian tube comprises the fimbriae, infundibulum, ampulla, isthmus and interstitium.

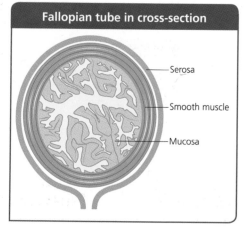

Fallopian tube in cross-section

Serosa

Smooth muscle

Mucosa

Figure 1.14 Cross-section of the fallopian tube, showing the three layers of the tubal wall: mucosa, muscular layer and serosa.

The internal mucosa contains ciliated and secretory cells. Both cell types aid in tubal transit.

> **Ciliary dysfunction in the fallopian tubes is associated with subfertility and ectopic implantation of pregnancies.** Subfertility and ectopic pregnancy occur as a result of the delay in transit of sperm to the oocyte and of the fertilised ovum to the uterus.

Function

The primary function of the fallopian tube is to facilitate the meeting of oocyte and sperm. At ovulation, the fimbriae contract rhythmically to sweep the oocyte into the duct. The oocyte then passes medially, aided by the peristaltic contractions of the smooth muscle of the tubal wall, into the infundibulum and then to the ampulla through the isthmus and onwards into the uterine body. If insemination occurs around the time of ovulation, sperm travel up through the uterus into the fallopian tubes to meet the oocyte.

Fertilisation occurs in the ampulla of the fallopian tube. The fertilised ovum, propelled by peristaltic contractions, travels to the uterus for implantation.

Fertilisation and transport are facilitated by three factors:

- tubal contractility
- ciliary movement
- tubal secretions

Peristaltic contractions propel the ovum along the fallopian tube (**Figure 1.15**). Tubal contractility is regulated by both changes in oestrogen and progesterone levels during the menstrual cycle and the sympathetic nervous system. Oestrogen stimulates tubal contractility, whereas progesterone has the opposite effect. Increasing progesterone levels after ovulation make the smooth muscle more responsive to sympathetic signals. Sympathetic stimulation relaxes the circular muscles of the isthmus, thereby allowing the passage of a fertilised ovum into the uterus.

Cilia are hair-like structures on the surface of the internal mucosa. They beat rhythmically to ensure the unidirectional travel of the ovum (see **Figure 1.15**).

Tubal secretions aid fertilisation by acting as lubricant and nourish the fertilised ovum before implantation.

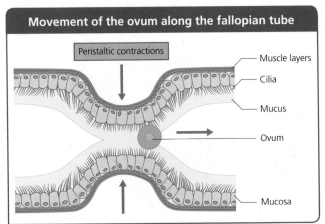

Movement of the ovum along the fallopian tube

Peristaltic contractions

Muscle layers
Cilia
Mucus
Ovum
Mucosa

Figure 1.15 Following fertilisation, the oocyte and pre-embryo are moved along the fallopian tube by peristaltic contractions of the muscular wall of the fallopian tube and wafting of the tubal cilia.

The uterus

Starter questions

The answer to the following question is on pages 74–75.

8.   Does the uterus return to its normal size following pregnancy?

The uterus is a hollow muscular organ located in the pelvis. It is the site of embryo implantation and is the organ within which the fetus develops.

Structure

The uterus lies anterior to the rectum and posterior to the bladder. Its position within the pelvis varies with distension of the bladder. For example, a full bladder will push it upwards and backwards, whereas emptying the bladder will return it to its resting position.

The position of the uterus is described in terms of version and flexion: version describes the position of the cervix in relation to the vagina and flexion describes the position of the uterine body in relation to the cervix (**Figure 1.16**). The most common resting position is anteverted, i.e. the cervix is tilted forward, and anteflexed, with the uterine body bent forward over the cervix.

> **One in five women have a retroverted (backwards tilting) uterus.** This is usually a normal variation but occasionally occurs when adhesions due to conditions such as pelvic inflammatory disease and endometriosis tether the uterus in this position. A fixed retroverted uterus can cause pelvic pain and dyspareunia. Retroversion also increases the risk of uterine perforation during procedures that involve instrumentation of the uterus.

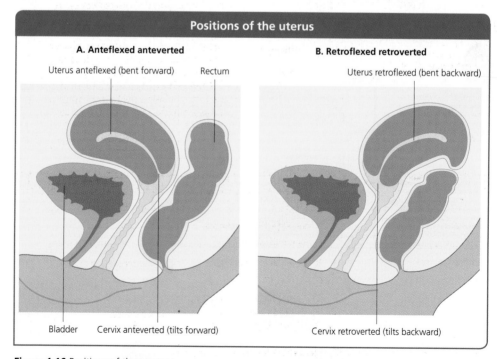

Positions of the uterus

A. Anteflexed anteverted

Uterus anteflexed (bent forward)   Rectum

Bladder   Cervix anteverted (tilts forward)

B. Retroflexed retroverted

Uterus retroflexed (bent backward)

Cervix retroverted (tilts backward)

Figure 1.16 Positions of the uterus.

The main supports of the uterus are the pelvic diaphragm, the transverse cervical ligaments and the uterosacral ligaments. These structures maintain uterine position. If they are torn during childbirth, uterine prolapse may result.

Anatomically, the uterus is divided into four sections (**Figure 1.17**):

- the fundus
- the uterine body
- the isthmus
- the cervix

Within the uterus, the internal cervical os opens into the uterine cavity, which is in direct continuation with the lumen of the right and left fallopian tubes. The anterior and posterior walls of the uterus are closely applied to each other, so the uterine cavity is very small. However, during pregnancy the capacity of the uterus increases from 6 mL to > 5 L at term.

The size and weight of the uterus varies considerably in response to oestrogen (**Table 1.7**). The uterus is at its smallest before puberty and after menopause, when oestrogen levels are low. During pregnancy, when oestrogen is abundant, the weight increases 20-fold to almost 1 kg.

> **The uterine cavity can be examined internally** by passing a fine camera (a hysteroscope) through the internal cervical os. Hysteroscopy can be used to visualise and therefore diagnose abnormalities of the endometrium (e.g. polyps) and provide visual guidance during treatments.

Arterial supply and venous drainage

The uterus is mainly supplied by the uterine artery, which arises from the anterior division of the internal iliac artery (see **Figure 1.9**). There is also a rich anastomotic connection with the ovarian vessels. Venous drainage of the uterus is via the uterine veins.

> **Embolisation of the uterine artery is used to shrink fibroids that cause troublesome bleeding or pressure-related symptoms.** A guide catheter is passed into the uterine artery under fluoroscopic guidance, and once in position, tiny embolisation beads < 1 mm in diameter are released to occlude the vessel. Collateral arterial supply ensures that the uterus itself does not become necrotic.

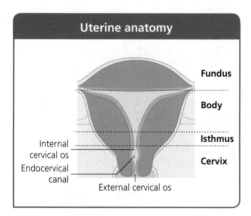

Uterine anatomy

Fundus
Body
Isthmus
Cervix
Internal cervical os
Endocervical canal
External cervical os

Figure 1.17 Uterine anatomy.

Hormonal effects on the uterus and cervix		
Characteristic	Oestrogen	Progesterone
Cervical mucus	Thinner, more abundant mucus	More viscous mucus
Tubal contractility	Increase in tubal contractility	Reduction in tubal contractility
Uterine contractility	Sensitises uterus to oxytocin	Reduces uterine contractility
Uterine size	Increases uterine size	No effect
Cervical consistency	Softens due to the increase in blood flow, accompanying oedema and relaxation of smooth muscle fibres	Firms as a result of reformation of collagen matrix

Table 1.7 Effects of oestrogen and progesterone on the uterus and cervix

Nerve supply

The inferior hypogastric plexuses and the pelvic splanchnic nerves innervate the uterus.

Lymphatic drainage

The fundus drains to the para-aortic lymph nodes. The uterine body and isthmus drain to the external iliac nodes (see **Table 1.5**).

Histology

The uterus is made up of three layers (**Figure 1.18**):

- serosa
- myometrium
- endometrium

The serosa is continuous with the peritoneum. It is a double layer of cells adherent to the myometrium.

The myometrium is composed of several layers of smooth muscle with fibres that crisscross each other. Running within this muscle layer are the arcuate vessels of the uterus. Contraction of muscle layers occurs during labour to dilate the cervix, and during menstruation to expel the sloughed endometrium. With each contraction, the fibres that encircle the blood vessels restrict flow within them.

The endometrium is made of columnar epithelium consisting of glandular cells. The functional layer matures in response to oestrogen and progesterone, but it is shed during menstruation if pregnancy does not occur.

Function

The uterus is the site of implantation of the embryo. Changes in the endometrium facilitate successful implantation of the blastocyst. They also allow the development of the placenta, which transfers oxygen, nutrients and waste products between the maternal and fetal circulations.

During gestation, the fetus develops within the uterine cavity. The uterus enlarges as a

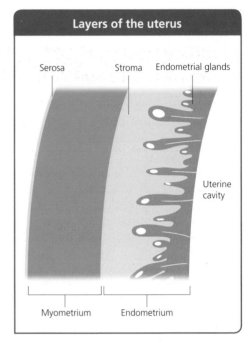

Layers of the uterus

Serosa — Stroma — Endometrial glands

Uterine cavity

Myometrium — Endometrium

Figure 1.18 The three layers of the uterus: the serosa, myometrium and endometrium.

consequence of hyperplasia and hypertrophy of the uterine smooth muscle cells that make up the myometrium. With the onset of labour, the uterus contracts to dilate the cervix and allow passage of the fetus through the birth canal. After delivery, uterine contractions continue; these facilitate delivery of the placenta and rapidly reduce the size of the uterus thus restricting vascular flow and hence blood loss.

Failure of the uterus to contract efficiently after birth, termed uterine atony, is the most common cause of post-partum haemorrhage. 'Rubbing up' a uterine contraction or carrying out bimanual uterine compression stimulates the myometrium to contract, thereby reducing bleeding caused by uterine atony.

The cervix

Starter questions

The answer to the following question is on page 75.

9.   Why is the cervix a common site for cancer?

The cervix forms the lowest part of the uterus and is composed of fibrous tissue. It is a dynamic structure that acts as a barrier between the uterus and the external environment.

It is cylindrical and 3 cm wide. Its distal end projects into the vagina. This divides the cervix into the upper portion, located above the vagina, and the lower portion, called the ectocervix, which is visible within the vagina. The vaginal recesses formed by the protrusion of the cervix into the upper end of the vagina are known as the fornices (**Table 1.8**).

The endocervical canal runs through the cervix and connects the vagina with the uterine cavity.

■ The distal opening within the vagina is the external os
■ The opening of the endocervical canal into the uterine cavity is the internal os

The cervix is divided into the ectocervix and the endocervix, which differ in their characteristics and functions (**Table 1.9**).

Vaginal fornices: anatomical relations		
Fornix	Anatomical relations	Pelvic space palpable
Anterior fornix	Formed by the reflection of the anterior vaginal wall and the cervix	Uterovesicular pouch
Posterior fornix	Formed by the reflection of the posterior vaginal wall and the cervix	Rectovaginal pouch
Lateral fornix (left and right)	Formed by the reflection of the lateral vaginal wall and the cervix	Ovarian fossa

Table 1.8 Anatomical relations of the vaginal fornices

The ectocervix and endocervix		
Characteristic	Ectocervix	Endocervix
Location	Portion of the cervix visible within the vagina	Canal between external cervical os and internal cervical os
Cell type	Non-keratinised stratified squamous epithelium	Columnar epithelium
Sensory innervation	Sparse	Abundant
Function	Protection against abrasion	Production of cervical mucus
Hormonal responsiveness	Minimal	Very responsive to oestrogen. Increasing oestrogen levels increase mucus production. High oestrogen levels predispose to ectopy
Appearance on examination	Pale pink	Dark pink

Table 1.9 Comparison of the ectocervix and endocervix

Arterial supply and venous drainage

Blood supply to the cervix is via the descending branch of the uterine artery (see **Figure 1.9**). Uterine arteries run in the lateral aspects of the cervix at the 3 and 9 o'clock positions. The corresponding veins run parallel to them and drain into the internal iliac veins.

Nerve supply

The nerve supply to the cervix is derived from the hypogastric plexus. Sensory innervation to the ectocervix is sparse, whereas autonomic and sensory nerve endings are abundant in the endocervix.

> **Because there are few nerve endings in the ectocervix, biopsy and cryotherapy involving only this outer surface of the cervix are often well tolerated without local anaesthesia.** However, the pain of dilating the endocervix may cause a reflex stimulation of the parasympathetic nervous system resulting in a vasovagal reaction.

Lymphatic drainage

The cervix drains to the internal and external iliac nodes (see **Table 1.5**).

Histology

The ectocervix and endocervix have different histological characteristics (see **Table 1.9**).

Ectocervix

The surface of the ectocervix is mainly comprised of stratified non-keratinising squamous epithelium. It is made up of the basal, intermediate and superficial layers (**Figure 1.19**).

The squamous epithelium is being constantly remodelled and renewed; its many layers protect the tissues underneath from abrasion. Basal cells form the source of new cells within the upper layers of the epithelium. As basal cells divide, they mature and migrate towards the surface of the epithelium, becoming larger and flatter, and start to produce glycogen.

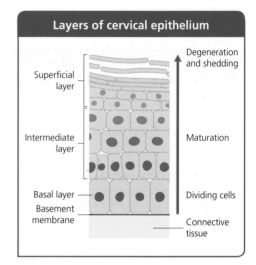

Layers of cervical epithelium

Superficial layer — Degeneration and shedding

Intermediate layer — Maturation

Basal layer — Dividing cells
Basement membrane — Connective tissue

Figure 1.19 Layers of cervical epithelium. Cells within squamous epithelium flatten as they mature.

> **In colposcopy, Lugol's iodine can be used to identify abnormal cells that have not undergone maturation.** Normal squamous cells contain glycogen in their cytoplasm and stain brown. Abnormal cells remain pink.

Endocervix

The surface of the endocervix consists of columnar epithelium. This is a single layer of glandular cells that produce mucus. This epithelium forms folds and crypts that line the endocervical canal. The crypts acts as reservoir for sperm, from which they are released up to two days after ejaculation, increasing the chances of fertilisation.

Squamocolumnar junction

The area where the squamous epithelium of the ectocervix meets the columnar epithelium of the endocervix is known as the squamocolumnar junction. Its location varies throughout a woman's life. Before puberty, it is located close to the external os. Higher oestrogen levels during the reproductive years cause the uterus and cervix to swell and elongate; this pushes the columnar epithelium out of the endocervical canal and onto the ectocervix (eversion), resulting in ectopy. The squamocolumnar junction therefore also moves out onto the ectocevix. On visual inspection, ectopy appears as a red area surrounding the external os. Cervical ectopy is a normal physiological process.

> **Increased oestrogen levels during pregnancy and use of the combined oral contraceptive pill make cervical ectopy more prominent.** The ectopy is more friable (susceptible to bleeding on contact) than mature squamous epithelium and tends to bleed, particularly during sexual intercourse.

The exposure of columnar epithelium to the acidic environment of the vagina causes these cells to transform into squamous epithelium by metaplasia. This process usually starts at the site of the original squamocolumnar junction and moves inwards towards the external os, thereby forming a new squamocolumnar junction. The zone between the original squamocolumnar junction formed in intrauterine life and the squamocolumnar junction formed by metaplasia is known as the transformation zone (**Figure 1.20**). This is the site of origin of > 90% of cervical cancers.

> **Persistent infection of immature metaplastic cells by oncogenic strains of human papillomavirus** causes them to transform into atypical cells with nuclear and cytoplasmic abnormalities. These may either regress with time or proliferate and progress into invasive cancer cells.

Function

The cervix acts as a barrier between the external environment and the uterus. The integrity of this seal changes in response to female sex hormones to allow passage of sperm between the vagina and the uterus or vice versa during labour to facilitate the delivery of the baby. The ectocervix protects against abrasion, and the endocervix produces cervical mucus (see **Table 1.9**).

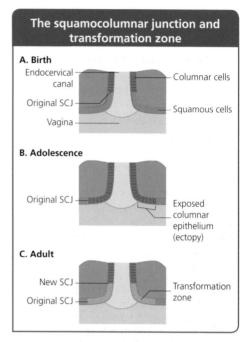

The squamocolumnar junction and transformation zone

A. Birth
- Endocervical canal
- Columnar cells
- Original SCJ
- Squamous cells
- Vagina

B. Adolescence
- Original SCJ
- Exposed columnar epithelium (ectopy)

C. Adult
- New SCJ
- Original SCJ
- Transformation zone

Figure 1.20 The squamocolumnar junction (SCJ) and the transformation zone. Exposed columnar epithelial cells undergo metaplasia in the transition zone forming a new squamocolumnar junction.

The glandular cells lining the endocervical canal produce a glycogen-rich mucus plug that acts as a physical barrier to pathogens. It is also rich in white blood cells, immunoglobulins and enzymes that augment its bactericidal properties.

In response to increasing levels of oestrogen, cervical mucus becomes thinner and more abundant halfway through the menstrual cycle, making it penetrable to sperm, aiding fertilisation. After ovulation, the mucus becomes more viscous and impregnable again. During pregnancy, the mucus remains viscous as a result of the continued action of progesterone. This maintains the barrier against ascending infections which could otherwise threaten the pregnancy.

Cervical mucus also contributes to vaginal lubrication, which reduces abrasion during penetrative intercourse. Prior to and during intercourse, sexual stimulation increases blood flow to the cervical glands increasing mucus production. The consistency of the cervix itself also changes in response to hormonal influences.

- In the non-pregnant state, the cervix is firm and non-compliant
- During pregnancy, the cervix become softer and more distensible
- With the forceful and regular contractions associated with the onset of labour, the cervix shortens and dilates to allow passage of the baby into the vaginal canal; this can lead to loss of the mucus plug ('show'), a sign that labour is imminent, which in some women may precede established labour by up to a week

The vagina

Starter questions

The answer to the following question is on page 75.

10. Do probiotic supplements prevent vaginal infections?

The vagina is a muscular tube connecting the uterus to the external environment. The vagina points upwards and backwards, and its anterior wall is shorter than its posterior wall (see **Figure 1.16**). On average, the vagina measures 7 cm in the absence of sexual arousal. With sexual arousal, the length and width of the vagina increases to accommodate the penis during penetrative intercourse.

Anterior to the vagina is the bladder and the urethra. Posterior to the vagina is the rectum.

Slow progress of the fetus through the vagina causes ischaemia as a consequence of compression of the soft tissues between the baby's head and the mother's pelvic bones. In areas of the world where access to caesarean delivery is limited, the prolonged compression of obstructed labour causes necrosis of these tissues. This leads to formation of a false passage (fistula) between the vagina and the bladder or rectum. The resulting constant urinary or bowel leakage and other health problems can leave women unable to work, and they may be shunned by their families and communities. Obstetric fistula is a major preventable cause of obstetric-related morbidity in poor resource settings.

Arterial supply and venous drainage

Blood supply to the vagina is via the uterine and vaginal arteries, which are branches of the internal iliac artery. Venous drainage is via the corresponding venous plexuses (see **Figure 1.9**).

Nerve supply

The upper vagina is supplied by parasympathetic nerves from the pelvic splanchnic nerves. The lower two thirds of the vagina are supplied by the pudendal nerve.

Lymphatic drainage

Lymphatic drainage is to the iliac and superficial inguinal nodes (see **Table 1.5**).

Histology

The vaginal wall consists of four layers.

- The mucosa is made up of stratified squamous epithelium
- The lamina propria is rich in elastic fibres
- The muscularis comprises an inner circular layer and an outer longitudinal layer of smooth muscle
- The adventitia consists of elastic fibres surrounded by loose connective tissue and a venous plexus that blends with the adventitia covering the bladder and rectum

The vaginal mucosa forms folds called rugae. The underlying muscle and the elastic lamina propria lining these folds allow the vagina to stretch and distend during delivery.

The vaginal mucosa is glandless. It is lubricated by secretions from the cervix and the Bartholin's glands. The latter are a pair of glands located just within the entrance to the vagina, at the 5 o'clock and 7 o'clock positions (**Figure 1.2**).

The duct of a Bartholin's gland can become blocked, thereby preventing release of its lubricating secretions. The resulting Bartholin's cyst presents as a painless swelling of the labia or lower vagina. Bartholin's cysts sometimes become infected, which causes pain as a result of localised inflammation and the accumulation of pus.

Function

The vagina connects the uterus with the external environment. Because of the close proximity to the anus, and the consequent potential exposure to faecal bacteria, the vagina is adapted to prevent ascending infection (**Table 1.10**). The vaginal epithelium is made up of stratified squamous epithelium that forms a tough physical barrier to pathogens. It is covered in a layer of adherent lactobacilli that break down glycogen made by the epithelial cells into lactic acid. This symbiotic relationship helps to maintain a low vaginal pH that is hostile to pathogens. Additionally, the lactobacilli form a further physical layer to protect the vagina and secrete antimicrobial substances such as hydrogen peroxide and bacteriocins that inhibit the growth of other bacteria.

During coitus, semen is deposited in the posterior fornix. Contractions of vaginal smooth muscle keep the pool of semen close to the cervix, thereby facilitating transport of sperm into the uterus.

Vaginal adaptations to prevent infection	
Characteristic	Adaptation
Vaginal pH	pH (3.5–4.5) inhibits growth of pathogenic bacteria
Microenvironment	Normal commensals (e.g. lactobacilli) inhibit growth of pathogenic bacteria
	Lactobacilli adhere to epithelium, forming a barrier against other bacteria
Cell types	Epithelial cells produce glycogen, which lactobacilli break down to form lactic acid
	Stratified squamous epithelium provides tough physical barrier to pathogens
	Thickening of epithelium in response to oestrogen provides protection against abrasion

Table 1.10 Vaginal adaptations to prevent infection

The vulva

Starter questions

The answer to the following question is on page 75.

11. Can examining the hymen determine whether a woman is a virgin?

The vulva is a collective term for the female external genitalia, which include:

- the mons pubis
- the labia majora
- the labia minora
- the clitoris

The introitus (vaginal orifice) and external urethral orifice are located in the vulva.

Structure

The mons pubis is the fatty pad that overlies the pubic symphysis and divides into the labia majora inferiorly. At puberty, the mons pubis becomes covered in thick terminal hairs.

The labia majora form the two outer folds of skin that cover the vaginal and urethral openings. The labia majora corresponds to the scrotum in males.

- The outer surface of the labia majora is pigmented and covered with sparse terminal hairs
- The inner surface of the labia majora is smooth and contains large sebaceous glands

The labia minora are the inner folds of labial skin. They correspond to the frenulum and foreskin in males. The upper part of the labia minora forms the clitoral hood and the clitoral glans. The folds of the labia minora extend laterally to the vestibule and join posteriorly in the midline in a fold of skin called the forchette.

The clitoris is the equivalent of the penis in the male, and is situated just below the division of the left and right labia minora. The clitoris consists of a cluster of erectile tissues and nerve endings.

Arterial supply and venous drainage

Blood supply to the vulva is via the paired pudendal arteries. Venous drainage is via the pudendal veins.

Nerve supply

The vulva has both sensory and parasympathetic innervation.

Sensory innervation to the anterior portion of the vulva is supplied by the ilioinguinal nerve and the genital branch of the genitofemoral nerve. The posterior portion of the vulva is supplied by the pudendal nerve and the posterior cutaneous nerve to the thigh (**Figure 1.21**).

A pudendal nerve block can be used to provide anaesthesia to the vulva during assisted vaginal delivery. Local anaesthetic is instilled 1 cm medial and 1 cm inferior to the ischial spine, thereby targeting the pudendal nerve as it enters the lesser sciatic foramen.

Lymphatic drainage

Lymphatic drainage is to the superficial inguinal nodes (see **Table 1.5**).

Histology

The labia are covered by stratified squamous epithelium. The skin of the labia contains both eccrine and apocrine sweat glands, which each have different characteristics (**Table 1.11**). Apocrine sweat glands are present only in the axillary and pubic areas.

Nerve supply to the vulva

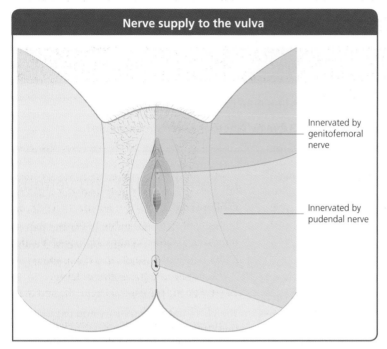

Innervated by genitofemoral nerve

Innervated by pudendal nerve

Figure 1.21 The genitofemoral nerve supplies the mons pubis and the medial aspect of the thigh. The pudendal nerve supplies the labia majora and minora and vaginal vestibule.

Apocrine and eccrine sweat glands

Characteristic	Apocrine sweat glands	Eccrine sweat glands
Location	All over the body; most numerous on hands and feet	Axilla and genital areas
Gland structure	Simple coiled tubular glands	Branched tubular glands
Opening	Open directly on to skin surface	Open into hair follicle
Secretion	Water (99% water, 1% salt)	Oily secretion that when degraded by bacteria produces an odour
Function	Thermoregulation and excretion	Secretion of chemicals that communicate sexual readiness

Table 1.11 Differences between apocrine and eccrine sweat glands

These modified sweat glands open into the base of hair follicles and produce a viscous oily secretion containing protein, lipids and androgens. This secretion, although initially odourless, is degraded by bacteria to produce a characteristic odour. Unlike eccrine sweat glands, which secrete in response to body temperature, apocrine sweat glands secrete in response to emotional stimuli such as anxiety, fear and sexual arousal.

Function

The vulva acts as sensory tissue during sexual intercourse; nerve endings are highly concentrated within the vulva and especially the clitoris. The labia and clitoris engorge with blood during sexual arousal.

The labia also directs the flow of urine during micturition and protects the clitoris, urethral orifice and internal female reproductive tract from trauma.

The perineum

Starter questions

The answer to the following question is on page 75.

12. Can perineal injury during childbirth be prevented?

The perineum is the most inferior part of the pelvic outlet. It is an anatomical region containing structures that support the urinary, genital and gastrointestinal organs from prolapse.

Structure

The perineum is a diamond-shaped region (**Figure 1.22**). Anteriorly, it is bound by the symphysis pubis; posteriorly, by the coccyx. Its lateral boundaries are the inferior pubic rami, the inferior ischial rami and the sacrotuberous ligaments. The pelvic floor, which consists of muscle fibres from the levator ani, coccygeus muscles and connective tissue which span the pelvic outlet, separates the perineum from the pelvic cavity.

The perineum is separated into the urogenital triangle anteriorly and the anal triangle posteriorly by a theoretical line drawn between the two ischial tuberosities.

- The urogenital triangle is associated with the external genitalia and the urethra; it contains the strong fascial layers supporting the external genitalia and the perineal muscles
- The anal triangle contains the anal aperture, the external anal sphincter and the ischioanal fossae; the ischioanal fossae contain fat and connective tissue that allow expansion of the anal canal on defecation

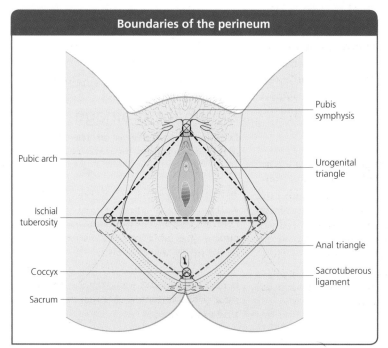

Boundaries of the perineum

Pubis symphysis

Pubic arch

Urogenital triangle

Ischial tuberosity

Anal triangle

Coccyx

Sacrotuberous ligament

Sacrum

Figure 1.22
Boundaries of the perineum. The perineum can be divided into the urogenital triangle and the anal triangle.

The perineal body

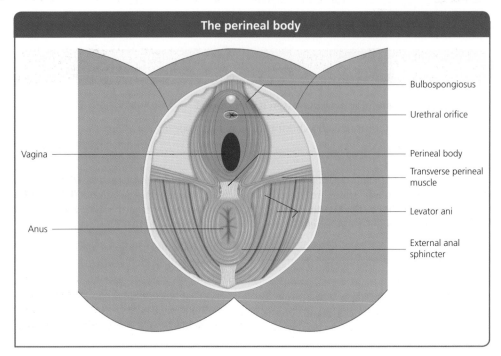

Bulbospongiosus

Urethral orifice

Vagina

Perineal body

Transverse perineal muscle

Levator ani

Anus

External anal sphincter

Figure 1.23 The perineal body forms the attachment of the muscles of the pelvic floor and perineum.

Perineal body

At the junction between the two anatomical triangles is the perineal body. The perineal body forms the attachment of the muscle fibres of the pelvic floor and the perineum, and lies just below the skin (**Figure 1.23**). The perineal body is formed from fibres from the levator ani, bulbospongiosus and transverse perineal muscles and the external anal sphincter. It forms the support between the external anal sphincter and the vagina.

Arterial supply and venous drainage

Blood is supplied to the perineum by the internal pudendal arteries. Venous drainage is via the pudendal veins.

Nerve supply

The pudendal nerve supplies the perineum.

Lymphatic drainage

Lymphatic drainage is to the superficial inguinal nodes.

The female urinary tract

The female urinary tract consists of the two kidneys, two ureters, the bladder and the urethra. Its primary function is to produce, store and eliminate fluid waste from the body.

Structure

The kidneys are paired retroperitoneal organs that excrete metabolic waste, excess ions and fluid, to produce urine. Urine drains via the ureters into the urinary bladder, where it is stored.

The ureters run parallel to the vertebral column and enter the pelvis at the level of the bifurcation of the iliac arteries. Within the pelvis, they run medial to the internal iliac artery and are crossed by the uterine arteries. Each ureter passes 2 cm lateral to the cervix as it turns medially to enter the posterolateral walls of the bladder.

The urethra conveys urine from the bladder to the exterior. The urethra passes through the urogenital triangle and opens into the external urethral orifice between the clitoris and the vagina. The flow of urine from the bladder into the urethra is controlled by muscles of the pelvic floor and the external and internal urethral sphincters.

> **The base of the bladder is related to the anterior vaginal wall.** Weakening of the fascia forming the pelvic floor can result in prolapse of the bladder into the vagina, i.e. a cystocoele.

Arterial supply and venous drainage

The kidneys are supplied by the renal arteries and drained by the renal veins. The ureters are supplied and drained by vessels along its course. The bladder is supplied by the superior and inferior vesical arteries and drains to the internal iliac veins.

Nerve supply

The kidney is supplied by the renal plexus. The bladder is supplied by the vesical nerve plexus. These plexuses contains parasympathetic, sympathetic and afferent sensory fibres.

Lymphatic drainage

The lymphatic vessels of the urinary tract drain to the various iliac nodes corresponding to their blood supply.

> **Urogynaecologists work closely with renal physicians and urologists to manage disorders affecting the urinary tract.** They focus on managing conditions associated with pelvic floor and bladder dysfunction in women.

Histology

The entire urinary tract is lined by transitional epithelium. In the bladder, the transitional epithelium falls into folds, known as ruggae, when it's empty. The ruggae allow the bladder to stretch as it fills. The bladder wall comprises three layers of smooth muscle known as the detrusor muscle. This muscle aids voiding.

Function

The urinary system allows the body to excrete excess fluid waste. Urine is made in the kidneys and stored in the bladder ready for voiding under voluntary control.

Micturition

Micturition (urination) is the voiding of urine from the bladder. The filling of the urinary bladder occurs passively, while micturition occurs under voluntary control (**Table 1.12** and **Figure 1.24**).

Filling and storing

Urine is transported to the bladder by gravity and peristaltic contractions of the smooth muscle within the walls of the ureters. The bladder fills passively at a rate of 1 mL/min. As the bladder distends (expands), the folds of the transitional epithelium flatten and the muscle fibres of the detrusor stretch passively. There is very little increase in intravesical pressure with bladder filling.

As the volume of urine increases, mechanoreceptors in the detrusor muscle are activated by stretch to send afferent impulses to the brain. The first sensation of bladder filling occurs when the bladder contains about 150 mL of urine. Micturition is inhibited voluntarily by constricting the external urethral sphincter.

Neural control of micturition				
Type of neural control	Action on detrusor muscle	Action on internal sphincter	Action on external sphincter	Function
Sympathetic	Relaxation	Constriction	None	Allows filling
Parasympathetic	Constriction	Relaxation	None	Allows emptying
Somatic	None	None	Constriction	Voluntary control

Table 1.12 Control of micturition by autonomic and somatic impulses

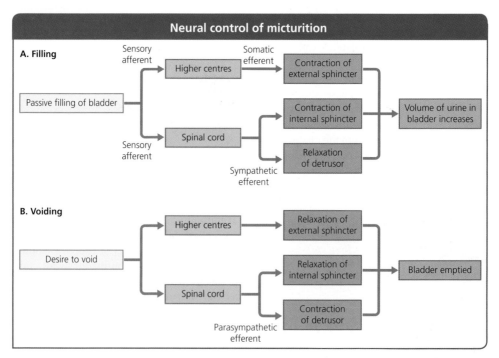

Figure 1.24 Neural control of micturition. Sympathetic impulses cause the detrusor to relax and the internal sphincter to contract. On micturition, parasympathetic impulses cause the detrusor to contract and the internal sphincter to relax. The external sphincter is relaxed under voluntary control.

Sympathetic impulses also signal the internal urethral sphincter to remain contracted and the detrusor muscle to relax (**Table 1.12**).

Voiding

To initiate voiding, voluntary relaxation of muscles of the pelvic floor and the external urethral sphincter leads to a decrease in intraurethral pressure. Higher centres release their inhibitory effect, and consequently parasympathetic impulses cause the detrusor muscle to contract and the internal urethral sphincter to relax. These actions lead to an increase in intravesical pressure.

Flow begins when the pressure in the bladder exceeds that in the urethra. After voiding, the pelvic floor muscles and external urethral sphincter contract, and further parasympathetic signals are inhibited by higher centres.

Symptoms of urgency and frequency are caused by overactivity of the detrusor muscle. This is treated by the use of anticholinergic agents that block muscarinic receptors, thereby reducing the sensitivity of the detrusor muscle to parasympathetic impulses.

The menstrual cycle

Starter questions

The answer to the following question is on page 75.

14. Do the menstrual cycles of women living together synchronise?

The menstrual cycle is a series of physiological events, coordinated by hormones from the hypothalamic-pituitary-ovarian axis, that occur between the start of one menses and the start of the next. In each cycle, changes within the ovaries lead to the release of an oocyte and prepare the endometrium for implantation, respectively (**Figure 1.25**).

The average length of the menstrual cycle is 28 days, with a normal range of 21–35 days. Considerable variation in cycle length may occur naturally around puberty and menopause. Menstruation occurs for 2–7 days of each cycle.

Hypothalamic–pituitary–ovarian axis

The hypothalamic–pituitary–ovarian axis controls the menstrual cycle (**Figure 1.5**). LH and FSH are produced by the anterior pituitary gland and act on the ovaries.

- LH promotes the production of oestrogen by the ovaries
- FSH promotes the growth of ovarian follicles

Inhibin is a by-product of follicle development and, along with oestrogen, inhibits secretion of gonadotropins from the anterior pituitary by negative feedback.

The ovarian hormones oestrogen and progesterone control endometrial changes throughout the cycle.

Ovarian cycle

The changes within the ovaries during the menstrual cycle are referred to as the ovarian cycle. It has three phases:

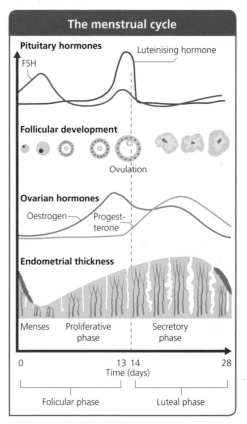

Figure 1.25 The menstrual cycle. Changes within the ovary and endometrium in response to changing levels of pituitary and ovarian hormones, respectively.

- follicular (days 1–13 in an average cycle)
- ovulatory (day 14)
- luteal (days 15–28)

Within each ovarian cycle a single developing follicle matures, releases an oocyte and differentiates into the corpus luteum. The granulosa cells within the follicle and corpus luteum secrete different ovarian hormones as the follicle progresses through the phases of the ovarian cycle; these hormones prepare the endometrium for a possible pregnancy.

Follicular phase

In each cycle, several of the follicles reach the secondary follicle stage. Up to this point maturation is independent of FSH, but stimulation by FSH is needed for the secondary follicles to mature into tertiary follicles. Typically, only one (the dominant follicle) reaches maturity. The rest degenerate and are reabsorbed into the ovary. The dominant follicle produces large amounts of oestrogen.

Ovulatory phase

The increasing levels of oestrogen produced by the follicle peak between days 12 and 14. This triggers a surge in secretion of LH by the anterior pituitary. In response, the primary oocyte within the dominant follicle completes its first meiotic division to generate a secondary oocyte and a polar body. Shortly afterwards, the follicle ruptures to release the mature oocyte (ovulation).

The mature oocyte that is released from the ovary into the reproductive tract is surrounded by an envelope of cumulus cells, the cumulus oophorus. These specialised granulosa cells nourish the oocyte. An unfertilised oocyte can survive for only 24 h after ovulation.

Luteal phase

After ovulation, the ruptured follicle collapses and forms the corpus luteum. Granulosa cells in the corpus luteum begin to secrete progesterone as well as oestrogen and relaxin. These hormones inhibit the release of FSH from the anterior pituitary, preventing further follicle development. If pregnancy does not occur, the corpus luteum degenerates and oestrogen and progesterone levels decrease. The luteal phase always lasts 14 days.

Variation in the length of the follicular phase determines the duration of a woman's menstrual cycle. The length of the luteal phase varies very little, so measurement of serum progesterone 7 days before the date of the next predicted menses reliably determines whether a woman has ovulated. In a woman with a 28-day cycle, this means measurement of progesterone on day 21.

Endometrial changes

The upper two thirds, or functional layer, of the endometrium is highly responsive to oestrogen and progesterone. These hormones stimulate changes in the endometrial structure that prepare it for a possible pregnancy:

- oestrogen stimulates endometrial growth
- progesterone matures the endometrium

The result is 3 phases of endometrial change:

- menstruation (days 1–5 in an average cycle)
- proliferative phase (days 5–14)
- secretory phase (days 15–28)

Menstruation

Decreasing levels of oestrogen and progesterone at the end of the preceding menstrual cycle lead to the death of cells within the functional layer of the endometrium. During menstruation, these cells are shed leaving only the thin basal layer.

Proliferative phase

In response to the increasing levels of oestrogen produced during the follicular phase the endometrium thickens, the number of endometrial glands and stromal cells increase, and new spiral arteries form. These changes lead to the development of a new functional layer. In addition, the endocervical glands start to produce increasing amounts of thin, sticky cervical mucus which is more penetrable to sperm.

Secretory phase

After ovulation, changes in the endometrium are driven by progesterone produced by the corpus luteum. Progesterone inhibits further proliferation of endometrial cells and causes the endometrium to differentiate and mature. As a result, the endometrial glands and arteries become coiled and intertwined, and the stroma becomes oedematous. These changes facilitate the production of a glycogen-rich secretion to nourish potential embryos.

Fertility and conception

Starter questions

The answer to the following question is on page 76.

15. When in the month is a woman most fertile?

At conception, male and female gametes containing a single set of chromosomes from each parent fuse to form a zygote that contains all the genetic material necessary to form a new individual. The male gamete (spermatozoon) is adapted to deliver this genetic material into the cytoplasm of the female oocyte. Problems transporting healthy spermatozoa to the oocyte can cause to subfertility.

Spermatogenesis

Spermatogenesis is the production of spermatozoa (sperm); it starts at puberty and continues throughout a man's life. Formation of a spermatozoon takes 70–80 days and occurs in several stages (**Figure 1.26**). Only one spermatozoon is needed to fertilise an ovum, but millions are produced to maximise the likelihood of success.

Spermatid production

Spermatozoa develop from germ cells known as spermatagonia, which line the seminiferous tubules in the testes. Spermatagonia continually divide by mitosis to produce an almost limitless supply of stem cells that divide by meiosis and differentiate into specialised cells called spermatozoa.

In response to stimulation by FSH, these cells grow and develop into primary spermatocytes. Primary spermatocytes undergo the first stage of meiotic division to form two equally sized daughter cells containing 23 chromosomes each (a haploid number). These daughter cells are known as secondary spermatocytes.

Each secondary spermatocyte undergoes a further meiotic division to form two spermatids of equal size. Each spermatid contains

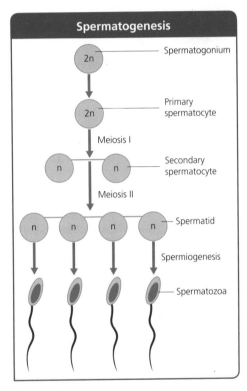

Figure 1.26 Spermatogenesis. Spermatozoa are formed from spermatogonia by mitosis and meiosis.

23 chromosomes. In contrast with oogenesis, in which a single mature oocyte is formed by meiotic division, meiosis in spermatogenesis results in four equally sized spermatids that remain connected to each other by a cytoplasmic bridge. These bridges arise due to the incomplete separation of the cell cytoplasm during cell division. They provide a way for haploid cells to continue to share the proteins coded on both sets of chromosomes.

Gametogenesis in males and females

Characteristic	Oogenesis	Spermatogenesis
Site	Ovarian cortex	Seminiferous tubules of the testes
Starts	In utero	At puberty
Development	Cyclical	Continuous
Hormonal control	FSH	FSH
Duration	Arrested for 12–50 years in meiosis I	70–80 days
Gamete production per meiosis	1 oocyte and 2 polar bodies	4 spermatids
Gamete production per cycle/per ejaculate	1	100–200 million
FSH, follicle-stimulating hormone.		

Table 1.13 Comparison of gametogenesis in males and females

This is essential for the differentiation of these cells into spermatozoa. These and other differences between oogenesis and spermatogenesis are summarised in **Table 1.13**.

Spermiogenesis

The final stage of spermatogenesis is spermiogenesis. During this stage, the spermatids develop specialised features that enable them to become mature spermatozoa able to self-propel and to penetrate the oocyte (**Table 1.14**).

Up until this stage, the spermatocytes and spermatids are symmetrical. During spermiogenesis, spermatids become polarised and are known as spermatozoa.

At one end the head forms (**Figure 1.27**). This comprises condensed nuclear material surrounded by a cap-like structure called the acrosome. The cytoplasm around the nucleus is minimal, so the head is almost all nuclear material. The acrosome is formed by fusion of enzyme-filled vesicles that, when released, help the spermatozoon penetrate the oocyte.

At the other end of the spermatid, the tail forms. The tail elongates to form a flagellum containing an axoneme, which is made up of several sets of microtubule bundles. The mitochondria migrate to form a sheath around the proximal part of the tail; they provide an energy source for motility.

Adaptations of spermatozoa

Adaptation	Function
Condensation of nuclear material	Tight packing of DNA reduces volume needed to transport genetic information
Tail	Rapidly propels spermatazoon through reproductive tract to meet oocyte
Abundant mitochondria	Provides energy for propulsion
Acrosome	Contains proteolytic enzymes that break down the corona radiata and zona pellucida to allow entry to the oocyte
Produced in large numbers	Increase chance that one viable sperm will find, fuse with and fertilise the oocyte
	Selection of most motile and healthy sperm
Ejaculated along with seminal fluid	Alkalinity of seminal fluid neutralises acidity of the vaginal environment to maintain viability of sperm

Table 1.14 Adaptations of spermatozoa to maximise the likelihood of fertilisation

Ejaculation

As new generations of spermatocytes form, successive generations of spermatids are pushed progressively towards the lumen of the tubule. Mature spermatozoa are released

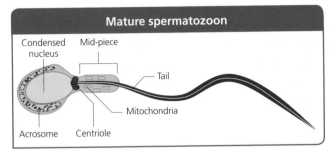

Figure 1.27 Structure of a mature spermatozoon. Spermatozoa are specialised to traverse the female reproductive tract and to fertilise ova.

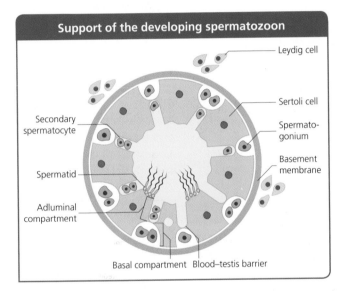

Figure 1.28 Support of the developing spermatozoon. Spermatozoa develop in the seminiferous tubules, supported by Sertoli and Leydig cells.

into the seminiferous tubules (**Figure 1.28**). At this stage, the spermatozoa are non-motile, so are transported, in testicular fluid secreted by the Sertoli cells, to the epididymis by peristaltic contractions of the seminferous tubules. Here, the spermatozoa become motile and are stored.

During ejaculation, the spermatozoa travel through the vas deferens and prostatic urethra. Here, they combine with seminal fluid to form semen. Seminal fluid is produced by the seminal vesicles, prostate and bulbourethral glands. It provides an nutritive and protective environment for the spermatozoa once within the female reproductive tract. Alkalis and prostaglandins within the semen neutralise the acidic environment within the vagina and suppress the immune response of the female body to foreign cells. An average ejaculate contains 2–5 mL of seminal fluid and 20–40 million sperm per millilitre.

> **Only sperm that pass through the epididymis are capable of fertilisation.** Surgical retrieval of sperm from the epididymis is used in assisted conception if the man is unable to ejaculate or if his sperm are unable to enter the semen (obstructive azoospermia).

Sexual intercourse

Arousal and sexually stimulating activity may initiate the sexual response cycle, a series of physical and emotional changes that occur in both male and female partners to prepare the body for sexual intercourse. It comprises four stages: excitement, plateau, orgasm and resolution (**Table 1.15**). Dysfunction can occur at any stage of the cycle, thereby reducing satisfaction with sexual activity.

Sexual dysfunction prevents people from experiencing satisfaction during sexual activity. For a woman, it encompasses a range of disorders that affect desire for sex, ability to become aroused and ability to achieve orgasm, as well as sometimes causing pain during intercourse. The causes of sexual dysfunction are often both physical and psychological; treatment requires an individualised multidisciplinary approach that targets both aspects.

Sexual response cycle	
Stage	**Features**
1 Excitement	Desire to have sex
	Increased heart rate and breathing rate
	Increased blood flow to genitals
2 Plateau	Intensified sexual pleasure
	Men: penile erection and withdrawal of testes into the scrotum
	Women: vaginal lubrication; engorgement of clitoris, vulva, vaginal walls and nipples
3 Orgasm	Peak of sexual pleasure
	Release of sexual tension
	Men: ejaculation
	Women: contraction of outer third of vagina
4 Resolution	Muscular relaxation
	Sense of well-being
	Fatigue
	Men: refractory period during which further erection and orgasm cannot recur
	Women: rapid return to orgasm phase, with multiple orgasms possible

Table 1.15 Masters and Johnson's four-stage sexual response cycle. This model describes the physiological changes which occur in sexual response. Although both men and women experience these stages during sexual activity, their duration and intensity, and the emotions they provoke, differ greatly between individuals.

Conception

Spermatozoa are able to fertilise an oocyte for up to 5 days after ejaculation into the vagina. This means that conception can occur if intercourse has occurred at any time in the 5 days before ovulation. Sperm compete to be the first to fertilise the oocyte. Sperm with poor motility or morphology move slower than normal healthy sperm, which are highly motile. This natural selection process ensures that the healthiest sperm fuses with the egg.

Semen analysis is used to evaluate male fertility. Factors determining semen quality include volume, sperm count, motility, morphology, pH and the proportion of live cells. An abnormal result is associated with a lower chance of pregnancy occurring naturally.

Transport of sperm

Once the spermatozoa enter the female reproductive tract, they must travel through the cervical canal, uterus and fallopian tubes to meet the oocyte. To complete this journey they must survive the physical stresses of ejaculation and contractions of the female reproductive tract, the acidic environment of the vagina, attack from the immune system and negotiate their way through the reproductive tract.

Semen coagulates to form a jelly-like substance shortly following ejaculation into the vagina. This prevents the immediate loss of the seminal fluid from the vagina. Over the course of the next 20 min, this liquefies to enable the spermatozoa to move more effectively.

Both seminal fluid and cervical mucus are alkaline. They neutralise the acidic environment within the vagina enabling sperm to survive.

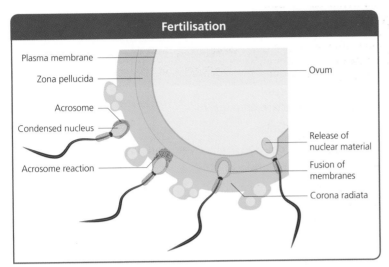

Figure 1.29 At fertilisation, the spermatazoon fuses with the oocyte, and nuclear material from the spematozoon enters the cytoplasm.

The passage of spermatozoa through the reproductive tract is aided by contractions of the uterus. These contractions produce negative pressure within the cavity to draw the sperm up the cervical canal. The spermatozoa also use their tails to propel themselves through the reproductive tract.

Fertilisation

Of the several million spermatazoa deposited in the vagina at ejaculation, only a few hundred reach the ampulla of the fallopian tube.

When these spermatozoa reach the cumulus oophorus of the oocyte, their acrosomes release lytic enzymes that break up the cumulus cells and penetrate the zona pellucida (**Figure 1.29**).

The first spermatozoon that reaches the underlying oocyte fuses with it. The spermatozoon then releases its nucleus into the cytoplasm of the oocyte. This triggers the release of cortical granules in the oocyte cell membrane. These granules contain enzymes that make the membrane tough and impenetrable to any more spermatozoa.

Pregnancy

Starter questions

Answers to the following questions are on page 76.

16. Why do babies hiccup in the womb?
17. Why do the majority of babies position themselves head down before birth?
18. Why do pregnant women feel breathless?
19. Why do women get cravings in pregnancy?

After fertilisation, the cells of the pre-embryo divide as it travels down the fallopian tube to the uterus. Here, it implants in the endometrium and becomes an embryo. Its outer membranes develop to form the placenta and amniotic sac.

Implantation inhibits menstruation. This ensures that the endometrium remains intact.

The embryo continues to develop and becomes a fetus after 8 weeks. On average, a full-term singleton pregnancy lasts 40 weeks from the mother's last menstrual period, so the fetus grows and develops in the uterus for 38 weeks, i.e. the period between mid-cycle fertilisation and birth.

Pregnancy is divided into three trimesters (**Table 1.16**):

■ In the first trimester (conception to week 12), the embryo starts to form all its organs

■ In the second trimester (weeks 13–27), the nervous system starts to mature and the fetus develops reflexes that enable it to respond to stimuli; also, hair and nails develop

■ In the third trimester (weeks 28 to birth), the fetus continues to grow and lays down the fat necessary to maintain body temperature; by 39 weeks, the lungs complete their development

By week 40, intrauterine development is complete and the fetus is ready to be born.

Development of the embryo

The pre-embryo produced by fertilisation travels to the uterus, where it implants in the endometrium as an embryo. Over the next

Structural and functional development of organs			
Anatomical structure	Development starts	Organogenesis completed	Functional development completed
Central nervous system	Week 3	Week 16	Adulthood
Heart	Week 3	Week 6	After birth
Limbs	Week 4	Week 8	After puberty
Face	Week 5	Week 12	Week 12
Respiratory system	Week 4	Week 16	After birth
Alimentary system	Week 5	Week 20	After birth
Internal genitalia	Week 7	Week 16	After puberty
External genitalia	Week 7	Week 16	After puberty

Table 1.16 Organ development by prenatal week

8 weeks, the embryo continues to grow, the placenta forms and the amniotic cavity surrounds the embryo to protect it.

Pre-embryo development

Immediately following fertilisation, the ovum completes the second meiotic division (**Figure 1.30**). Nuclear membranes reform around the two sets of haploid chromosomes, thereby forming a female pronucleus and a male pronucleus. At the first cleavage division, the male and female chromosomes come together on the mitotic spindle. This creates a pre-embryo with 23 pairs of chromosomes (23 from the mother and 23 from the father). This process occurs within 30 h of fertilisation.

Subsequent cleavages (rounds of mitotic division) occur in quick succession. This produces multiple daughter cells; each cell splits in two, so each cleavage doubles the number of cells. During this early stage, cleavage is controlled by maternally-derived proteins and RNA stored in the egg during oogenesis. The paternal genetic material is silent (i.e. does not produce gene transcripts or proteins). When the pre-embryo reaches the 4–8-cell stage, both sets of genes become active (maternal to zygotic transition). Problems arising during this transition result in embryonic loss.

> **Approximately 70% of conceptions do not result in a live birth:** 30% of pregnancies are lost prior to implantation, 30% following implantation, but prior to a missed period and 10% are clinically-recognised miscarriages (occur after a missed period). The majority of losses occur due to chromosomal abnormalities caused by errors in meiosis.

Morula formation

Once the pre-embryo has 16 cells, it begins to compact. The cells flatten and increase

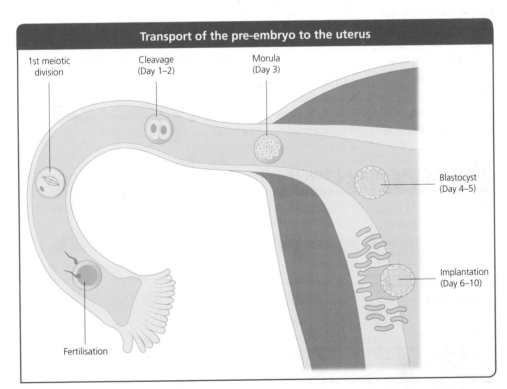

Transport of the pre-embryo to the uterus

1st meiotic division

Cleavage (Day 1–2)

Morula (Day 3)

Blastocyst (Day 4–5)

Implantation (Day 6–10)

Fertilisation

Figure 1.30 Transport of the pre-embryo to the uterus. It is transported along the fallopian tube and implants in the endometrium at day 6.

intercellular connections to form a morula. During this stage, the cells are able to differentiate into any tissue, i.e. they are totipotent.

At 4–5 days after fertilisation the morula starts to develop a cavity, forming a hollow ball of cells known as a blastocyst. It is only after this stage that the cells start to differentiate, i.e. become more specialised (**Figure 1.31**). The blastocyst has two layers:

- The outer cells differentiate to form a watertight epithelial layer known as the trophoblast; the trophoblast gives rise to the extraembryonic membrane that forms the amniotic sac and the placenta
- The inner cells remain totipotent and cluster to form a clump of cells on the inside wall of the blastocyst called the inner cell mass; these cells give rise to the fetus

During these first 4–5 days of development the pre-embryo simultaneously travels along the fallopian tubes to the uterus aided by peristaltic contractions. It is nourished by the secretion of glandular cells lining the fallopian tube.

Implantation

About 6 days after fertilisation, the blastocyst attaches to and buries itself in the endometrium (implantation) (**Figure 1.32**). This process takes 3–5 days.

During this time, the trophoblast cells release proteolytic enzymes that allow the blastocyst to invade the endometrium. A sublayer of the trophoblast, the basal cytotrophoblast, rapidly divides to give rise to a multinucleate layer of cells known as the syncytiotrophoblast. These cells interlock with the maternal endometrium to form the placenta.

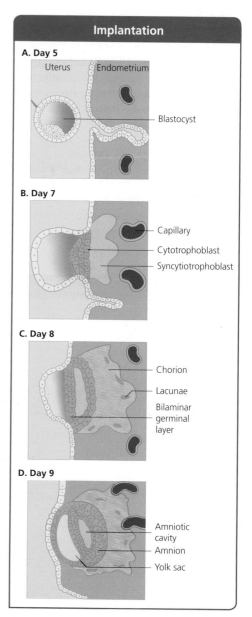

Implantation

A. Day 5
Uterus | Endometrium
Blastocyst

B. Day 7
Capillary
Cytotrophoblast
Syncytiotrophoblast

C. Day 8
Chorion
Lacunae
Bilaminar germinal layer

D. Day 9
Amniotic cavity
Amnion
Yolk sac

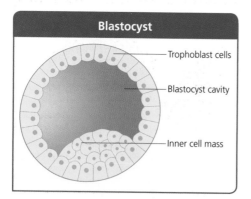

Blastocyst

Trophoblast cells
Blastocyst cavity
Inner cell mass

Figure 1.31 The embryo differentiates into a blastocyst consisting of an inner cell mass and a shell of trophoblast cells.

Figure 1.32 At implantation, the blastocyst releases proteolytic enzymes to embed itself in the endometrium.

Development of the germ layers

The inner cell mass starts to differentiate from the 10th day after conception. A bilaminar disc is formed, initially composed of embryonic ectoderm and endoderm.

- The ectoderm gives rise to the skin and neural structures
- The endoderm gives rise to the lining of the gut, the thyroid, the parathyroid, the respiratory tract, the liver and the pancreas

Between these two layers forms a third layer, the mesoderm. The mesoderm gives rise to bones, muscle, cartilage, subcutaneous tissue and the genitourinary organs.

All anatomical structures originate from these three layers, which are known as the germ layers (**Table 1.17**).

Folding

Initially, the germ layers form a flat circular disc. Disproportionate growth of the ectoderm means that the embryo folds in on itself, both longitudinally and transversely, to form a cylinder with a head and a tail fold (**Figure 1.33**). As a result of this folding:

- the ectoderm becomes the external surface of the embryo
- the endoderm becomes the internal surface
- the amniotic sac surrounds the whole embryo

Embryological origins of anatomical structures		
Germ layer	Component of germ layer	Anatomical structures
Ectoderm	Epidermis	Skin and hair
	Neural tube	Brain and spinal cord
	Neural crest	Peripheral nervous system
Endoderm	Primitive gut	Lung, liver, pancreas and gastrointestinal tract
Mesoderm	Paraxial	Skeleton, muscles and subcutaneous tissue
	Intermediate	Genitourinary tracts
	Lateral	Connective tissue of body wall, heart and blood vessels

Table 1.17 The embryological origins of all anatomical structures: the three germ layers

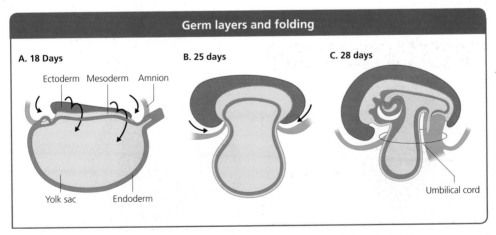

Germ layers and folding

A. 18 Days

Ectoderm Mesoderm Amnion

Yolk sac   Endoderm

B. 25 days

C. 28 days

Umbilical cord

Figure 1.33 Germ layers and folding. By day 25, the disproportionate growth of the ectoderm causes the embryo to form a cylinder with a head and a tail fold. The endoderm forms the yolk sac and the internal organs of the embryo. The yolk sac regresses and disappears by the 10th week of development.

Amnion and chorion

Extraembryonic membranes, known as the chorion and amnion, develop between weeks 2 and 12 to support the growing embryo.

- The chorion is the outer membrane; it develops from the trophoblast and becomes the fetal portion of the placenta and the outer layer of the amniotic sac
- The amnion is the inner membrane; it develops from the inner cell mass and forms the inner layer of the amniotic sac

Formation of the amniotic sac

The amniotic sac provides a protective environment in which the fetus can grow.

Amniotic cavity

This forms from the amnion that initially surrounds and protects the embryo (see **Figure 1.34**). When the inner cell mass differentiates into a bilaminar disc consisting of ectoderm and endoderm a small sac starts to form between the cytotrophoblast and the newly differentiated tissues. This is the amniotic cavity. The amniotic epithelium forming the roof and walls of the amniotic cavity are derived from the cytotrophoblast. The base of the amniotic cavity is the embryonic ectoderm.

Formation of the amniotic membrane

A second cavity (the extra-embryonic coelom) separates the amnion from the chorion

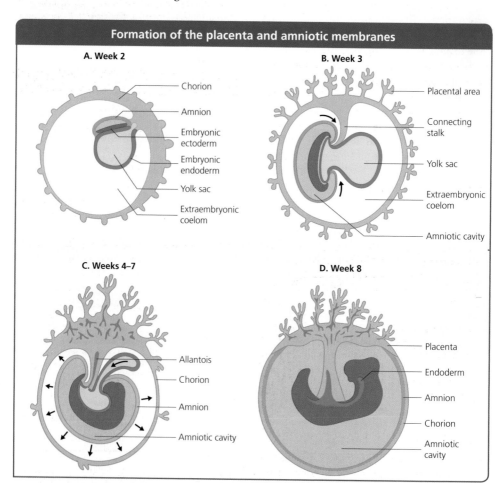

Formation of the placenta and amniotic membranes

A. Week 2 — Chorion, Amnion, Embryonic ectoderm, Embryonic endoderm, Yolk sac, Extraembryonic coelom

B. Week 3 — Placental area, Connecting stalk, Yolk sac, Extraembryonic coelom, Amniotic cavity

C. Weeks 4–7 — Allantois, Chorion, Amnion, Amniotic cavity

D. Week 8 — Placenta, Endoderm, Amnion, Chorion, Amniotic cavity

Figure 1.34 Formation of the placenta and amniotic membranes. The amnion and chorion form from the cytotrophoblast to give rise to the placenta and amniotic sac. The yolk sac shrinks as the embryo grows, disappearing by week 10. The allantois forms the umbilical arteries and veins.

until 14 weeks. As the pregnancy progresses, the amniotic space enlarges. This obliterates the extraembryonic coelom and leads to fusion of the amnion and chorion. A second sac, known as the the yolk sac, is simultaneously formed from the cells of the embryonic endoderm. It provides nutrients for the growing embryo until the placenta is established. It starts to disappear from the 10th week.

Amniotic fluid

The fluid in the amniotic cavity:

- cushions the fetus
- helps prevent compression of the umbilical cord
- gives the fetus room to grow and move

The volume of amniotic fluid increases during pregnancy, reaching 900–1000 mL in late pregnancy.

In the first trimester, water and solutes are able to pass freely through the fetal skin. Water and other solutes can also diffuse through the amniotic membrane covering the placenta.

By the second trimester, the fetal skin becomes keratinised and impermeable. From this time onward any increase in amniotic fluid volume is due to fetal urination. The fetus eliminates this fluid by swallowing and re-excreting it. At term, the fetus swallows and re-excretes 500 mL of fluid per day.

> **The volume of amniotic fluid provides information about fetal well-being.** In growth-restricted fetuses, chronic hypoxia due to impaired placental transfer leads to shunting of blood away from the kidneys to other vital organs. This causes reduced urine output and low amniotic fluid levels (oligohydramnios). Ultrasound measurements of the volume of amniotic fluid enable early recognition of impending placental failure and enable timely intervention or delivery.

Formation of the placenta

The placenta is specially adapted for the efficient delivery of oxygen and nutrients from mother to fetus, and the passage of waste products from fetus to mother (**Table 1.18**). The placenta is an organ with both maternal and fetal components.

- The maternal portion is known as the decidua basalis
- The fetal portion is known as the chorion (**Figure 1.35**)

The two portions are held in close contact by villi that grow from the fetal portion of the placenta into the decidua basalis.

The placenta forms between 2 and 12 weeks. Placental growth continues, with further branching of the villous trees and formation of new villi, until term.

Formation

In early pregnancy, lacunae ('lakes') form within the syncytiotrophoblast (**Figure 1.35**). These join to become the intervillous spaces into which maternal blood flows as the

Adaptations of the placenta	
Property	Adaptation
Surface area	Large surface area created by multiple branching villi, to maximise area available for transfer
Capillary density	High density of capillaries in areas in which exchange occurs, to maximise transport along concentration gradients
Diffusion distance	Direct contact between villi and maternal blood to minimise diffusion distance
Maternal blood flow	Large volume blood flow to placenta to maximise transfer
Changes with gestation	Surface area, capillary density and maternal blood flow increase to cope with the increasing demands of the growing fetus
	Diffusion distances decrease as a result of reduction in the villous stroma, thickness of the trophoblast layer and distance between the capillary and the villus wall

Table 1.18 Adaptations of the placenta for efficient feto-maternal transfer

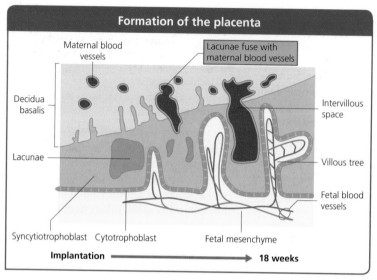

Formation of the placenta

Maternal blood vessels

Lacunae fuse with maternal blood vessels

Decidua basalis

Lacunae

Intervillous space

Villous tree

Fetal blood vessels

Syncytiotrophoblast   Cytotrophoblast

Fetal mesenchyme

Implantation ──────────────► 18 weeks

Figure 1.35 The placenta forms from the interconnection of the decidua basalis and the fetal chorionic villi. Lacunae within the synctiotrophoblast fuse with the maternal blood vessels to form the intervillous spaces. Villous trees, specialised for efficient exchange between the maternal and fetal blood, develop from the columns of synctiotrophoblast which separate the intervillous spaces.

maternal vessels become remodelled (see below). This interconnection allows the maternal blood to come into direct contact with the syncytiotrophoblast.

To enable efficient exchange at these points of contact, a network of villous trees develop to increase the surface area available. The villous trees develop from columns of syncytiotrophoblast that separate the intervillous spaces. These early villi contain a core of mesenchymal tissue, which develops into embryonic capillaries (**Figure 1.35**).

At the tips of the terminal villi are specialised membranes for solute exchange; these are known as vasculosyncytial membranes. Here, the embryonic capillary endothelium is fused to the syncytiotrophoblast. This reduces the diffusion distance between embryonic and maternal blood to $< 0.5\ \mu m$.

Remodelling the maternal blood vessels

A series of changes to the endometrial vasculature occurs to increase the maternal blood flow to the placenta. Groups of cytotrophoblastic cells invade the spiral arteries of the endometrium (**Figure 1.36**). These cells replace the endothelium and destroy the muscular and elastic walls of the arteries. The weakened arterial walls cause the vessels to dilate and the resistance within them to decrease. This results in the low-pressure, high-volume flow of maternal blood through the placenta. Blood flow into the extravillous spaces is seen by

11 weeks. Remodelling is thought to continue until 18 weeks of pregnancy.

> **Impaired remodelling of the spiral arteries** causes a range of placental pathologies, such as pre-eclampsia.

Endocrine changes

The placenta also acts as an endocrine organ, secreting numerous hormones to support the pregnancy (**Figure 1.37**). Hormones secreted from the placenta are responsible for the physiological and anatomical changes in pregnancy.

Secretion of human chorionic gonadotrophin (hCG) from the cytotrophoblasts starts within 48 h of implantation. hCG prevents the regression of the corpus luteum and signals it to enlarge. As a result, the corpus luteum continues to secrete progesterone, ensuring the endometrium is not shed.

> **Secretion of hCG leads to the retention of the endometrium.** Because the endometrium is not shed through menstruation, the first sign of pregnancy is often a missed period. Exponentially increasing levels of hCG in the first trimester, and renal excretion of hCG, mean that hCG can be detected in the urine from 2 weeks after fertilisation. This forms the basis of the urinary pregnancy test.

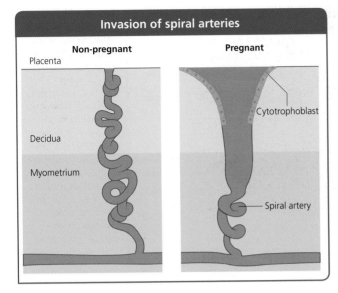

Figure 1.36 Invasion of spiral arteries by cytotrophoblast cells, which results in low-pressure, high-volume blood flow to the placenta.

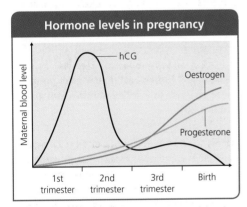

Figure 1.37 Hormone levels in pregnancy. Human chorionic gonadotrophin (hCG) is produced by the cytotrophoblast to maintain the corpus luteum. From the 5th week of pregnancy, the placenta produces oestrogen and progesterone.

From the 5th week of pregnancy, the placenta starts to produce oestrogens and progesterone, which mediate the changes in the mother's body required to meet the demands of the growing fetus and prepare the body for labour and delivery. Placental production of oestrogen and progesterone requires a series of chemical conversions in both the fetus and the placenta.

■ The placenta converts cholesterol to progesterone

■ Progesterone is converted by the fetal adrenal glands and liver to the androgen dehydroepiandrosterone sulphate (DHEA-S)
■ DHEA-S is transported back to the placenta, via fetal blood, to be converted to oestrogens

Organogenesis
Development of the nervous system

The neural tube is the precursor of the brain and spinal cord (**Figure 1.38**). It is formed by the folding of a thickening of the dorsal ectoderm called the neural plate.

■ The brain develops at the cranial end of the neural tube
■ The spinal cord develops from the caudal end

> **Neural tube defects, such as anencephaly and spina bifida, occur because of the incomplete closure of the neural tube during development.** Folic acid supplementation reduces the incidence of neural tube defects.

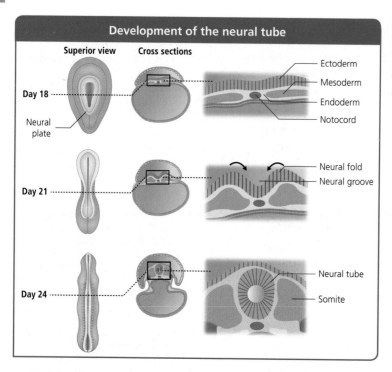

Development of the neural tube

Superior view   Cross sections

Day 18

Neural plate

Ectoderm
Mesoderm
Endoderm
Notocord

Day 21

Neural fold
Neural groove

Day 24

Neural tube
Somite

Figure 1.38 Development of the neural tube. The neural tube folds to form the spinal cord and the brain.

Development of the head and neck

The head and neck are formed from the frontonasal prominences and the pharyngeal arches (a series of folds of tissue derived from all three germ layers). Each arch has a cartilaginous bone, corresponding muscles, an aortic blood supply and innervation by a cranial nerve (**Table 1.19**).

The pharyngeal arches are separated by grooves. The internal surfaces of these grooves are known as pharyngeal pouches. These give rise to a series of tubes and glands (**Table 1.20**).

Face

The face develops from the frontonasal prominences and the first pharyngeal arch (**Figure 1.39**).

■ The frontonasal prominences give rise to the forehead, nose and mid-section of the lip (philtrum)

Pharyngeal arch derivatives

Arch*	Skeletal derivative	Muscle derivative	Innervation	Blood supply
1st	Facial bones and malleus, incus of the middle ear	Muscles of mastication	Trigeminal nerve (CN V)	Maxillary artery
2nd	Stapes and part of the hyoid	Muscles of facial expression	Facial nerve (VII)	Stapedial and hyoid artery
3rd	Part of the hyoid	Stylopharyngeus	Glossopharyngeal nerve (XI)	Internal carotid
4th and 6th	Thyroid and cricoid cartilages	Muscles of the larynx and pharynx	Vagus nerve (X)	Right subclavian and aorta

*No structures are derived from the 5th arch. CN, cranial nerve.

Table 1.19 Pharyngeal arch derivatives and their innervation and blood supply

Pharyngeal pouch derivatives	
Pharyngeal pouch	Organ
1st	Auditory canal and middle ear
2nd	Palatine tonsils
3rd	Inferior parathyroids and thymus
4th	Superior parathryoids and C cells of the thyroid

Table 1.20 Organs of the pharyngeal pouches

■ The first pharyngeal arch gives rise to the remaining features, which make up the lower two thirds of the face

The philtrum is formed by fusion of the medial nasal prominences. The lateral nasal prominences merge with the maxillary processes and the newly formed philtrum to form the midface.

Palate

The palate is the roof of the mouth, separating the nasal cavity from the oral cavity. It has roles in both feeding and speech. During suckling, babies form a seal around the nipple or teat by pressing it up against the palate, producing a vacuum that allows muscular motions of the jaw and tongue to draw milk into their mouths. During normal speech, the palate regulates the flow of air between the nose and the mouth. The ability to close off the nasal cavity from the mouth means that more air and therefore sound is directed from the mouth; this enables us to make consonant sounds.

The palate is formed in two parts: the primary palate and the secondary palate. The primary palate forms at the same time as the

external face, from the posterior extension of the intermaxillary prominence.

As the face grows, the primary palate becomes too short to adequately separate the oral and nasal cavities. The palatal shelves form from the maxillary processes on either side. They grow medially and fuse in the midline and become the secondary palate. Simultaneously, the secondary palate fuses with the primary palate to form one continuous sheet of tissue: the definitive palate.

Failures of the nasal prominences to merge or the palatal shelves to fuse result in clefts of the palate, the lip or both. These can cause difficulties with feeding and speech. The likelihood of a cleft occurring is increased if:

■ one or both parents, or other family members, have a cleft

■ there is poor maternal nutrition, folic acid deficiency, obesity, smoking, alcohol consumption, or use of drugs such as phenytoin and methotrexate

■ the baby has an underlying genetic condition, e.g. Pierre Robin sequence, DiGeorge syndrome (deletion of chromosome 22)

Usually no specific cause is identified. Preconception counselling can help women reduce the chance of a cleft developing.

Development of the fetal cardiovascular system

The heart is one of the first organs to develop. A fetal heartbeat can be detected by the 22nd day of intrauterine life.

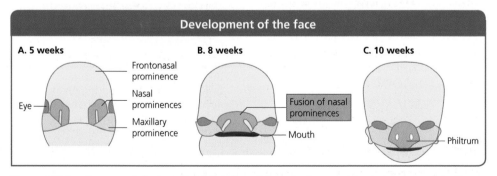

Development of the face

A. 5 weeks — Frontonasal prominence, Nasal prominences, Maxillary prominence, Eye

B. 8 weeks — Fusion of nasal prominences, Mouth

C. 10 weeks — Philtrum

Figure 1.39 Development of the face. The face is formed from the frontonasal prominences and the first pharyngeal arch.

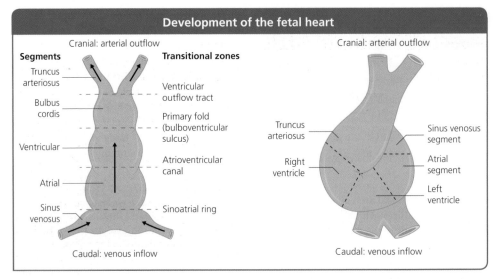

Figure 1.40 Development of the fetal heart. Rotation of the fused endocardial tubes leads to the position of the atria and ventricles at birth.

The heart is formed by fusion of the two endocardial tubes to form a single tract (**Figure 1.40**). The resulting heart tube differentiates into segments known as the truncus arteriosus, bulbus cordis, primitive ventricle, primitive atrium and sinus venosus.

The truncus arteriosus forms the ascending aorta and the pulmonary trunk. Growth of the primitive ventricle causes the tube to loop back on itself to form an 'S' shape. The atrium then moves upwards and to the left to lie above and in front of the ventricle.

Overlapping septa then form in the atrium and ventricle to separate the right and left sides of the heart. Before birth, the overlapping edges of the atrial septa form a one-way valve that allows the shunting of blood from the right side of the heart to the left, via the foramen ovale. At birth, increased pressure from the left side presses the two edges of the overlapping septa together, closing the shunt and separating the right and left atria.

Development of the alimentary system

By the 3rd week of gestation, a primitive gut tube extends from the buccopharyngeal membrane, an embryonic structure that covers the developing mouth and pharynx, to the cloacal membrane, which covers the developing rectum and urogenital tracts. The gut tube is divided into three regions:

- the foregut
- the midgut
- the hindgut

All organs of the alimentary system derive from these regions (**Table 1.21**). Each region has its own blood supply and lymphatic drainage.

Omphacele and gastroschisis are congenital defects of the anterior abdominal wall. They differ in terms of their pathology and associated conditions.

An omphalocele is a consequence of failure of the midgut to return to the abdominal cavity; it remains outside the abdomen, enclosed in a peritoneal sac. This protrusion (herniation) is located in the midline, through the umbilicus. Omphaloceles are associated with cardiac and neural tube defects.

In gastroschisis, there is a failure of the abdominal wall to completely fuse. This leads to the protrusion of abdominal contents through the defect. It differs from an omphacele in that the abdominal contents are not covered by peritoneum and the herniation occurs lateral to the umbilicus. Gastroschisis has no associations with other birth defects.

Embryological origins of organs of the alimentary canal	
Section of embryonic gut	**Organs**
Foregut	Oesophagus, upper duodenum, stomach, liver and pancreas
Midgut	Lower duodenum, small intestine and proximal two thirds of transverse colon
Hindgut	Distal third of transverse colon, descending colon and rectum

Table 1.21 Embryological origins of the alimentary canal: the foregut, midgut and hindgut

The midgut grows far more rapidly than the rest of the tube. Therefore much of the midgut is herniated through the abdomen at the umbilicus during the first trimester. From 11 weeks, the midgut rotates 90°, thereby moving the duodenum, jejunum and ileum to the right and the distal ileum, caecum and ascending colon to the left, and returns to the abdomen. Within the abdomen, the gut continues to rotate until it reaches its final position (**Figure 1.41**).

All the nutritional requirements of the fetus are met by uptake of nutrients via the placenta. However, the digestive system must be ready to absorb nutrients and water immediately after birth. Passage of food and fluids through the digestive tract requires autonomic control. Swallowing and gut movement are visible in fetuses from 12 weeks of gestation.

> **Swallowing of amniotic fluid is essential for the maintenance of levels of amniotic fluid.** Gastrointestinal abnormalities that prevent swallowing, such as duodenal and oesophageal atresia, are a cause of an excess of amniotic fluid (polyhydramnios).
>
> In contrast, bilateral renal agenesis results in a deficiency of amniotic fluid (oligohydramnios). The absence of kidneys means that the volume of amniotic fluid freely swallowed by the fetus is not replaced by the volume of urine voided during micturition.

Development of the genitourinary system

The urinary and genital systems develop in close conjunction (see page 9 for a description of the development of the female reproductive tract).

Kidney development occurs in three stages between the 3rd and 4th week of gestation. The first two stages are development of first the pronephros and then the mesonephros. These structures regress, and it is only the metanephros, which develops in the last stage, going on to form the functional kidney. The metanephros is formed from two embryological structures:

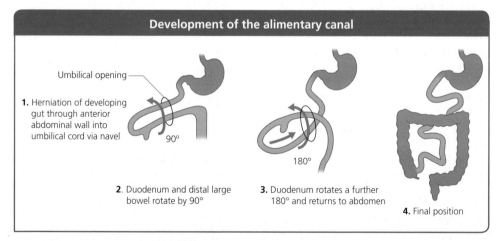

Development of the alimentary canal

Umbilical opening

1. Herniation of developing gut through anterior abdominal wall into umbilical cord via navel

90°

180°

2. Duodenum and distal large bowel rotate by 90°

3. Duodenum rotates a further 180° and returns to abdomen

4. Final position

Figure 1.41 Development of the alimentary canal. The position of the midgut and hindgut structures within the abdominal cavity are the result of rotation during development.

- the ureteric bud, which grows upwards from the cloaca to form the ureter, renal pelvis and renal calyces
- the metanephric mesoderm, which forms the renal parenchyma and collecting duct systems

The metanephros develops in the sacral region. Over the next few weeks, the kidney 'ascends' to sit in the lumbar area. This is a consequence of differential growth in the sacral and lumbar regions rather than true migration.

> **A failure of the kidneys to ascend during development causes anatomical variants.** The most common variant is horseshoe kidneys, which are present in 1 in 500 people. Horseshoe kidneys are prevented from ascending by their fusion in the midline. Up to 25% of people with a horseshoe kidney also have chromosomal abnormalities or malformations of other genitourinary structures.

The hindgut and the genitourinary tract share a common opening, known as the cloaca, until the 5th week of gestation. A band of tissue known as the urorectal septum forms from the 5th week to separate the urogenital membrane and the anal membrane. The bladder, the urethra and in females the lower part of the vagina are all formed from the ventral portion of the cloaca, the urogenital membrane.

Fetal adaptations to intrauterine life and changes at birth

The fetus relies on the placenta for fulfilment of all its respiratory and metabolic needs. Both the fetus and the placenta are adapted to ensure the efficient transfer of respiratory gases and other substances. At birth, various changes occur to enable the neonate to survive without a placenta.

Fetal gas exchange and changes at birth

Less oxygen is available to a fetus in utero than to a baby after birth. Fetal circulation is adapted to facilitate efficient gas exchange in utero. The site of gas exchange switches to the lungs at birth.

Placental gas exchange

The exchange of oxygen and carbon dioxide between the maternal and fetal circulations occurs in the placenta by diffusion down the concentration gradient of each gas. The rate of gaseous exchange depends on the relative concentration of each gas on the maternal and fetal side of the placenta. At the placental surface, maternal blood releases oxygen. The oxygen binds to haemoglobin in fetal red blood cells.

Fetal red blood cells contain a unique form of haemoglobin with a higher affinity for oxygen than adult haemoglobin (**Figure 1.42**). This enables oxygen loading of fetal red blood cells to occur at lower oxygen concentrations. However, it also means that less oxygen dissociates from haemoglobin at a given tissue oxygen concentration. Therefore to ensure efficient delivery of oxygen to fetal tissues:

- fetal red blood cells make up a greater percentage of blood volume (haematocrit)
- fetal haemoglobin has an exaggerated response to acidic pH (the Bohr effect)

Gas exchange in fetal tissues

Dissolved carbon dioxide in fetal tissues ionises to form hydrogen ions (H^+) and bicarbonate ions (HCO_3^-). When fetal haemoglobin binds H^+ ions, its affinity for oxygen decreases. This shifts the oxygen dissociation curve to the right, favouring the release of oxygen bound to fetal haemoglobin. This deoxygenation increases the ability of the haemoglobin to carry carbon dioxide.

> **The oxygen dissociation curve is a plot of percentage oxygen saturation at any given oxygen concentration.** The dissociation curve for fetal haemoglobin is shifted to the left compared with that for adult haemoglobin. This enables the fetus to obtain oxygen from the maternal circulation.

In hypoxia, oxygen levels decrease and carbon dioxide accumulates. The reduction in oxygen causes the tissues to switch

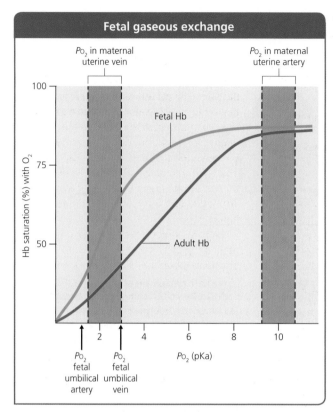

Figure 1.42 Fetal gaseous exchange. Fetal haemoglobin has a higher affinity for oxygen, shifting the dissociation curve to the left.

to anaerobic respiration, which produces lactic acid. Therefore hypoxia produces a mixed respiratory and metabolic acidosis. To compensate for acute acidosis, the oxygen dissociation curve shifts to the right, so that more oxygen is released and more haemoglobin becomes available to buffer the H+ ions.

> **Measurements of fetal scalp pH during labour provide an indication of fetal well-being.** Fetuses are normally able to maintain their pH within a tight range. If a fetus cannot compensate for the acidosis associated with acute hypoxia, the pH of the fetal blood decreases.

Throughout gestation, production of fetal haemoglobin declines and that of adult haemoglobin increases. At birth, fetal haemoglobin makes up 50–95% of the infant's haemoglobin. The switch to adult haemoglobin production is complete by 6 months of age.

Initiation of breathing

At birth, the initiation of breathing depends on the infant's ability to respond to a number of stimuli. This requires:

- an intact nervous system
- a respiratory centre sufficiently mature to respond to chemical and mechanical stimuli
- lungs mature enough to inflate efficiently

The initiation of breathing is integral to the profound alterations in the fetal circulation that allow gaseous exchange to occur in the lungs.

Irregular breathing movements are visible in fetuses from 11 weeks' gestation. These become more regular as pregnancy progresses, and are a sign of an intact central nervous system. Breathing movements reduce in frequency just before birth. Fetal breathing movements aid the flow of lung fluid to and from the amniotic cavity, and increase the tone of respiratory muscles in preparation for birth (**Figure 1.43**).

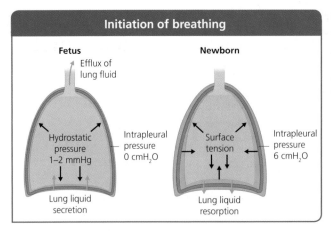

Figure 1.43 Initiation of breathing. Fetal breathing movements help move amniotic fluid in and out of the lungs. After birth, fluid is pushed into the vascular space and the lungs fill with air. To prevent the lungs collapsing during exhalation, surfactant is produced to increase surface tension.

At birth, tactile and cold stimuli, along with stimuli caused by hypoxia and hypercapnia from the rapid reduction of blood flow to and from the placenta, act centrally to trigger an increase in breathing movements. As the first breath is taken, fluid is pushed across the alveolar walls into the capillaries and lymphatics of the lung parenchyma (see **Figure 1.43**). Large intrathoracic pressures are required to overcome the pressure of the viscous lung fluid.

About 40 mL of air enters the lungs in the first breath. Half of this is expelled during exhalation. The remainder forms the residual volume. Functional residual capacity, i.e. the volume of air present at the end of quiet breathing, is established within a few breaths.

Maintenance of regular breathing depends on the ability of the lung to remain inflated at the end of expiration. From 24 weeks, type 2 pneumocytes (alveolar cells) start to make pulmonary surfactant. Surfactant is a mixture of phospholipids and proteins that help maintain the surface tension of the alveolar walls at low lung volumes. This surface tension prevents the alveoli from collapsing after exhalation (**Figure 1.43**).

The production of surfactant is triggered by release of cortisol from the fetal adrenal glands. Cortisol production increases gradually throughout gestation, and increases dramatically in response to the stress of labour.

Preterm babies are at particular risk of difficulty establishing regular breathing. Corticosteroid injections are given to pregnant women in whom preterm delivery is imminent, to boost the baby's surfactant production before birth. This intervention reduces the risk of neonatal respiratory distress syndrome for up to a week after administration.

In utero, blood flow is diverted away from the pulmonary vasculature. When the umbilical cord is clamped, placental circulation ceases and there is a decrease in pressure in the right side of the heart triggering a series of events that divert blood into the pulmonary vasculature.

With the start of breathing, the arterial partial pressure of oxygen increases rapidly and that of carbon dioxide decreases. This triggers relaxation of the arterioles within the pulmonary vascular bed, thereby enabling a large increase in pulmonary blood flow. These changes mean that changes in ventilation are matched by changes in perfusion (**Table 1.22**).

Fetal circulation and changes at birth

The fetus receives oxygenated blood from the placenta via the umbilical vein (**Figure 1.44**).

Fetal respiratory system: changes after birth			
Component of the cardio-respiratory system	Changes in utero	Changes after birth	Trigger for changes after birth
Lungs and chest wall	Increase in production of surfactant Increase in respiratory muscle tone Increase in breathing movements in second trimester	Fluid is pushed out of lungs by breathing movements Lungs become inflated with air Surfactant prevents alveolar collapse	Hypoxia Hypercapnia Cold Light Tactile stimuli
Pulmonary circulation	Diversion of blood away from the pulmonary circulation	Diversion of blood into pulmonary circulation Relaxation of pulmonary arterioles	Closure of foramen ovale and ductus arteriosus Positive feedback from increasing po_2 and decreasing pco_2 in pulmonary vasculature
Oxygen-carrying capacity of blood	Predominance of fetal haemoglobin	Gradual switch from fetal to adult haemoglobin	Changes in the ratio of fetal to adult haemoglobin production start before birth

Table 1.22 Changes to the fetal respiratory system to prepare for the switch of gas exchange from the placenta to the lungs

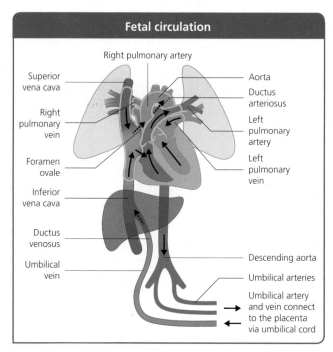

Figure 1.44 The fetal circulation is adapted to receive oxygenated blood from the umbilical vein and bypass the lungs.

Newly oxygenated blood mixes with deoxygenated blood from the inferior cava by bypassing the liver via the ductus venosus. This blood is joined by deoxygenated blood from the superior vena cava as it enters the right atrium.

Pressure in the right atrium is higher than in the left atrium. This pressure differential causes most of the blood to pass through the patent foramen ovale into the left atrium, thereby bypassing the pulmonary circulation. Some of the blood enters the right ventricle and passes through the pulmonary trunk. This blood is diverted to the aorta by the ductus arteriosus, again avoiding the pulmonary circulation.

Blood from the left ventricle (and the right ventricle via the ductus arteriosus) enters the aorta to pass into the fetal circulation. Deoxygenated blood from the body returns to the placenta via the umbilical arteries.

Table 1.23 summarises the changes in the fetal circulation at birth. Immediately after birth, the umbilical arteries spasm in response to the difference in temperature between the outside world and the uterine environment. This greatly reduces venous return to the heart. Consequently, pressure in the right atrium decreases, thereby closing the foramen ovale.

With the baby's first breath, resistance in the pulmonary circulation decreases. Blood from the right atrium now preferentially enters the right ventricle, thereby redistributing blood flow into the pulmonary arteries. The ductus arteriosus, which previously diverted blood into the aorta, also closes.

These changes occur rapidly. In healthy infants, the foramen ovale and ductus arteriosus close functionally within the first few hours after delivery. Permanent closure of these shunts by fibrosis is completed 4–6 weeks later.

> In the fetus, the ductus arteriosus remains patent because of the action of prostaglandins. Prostaglandins cause dilation of the smooth muscle of the vessel walls. After birth, prostaglandin levels decrease rapidly, leading to closure of the ductus arteriosus. Prostaglandin synthetase inhibitors, such as indomethacin, are used therapeutically to accelerate closure of the ductus arteriosus in newborns.

Maternal adaptions in pregnancy

During pregnancy, the female body undergoes various adaptations to cope with the

Fetal circulation: changes at birth				
Structure	Before birth	After birth	Name in adults	Effect of closure
Umbilical vein	Carries oxygenated blood from placenta	Becomes obliterated	Ligamentum teres	Reduction in oxygen tension after loss of blood flow from placenta triggers initiation of breathing Decrease in blood flow to right side of heart closes foramen ovale
Umbilical artery	Returns deoxygenated blood to placenta	Becomes obliterated	Medial umbilical ligament	Hypercapnia at birth triggers breathing
Ductus venosus	Shunts oxygenated blood from umbilical vein directly into inferior vena cava	Degenerates	Ligamentum venosum	Only deoxygenated blood enters inferior vena cava
Foramen ovale	Shunts mixed blood from right atrium to left side of heart	Closes, leaving a small depression	Fossa ovalis	Isolates oxygenated and deoxygenated blood to separate sides of heart
Ductus arteriosus	Shunts blood leaving the right ventricle into the aorta	Constricts	Ligamentum arteriosum	Blood from right ventricle enters pulmonary circulation

Table 1.23 Changes in the fetal circulation at birth

increased demands of supporting a growing fetus. These include:

- increase in minute ventilation
- increase in blood volume and cardiac output
- increase in clotting ability of the blood
- maturation of breast tissue
- enlargement of the uterus

These changes are mediated by increasing levels of oestrogen and progesterone.

Cardiovascular system

Changes to maternal cardiovascular physiology are evident from the 4th week of pregnancy (**Table 1.24**). These changes are required to meet the increasing metabolic demands of the growing fetus and developing organs. They also protect the mother from the effects of blood loss at delivery.

Blood plasma

Plasma volume increases by 45% during the first half of pregnancy to meet the increasing metabolic demands from the growing fetus and the maternal organs, e.g. uterus, breast, skin. This change is caused by increased activation of the renin–angiotensin–aldosterone system. During pregnancy, the level of renin produced by maternal kidney, ovary and decidua increases. Oestrogen stimulates the production of angiotensinogen from the liver, while progesterone inhibits aldosterone binding to mineralocorticoid receptors leading to an increase in aldosterone production. These changes lead to sodium and water retention by the kidney. Minimal further change in plasma volume occurs from 28 weeks' gestation.

Blood volume

The number of red blood cells increases in conjunction with the increase in plasma volume; together they cause an increase in blood volume that protects the mother from the effects of blood loss during delivery. Red blood cell mass (the total number of red blood cells in circulation) increases steadily in response to increased erythropoietin production by the kidney. This increases the oxygen carrying capacity of the blood. However, in contrast to the great increase in plasma volume, red blood cell mass increases by only 20%. Therefore haematocrit and relative haemoglobin levels decrease; a 20% decrease in haemoglobin concentration is normal. This phenomenon is known as physiological anaemia of pregnancy.

The increase in blood volume in pregnancy can mask signs of hypovolaemia. Tachycardia and hypotension are signs of massive blood loss, but do not commonly occur until the woman has lost >30% of her blood volume, i.e. nearly 2 L of blood.

> **Massive haemorrhage increases the risk of disseminated intravascular coagulopathy and is a major cause of maternal death.** The cause of bleeding must be identified and corrected rapidly, and fluids replaced accordingly.

Haemodynamic variables: changes in pregnancy			
Variable	First trimester	Second trimester	Third trimester
Pulse rate	+	++	+++
Systolic blood pressure	↓	No change	No change
Diastolic blood pressure	↓	↓	Returned to prepregnancy levels
Blood volume	+	++	+++
Cardiac output	No change	+++	+++
Systemic vascular resistance	↓	↓	↓
Haematocrit	↓	↓	↓
+, small increase; ++, moderate increase; +++, large increase.			

Table 1.24 Changes in mean haemodynamic variables in pregnancy

Cardiac output

In response to increased blood volume (preload), the stroke volume (the amount of blood ejected from the heart) increases. This is accompanied by an increase in heart rate from 80–90 beats/min. Together, these changes account for an increase in the cardiac output from 4.5 L at the beginning of pregnancy to 6 L by the end. This increases the volume of oxygenated blood reaching the tissues. Because oxygen demand increases only slightly, the arteriovenous oxygen gradient decreases in pregnancy. Much of this increased blood flow goes to the kidneys, skin and breasts in early pregnancy. Blood flow to the uterus increases throughout pregnancy, and at term it receives 400 mL of blood a minute.

Peripheral vascular resistance

Increased levels of oestrogen and progesterone cause vasodilation and a reduction in peripheral vascular resistance. As a result, both systolic and diastolic blood pressure decrease in the first trimester. Increases in the cardiac output mean that despite a reduction in peripheral vascular resistance, blood pressure returns to prepregnancy levels by the second trimester.

By 20 weeks' gestation, the enlarging uterus can compress the descending aorta and inferior vena cava when the mother is supine (lying on her back). Compression of the vena cava decreases venous return and therefore blood pressure. Compression of the aorta further reduces blood flow to the uterus. Both factors lead to decreased placental perfusion and maternal hypotension.

For cardiopulmonary resuscitation, pregnant women are placed in the left lateral position using a wedge. This reduces compression of the vena cava by the pregnant uterus, thereby helping restore venous return to the heart and facilitating resuscitation. Perimortem caesarean delivery should be carried out within 4 min of cardiac arrest to reduce the risk of hypoxic brain injury to both mother and baby.

Coagulation

High levels of oestrogen during pregnancy induce a hypercoagulable state, i.e. an increased tendency for blood clotting (**Table 1.25**). This aids haemostasis after delivery, thereby minimising post-partum blood loss. There is also an increase in platelet production, but increased platelet consumption and increased plasma volume mean that platelet levels decrease towards term.

Pregnant women are 20 times more likely to develop a venous thromboembolism. This is a leading cause of maternal mortality. To reduce the risk of DVT during a long-haul flight, pregnant women are advised to keep well hydrated, take regular walks whilst on the aeroplane and to wear graduated compression stockings.

Coagulation factors: changes in pregnancy	
Factor(s)	Change in pregnancy
Factors II, VII, VIII, IX, X, XII and fibrinogen	↑
Protein S	↓
Protein C and antithrombin III	No change
Von Willebrand's factor	↑
Plasminogen	↑
D-dimer	↑
Bleeding time and prothrombin times	No change

Table 1.25 Changes in coagulation factors in pregnancy

Respiratory system

During pregnancy, the oxygen requirements of the fetus and the increased metabolic activity of the mother's organs mean that there is an increased requirement for oxygen. The respiratory system meets this requirement by increasing the amount of air inhaled (minute ventilation, i.e. the volume of air inhaled in 1 minute).

Respiratory variables: changes in pregnancy	
Variable	Change in pregnancy
Respiratory rate	↑
Peak flow	No change
Arterial oxygen concentration	↑
Arterial carbon dioxide concentration	↓
Tidal volume	↑
Minute ventilation	↑
Vital capacity	No change
Functional residual capacity	↓

Table 1.26 Changes in respiratory variables in pregnancy

Physiological changes in ventilation, summarised in **Table 1.26**, are mediated by hormones. For example, progesterone:

- stimulates respiratory centres directly
- increases the sensitivity of chemoreceptors to CO_2, leading to a small increase in respiratory rate
- promotes relaxation of the bronchial and tracheal smooth muscle

Relaxin causes progressive relaxation of the ligamentous attachment of the ribs, thereby increasing chest circumference. This allows an increase in tidal volume with minimal change in respiratory effort.

By the end of the third trimester, the uterus lies underneath the diaphragm, reducing the functional residual capacity. Lung compliance and peak flow remain unchanged.

Pregnancy has variable effects on asthma. During pregnancy, one third of women with asthma will get worse, one third will feel better and one third will show no change in symptoms. Peak flow is unaffected by pregnancy; therefore changes in peak flow remain reliable measures of the severity of an exacerbation of asthma.

Changes in the respiratory system also trigger the production of 2,3-diphosphoglycerate (2,3-DPG), which increases oxygen transfer in the periphery. Production of 2,3-DPG is triggered by the increase in secretion of bicarbonate to compensate for the respiratory alkalosis caused by increased minute ventilation. 2,3-DPG in the blood shifts the oxygen dissociation curve to the right, favouring unloading of oxygen in the periphery and aiding placental oxygen transfer.

Renal system

Profound changes occur in the renal system during pregnancy to cope with the increased blood volumes needed to meet the demands of the growing fetus and the maternal organs.

In pregnancy, increases in renal blood flow cause an increase in the excretion of waste products. This typically causes levels of serum creatinine and urea to fall. Therefore, normal test results for creatinine and urea in non-pregnant women can indicate significant renal impairment in pregnancy.

There are several changes in the renal system during pregnancy.

- The kidneys increase by 1 cm in length as a result of increased renal vascular and interstitial volume
- The ureters dilate, partly as a consequence of smooth muscle relaxation in response to progesterone and pressure from the enlarging uterus; this increases urinary stasis within the ureters making pregnant women more prone to upper urinary tract infections (pyelonephritis)
- Renal blood flow and glomerular filtration rate increase, because of the increase in cardiac output; these effects lead to decreases in urea, creatinine and bicarbonate levels
- The activity of renin-angiotensin, aldosterone and progesterone increases in pregnancy; this leads to water retention and a resultant decrease in plasma osmolality

Renal variables: changes in pregnancy		
Variable	Change in pregnancy	Normal values in pregnancy
Kidney size	↑	10–12 cm
Ureteric diameter	↑	Right greater than left because of position of uterus
Renal blood flow	↑	700 mL/min
Glomerular filtration rate	↑	140 mL/min per 1.73 m^2
Serum creatinine	↓	35–75 µmol/L
Serum urea	↓	1.0–3.8 mmol/L

Table 1.27 Changes in renal variables in pregnancy

The effects of pregnancy on renal variables are summarised in **Table 1.27**.

Excess sugar in the urine (glycosuria) is common in pregnancy and is not necessarily a sign of diabetes. Increases in glomerular filtration rate increase the amount of glucose reaching the kidneys at any given time. This reduces the capacity of the renal tubules to reabsorb glucose. Serum glucose levels following a glucose load (oral glucose tolerance test) are used instead for screening for diabetes in pregnancy.

Nutrition

During pregnancy, energy requirements from the growing fetus and maternal organs increase with each trimester. By the third trimester, pregnant women require an extra 300 calories (1250 kJ) a day to meet the demands of pregnancy.

Carbohydrate metabolism

This is altered in pregnancy to favour transfer of glucose to the fetus. Glucose is transferred into the fetal circulation by carrier proteins in the villous membranes (facilitated diffusion) in the placenta. To maintain high levels of maternal plasma glucose, the anti-insulin effects of two placental-derived hormones reprogramme the body's response to insulin. Human placental lactogen and human placental growth hormone:

- decrease maternal insulin sensitivity
- decrease maternal glucose use
- stimulate lipolysis

Maternal insulin does not cross the placenta, but glucose can move freely. Chronic hyperglycaemia associated with maternal diabetes therefore leads to an increase in fetal insulin production. Fetal hyperinsulinaemia predisposes infants to hypoglycaemia once placental transfer of glucose ceases at birth.

Iron

The requirement for iron is increased in pregnancy, to meet the need for increased production of red blood cells. Pregnant women need an additional 4 mg of iron daily. This requirement cannot be met by increased absorption of iron from the diet alone, so stored iron is mobilised from ferritin molecules.

In women with low iron stores or who are already anaemic, pregnancy rapidly causes symptoms of anaemia, e.g. dizziness, fatigue and breathlessness. Iron supplementation increases serum iron concentration and over the course of a few weeks increases haemoglobin levels.

Labour and the puerperium

Starter questions

Answers to the following questions are on page 76.

20. Why do women have painful labours?
21. Can eating certain foods induce labour?

During pregnancy, there is a dynamic balance between factors that inhibit uterine contractility, such as progesterone, and those that stimulate uterine activity, such as prostaglandins and oxytocin. For delivery to occur, two changes in the reproductive tract have to take place:

■ the uterus must become capable of regular synchronised contractions
■ the structure of the cervix must change to allow dilation and passage of the fetus

The forceful uterine contractions of labour expel the fetus and the placenta. Labour is divided into three stages.

■ The first stage is onset of regular painful contractions and dilation of the cervix
■ The second stage is passage of the fetus through the vaginal canal, resulting in its delivery
■ The third stage, expulsion of the placenta, occurs rapidly thereafter

The puerperium follows delivery; it is the period in which the reproductive organs return to their non-pregnant state. Changes in the breast during pregnancy facilitate lactation, enabling the mother to produce milk to feed the baby following delivery (see page 71).

First stage of labour

During the first stage of labour, regular uterine contractions force the fetus against the cervix, causing progressive shortening and subsequent dilation of the cervix. By the end of the first stage of labour, the cervix dilates enough for the widest point of the presenting (leading) part of the fetus to pass through. On vaginal examination, the cervix will no longer be felt in front of the fetus.

Uterine contractions

The uterus is naturally contractile. As the pregnant uterus expands, the muscle fibres of the myometrium are stretched but contractility does not increase. Throughout pregnancy, progesterone inhibits myometrial contractility. This inhibition functions as a physiological 'brake', which is overridden by the complex interactions of multiple factors that trigger labour.

The progesterone antagonist mifepristone is used to prime the uterus for contractions. It is used, in conjunction with the synthetic prostaglandin misoprostol, to induce delivery after fetal demise. These drugs cause strong contractions. Because they are given orally or vaginally their absorption, and therefore the strength and duration of the resulting contractions, cannot be easily controlled. Contractions that are too frequent cause hypoxia in a live fetus and therefore these drugs are not commonly used to augment contractions in live pregnancies.

The uterine muscle undergoes multiple changes to make it capable of producing rhythmic contractions. These changes occur in response to increasing levels of corticotrophin-releasing hormone and oestrogen.

■ The density of calcium channels and gap junctions increases, making the myocytes more sensitive to depolarisation

- Myocytes transmit action potentials more readily
- Oestrogen also stimulates production of uterotonic substances, such as oxytocin and prostaglandins, that trigger contractions

Labour is induced artificially by the use of intravaginal prostaglandins. This softens the cervix and causes mild uterine contractions. In most women undergoing induction of labour, oxytocin must also be given to augment the frequency and force of these contractions. Oxytocin has a short half-life, so its action can be easily titrated during intravenous administration.

Placental blood flow decreases as a result of the occlusion of the spiral arteries during uterine contraction. When the uterus relaxes between contractions, large volumes of maternal blood enter the intervillous spaces, thereby increasing gaseous transfer. If the contractions become too frequent, or the time between contractions decreases, less gas exchange can occur, leading to fetal hypoxia.

Cervical dilation

Before labour, the cervix is firm and 3–4 cm long. To enable the passage of the fetus, the cervix must shorten and dilate (**Figure 1.45**).

The first stage of labour has two stages.

- During the latent stage, the cervix thins and begins to dilate
- The established stage begins when the cervix dilates to 4 cm and ends when the cervix is fully dilated at 10 cm

First, the cervix becomes soft and pliable. Prostaglandins and relaxin mediate this cervical ripening. These factors cause the connective tissue of the cervix to be remodelled; collagen and elastin fibres in the cervix are enzymatically degraded, softening the cervix. During this process, the junction between the amniotic membranes and the decidua basalis weakens, which releases an adhesive protein known as fetal fibronectin into the vagina.

The presence of fetal fibronectin in vaginal fluids is associated with imminent delivery. Women presenting with threatened preterm labour can be triaged according to whether or not fetal fibronectin is detected. If fibronectin is present, the risk of preterm delivery is increased; the mother is offered potent corticosteroids to help mature the fetal lungs in preparation for an early delivery.

Uterine contractions force the presenting part, most commonly the head, against the

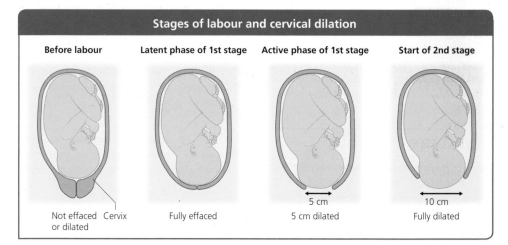

Stages of labour and cervical dilation

| Before labour | Latent phase of 1st stage | Active phase of 1st stage | Start of 2nd stage |

Not effaced Cervix
or dilated

Fully effaced

5 cm
5 cm dilated

10 cm
Fully dilated

Figure 1.45 Stages of labour and cervical dilation. In the first stage of labour, the cervix shortens, effaces and dilates. When the cervix is fully dilated, the fetus descends along the vaginal canal.

cervix, which leads to shortening and thinning of the cervical canal. When the cervix thins to the thickness of the adjacent lower segment of the uterus, it is termed fully effaced. Further contractions enable the fetus to descend in the pelvic cavity, thereby dilating the cervix further. The cervix is said to be fully dilated when no further cervix can be felt around the presenting part.

Second stage of labour

The second stage of labour is divided into:

- the passive phase, when the fetal head is pushed only by uterine contractions down through the pelvis
- the active phase, when the passage of the fetal head is assisted by both uterine contractions and voluntary pushing by the mother

During the passage of the fetus through the birth canal the direction of the fetal head changes to negotiate the bends imposed by the bony pelvis. These movements are known as the cardinal movements of labour. Typically, the fetal head flexes (bends forwards) and rotates into a position where the smallest diameter will pass through the bend. If the presenting diameter is too large, no further descent occurs and delivery needs to be assisted (see Chapter 7). Passage of the fetal head down the birth canal depends on three factors.

- Power: the expulsive force supplied by uterine contraction and in the second stage by voluntary pushing by the mother
- Passage: the diameter of the birth canal
- Passenger: position, flexion and size of the fetal head affect the rate of descent

Both mother and fetus have anatomical adaptions to facilitate the passage of the fetus down the birth canal.

Maternal adaptions

The shape of the female pelvis is adapted to enable upright walking and to allow the passage of a fetus with a large, well-developed brain. It is wider and shallower than the male pelvis.

The pelvic inlet is bounded by the symphysis pubis anteriorly, the iliopectineal line laterally and the sacral promontory posteriorly (**Figure 1.46**). At its inlet, the transverse diameter is wider than its anterior diameter (**Table 1.28**). The outlet is formed by the lowest point of the pelvic arch, the tip of the coccyx, the ischial tuberosities and the surrounding ligaments. It is narrower in its transverse diameter than its anteroposterior diameter. The fetal head must negotiate this series of bends to pass through the pelvis.

Fetal adaptions

The bones of the fetal cranium overlap (are moulded) to aid the passage of the fetal head as it is squeezed through the birth canal. This reduces the diameter of the fetal head, facilitating descent.

The degree of flexion of the fetal head determines which part of the head is lowest,

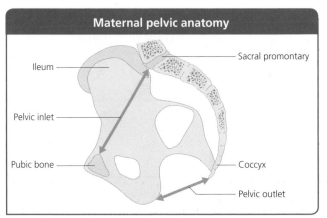

Maternal pelvic anatomy

Ileum

Pelvic inlet

Pubic bone

Sacral promontary

Coccyx

Pelvic outlet

Figure 1.46 Maternal pelvic anatomy. The pelvis is a bony structure with an inlet and an outlet.

Maternal pelvic measurements			
Plane	Anteroposterior (cm)	Oblique (cm)	Transverse (cm)
Pelvic inlet	11	12	13
Mid pelvis	12	12	12
Pelvic outlet	13	12	11

Table 1.28 Measurements of the maternal pelvis. The different diameters at each level impose a series of bends that encourage rotation and flexion of the fetal head with descent

Fetal head diameters presenting in labour		
Presentation	Presenting diameter	Diameter (cm)
Fully flexed vertex	Suboccipitobregmatic	9.5
Deflexed vertex (occipitoposterior)	Suboccipital frontal	12.5
Brow	Mentovertical	13.5
Face	Submentobregmatic	9.5

Table 1.29 Fetal head diameters presenting in labour. Larger presenting diameters are associated with a higher risk of obstructed labour.

and therefore the width that needs to pass through the birth canal. When the head is fully flexed, the presenting diameter is at its smallest (**Table 1.29**). This diameter is measured from the suboccipital region to the bregma (the point at which the coronal and sagittal sutures meet), i.e. the suboccipito-bregmatic diameter (**Figure 1.47**).

> **Malpresentation of the fetal head can cause prolonged labour.** If the head becomes deflexed, larger diameters present. If there is insufficient space for the fetal head to pass through or the head does not return to the flexed position, no further descent occurs and delivery must be assisted.

Cardinal movements

The cardinal movements are the series of movements the fetal head makes as it negotiates its way through the birth canal. They occur as the leading part of the head is pushed against the bends in the canal (**Figure 1.48**). The movements are:

1. Engagement
2. Descent (of the head through the pelvis)

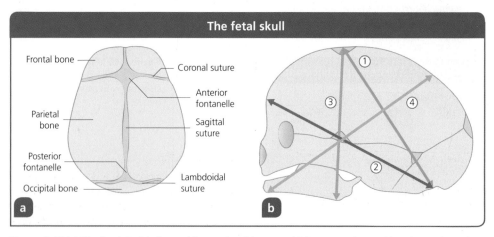

Figure 1.47 (a) The fetal skull is formed from several bones, which can overlap and bend to reduce the overall diameter of the head to aid descent. (b) The fetal head diameters. ①, Suboccipitobregmatic; ②, suboccipital frontal; ③, submentobregmatic; ④, mentovertical.

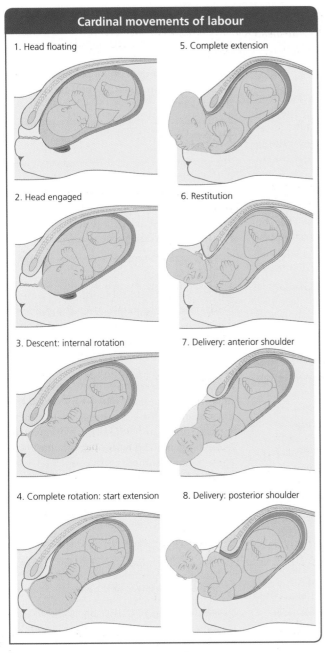

Cardinal movements of labour

1. Head floating

2. Head engaged

3. Descent: internal rotation

4. Complete rotation: start extension

5. Complete extension

6. Restitution

7. Delivery: anterior shoulder

8. Delivery: posterior shoulder

Figure 1.48 The cardinal movements of labour During labour, the fetus must negotiate a series of bends to pass through the inlet and outlet formed by the bony pelvis.

3. Flexion (of the head on to the chest)
4. Internal rotation
5. Extension
6. Restitution and external rotation
7. Expulsion

Engagement

The fetus is engaged when the widest parts of its head have passed the pelvic inlet. The lowest part of the fetal head, known as the vertex, can be felt 1 cm above the ischial spines.

Descent

Downward movement of the fetal head occurs with uterine contractions.

Flexion

Descent is most efficient when the fetal head is flexed. Uterine contractions force the fetal head forwards as it presses against the lower segment of the uterus. This ensures that the smallest diameter of the head passes through the birth canal.

Internal rotation

The fetal head gradually rotates so that the occiput can pass below the symphysis pubis. By rotating to this position, the fetal head maintains the smallest presenting diameter.

Extension

Further contractions aided by voluntary pushing from the mother force the occiput under the symphysis pubis. This causes extension of the fetal head as the birth canal curves upwards. The head delivers through the vaginal introitus by extension. The occiput delivers first, and is followed by the bregma, forehead, nose and then chin.

Restitution and external rotation

As the head delivers, it rotates back to the position in which it entered the birth canal, so that the anterior shoulder lies under the symphysis pubis and the posterior shoulder lies in front of the sacral promontory.

Expulsion

Birth is completed with delivery of the anterior shoulder and lateral flexion of the head to facilitate delivery of the posterior shoulder.

Third stage of labour

Within 30 min of birth, contractions of the uterus rapidly decrease its size and cause the placenta to be expelled. With each contraction, the muscle fibres of the uterus shorten rather than returning to their original length. Shrinkage of the uterine wall shears the placenta away from its attachments.

Fibrinous thrombi form to plug the exposed sinuses in the decidua basalis, thereby achieving haemostasis, preventing further bleeding. The formation of a retroplacental clot aids detachment of the placenta. Further contraction of the uterus expels the placenta from the uterus.

Puerperium

The puerperium is the 6-week interval after delivery, in which the physiological and anatomical changes of pregnancy are reversed and the reproductive organs returns to its non-pregnant state. Milk production (lactation) also starts during this time.

Uterus

The uterus starts to return to its non-pregnant state immediately after the placenta is delivered. This process, which involves shortening of the muscle fibres and death of excess myometrial cells, is known as involution. Oxytocin continues to be released from the posterior pituitary, stimulating ongoing contractions of the uterus, several days after delivery to compress the myometrial fibres and maintain haemostasis. Excess myometrial cells undergo autolysis. The decidua is shed and is replaced with new endometrium. The resultant vaginal loss, consisting of decidual and trophoblastic debris, is known as lochia. The lochia gradually decreases in volume and becomes less blood-stained.

Palpation of the size of the uterus enables assessment of the rate of involution. Normally, the fundus descends by 1–2 cm daily and is not palpable over the pelvic brim by 2 weeks after birth. Failure of the uterus to involute can be caused by retained placental fragments and infection.

Menstruation resumes in non-breastfeeding women about 8 weeks after birth. In breastfeeding women, prolactin inhibits FSH secretion and prevents ovulation. The onset of menstruation is delayed as a result.

Lactation

Lactation is the secretion of milk from mammary glands in the breasts. Breast milk provides babies with passive immunity as a result of the transfer of immune cells and antibodies in the breast milk, and nourishment after delivery in the form of sugars, fats and protein.

Mammogenesis

During pregnancy, oestrogen, progesterone and prolactin stimulate the breasts to enlarge. This process is mammogenesis and is due to increased fat deposition, increased blood flow and growth and differentiation of the mammary glands. Before pregnancy, breast tissue is predominantly adipose tissue. Increasing levels of oestrogen stimulate differentiation of epithelial cells into mature functional lobular-alveolar ductal units, which are glandular structures capable of producing and secreting milk.

Milk secretion

From 20 weeks onwards, the breasts are capable of secreting milk. This is inhibited by progesterone during pregnancy. The dramatic decrease in hormone levels after expulsion of the placenta lifts this inhibition. In the first few days after delivery, colostrum is produced. It is a thick, yellow fluid, rich in proteins, antibodies and growth factors. The antibodies in colostrum provide the newborn baby with passive immunity, and the growth factors help to mature the baby's immature digestive system. A few days later, the secretion of a more watery, energy-rich milk starts to occur as more lactose is incorporated into the milk by the mammary gland.

Suckling

Milk production and secretion is stimulated by suckling. Lactation works in a supply-and-demand manner. Without the stimulation of suckling, milk production quickly ceases. Sensory signals from suckling are transmitted to the hypothalamus to stimulate release of oxytocin and prolactin from the pituitary.

Prolactin stimulates milk synthesis. Oxytocin stimulates contraction of the myoepithelial cells that surround the alveoli. This forces milk from the alveoli into the ducts carrying milk to the nipple.

Cardiovascular system

Cardiac output increases in the immediate puerperium. This effect is caused by an increase in venous return as blood from the placenta returns to the central circulation, reduction in caval compression and movement of the excess extracellular fluid into the vascular compartment.

> **The immediate puerperium is the time of greatest risk for women with heart conditions such as aortic stenosis.** These women are unable to compensate for the sudden increase in venous return by increasing their stroke volume, and they may develop heart failure as a consequence.

Excess fluid starts to be lost within 12 h of delivery. Declining levels of aldosterone and oxytocin lead to a decrease in tubular reabsorption of fluid, resulting in a massive increase in urinary output between 2 and 5 days after delivery. Urinary output increases to 3000 mL/day.

Menopause

Starter questions

Answers to the following questions are on pages 76–77.

22. Is it possible for a woman to conceive after she has gone through the menopause?

23. How does menopause affect sexual function?

Menopause is the permanent cessation of menstruation. In the UK, the average age of a woman's final period is 51 years. Clinically, women are described as post-menopausal if they have not had a period in over a year. Physiologically, this coincides with depletion of all the follicles within the ovaries and the resulting cessation of production of oestrogen and progesterone by these organs. This leads to a dramatic decrease in the level of circulating oestrogens. Oestrogens are still produced at low levels locally by the adipose tissue, bone and brain.

Perimenopause

Up to 5 years before periods cease, changes start to occur that mark the transition between the premenopausal state and the menopausal state; this time is known as the perimenopause. As ovarian reserve declines, levels of LH and FSH increase to try to maintain levels of oestrogen despite the reduction in the number of follicles available to produce it. This can lead to large fluctuations in GnRH levels which may be responsible for the menopausal symptoms, for example hot flushes, night sweats and mood changes, that many women experience at this time. Fertility also declines in the perimenopause.

Urogenital changes

As oestrogen levels decrease, the uterus and ovaries shrink and the vaginal mucosa thins, becomes less elastic and less vascular. These changes mean that the vagina shortens. The fornices almost completely disappear, making the cervix nearly flush with the superior end of the vagina.

Maturation of the vaginal epithelium depends on oestrogen. After the menopause, the intermediate and superficial layers of epithelium do not mature to form multiple layers of flat cells. As a consequence, the epithelium becomes thin and atrophic and susceptible to trauma. Therefore dyspareunia can be a problem in older women.

The normal flora that helps to maintain a healthy vaginal pH of 3.5–4.5 decreases. As a result, vaginal pH increases to 5–7.5. This more alkaline environment allows the overgrowth of pathogenic bacteria and make post-menopausal women more prone to vaginal infections.

The urethra and bladder are also sensitive to oestrogens. With a decrease in oestrogen, the urethral mucosa thins and periurethral collagen decreases. Older women have reduced urinary flow rates, higher residual volumes after voiding and decreased detrusor pressures. Therefore post-menopausal women are more prone to urinary tract infections.

Thinning of the urethral mucosa predisposes post-menopausal women to stress incontinence. Continence is maintained by the integrity of the urethral valves. Thinning of the mucosa means that the folds forming these valves can no longer maintain a watertight seal when there is a rise in intra-abdominal pressure, for example with coughing, laughter or movement.

Vasomotor changes

Hot flushes are one of the most characteristic and troublesome symptoms associated with the menopause. It is unclear why they occur. Disturbances of the temperature-regulating mechanism within the hypothalamus in response to decreasing oestrogen levels have been suggested to play a role. During a hot flush, there is a sudden sensation of warmth, which may be accompanied by sweating or reddening of the skin. Hot flushes may be spontaneous or triggered by stress, changes in temperature, or caffeine or alcohol consumption.

> **Selective noradrenaline (norepinephrine) reuptake inhibitors such as venlafaxine are effective in reducing vasomotor symptoms.** These drugs help to increase the availability of neurotransmitters that regulate thermoregulation.

Systemic changes

Low oestrogen levels also lead to the long-term effects of the menopause, the most serious of which are bone thinning and increased cardiovascular risk.

Ageing is associated with increased bone loss. This is accelerated after the menopause. Oestrogen deficiency leads to an increase in bone resorption. This is not accompanied by a sufficient compensatory increase in bone formation. Rapid bone loss occurs in the vertebrae, pelvis and wrist bones for about 10 years after the menopause. Bone mineral density declines to around 70% of premenopausal levels after 10 years. After this period of rapid bone loss, it starts to slow. These changes predispose older women to fractures of the vertebrae, hips and distal forearms.

Postmenopausal women have an increased risk of cardiovascular disease. Low oestrogen levels are responsible for a redistribution of body fat, increased blood pressure, reduced glucose tolerance, altered lipid metabolism, endothelial dysfunction and vascular inflammation. Together, these factors serve to greatly increase a woman's risk of cardiovascular and cerebrovascular events after the menopause.

Answers to starter questions

1. Our genes determine our biological sex, the anatomy of our reproductive system and secondary sexual characteristics we display. Gender identity is influenced by both biological and social factors; transgender individuals, for example, do not identify with their biological sex.

2. Some foods, e.g. soy products, are naturally high in plant oestrogens, but it is unlikely that eating them is harmful to women with functioning reproductive organs. Supplements containing plant oestrogens are marketed to help with troublesome menopausal symptoms or managing premenstrual syndrome, but there is insufficient evidence on whether they are beneficial or harmful.

3. A baby's biological sex is determined by the number and type of their sex chromosomes, their gonads, hormones and internal and external reproductive anatomy. Disruption to sex organ development can lead to a mismatch between internal and external genitalia. Deficiencies or insensitivity to male hormones can cause ambiguous genitalia in genetic males, while exposure to excess male hormones can also lead to ambiguous genitalia in genetic females.

4. Over the last century the average age of first menstruation has lowered by almost 5 years. Breast bud and pubic hair development are also occurring earlier. It is thought that decreased rates of childhood disease, better nutrition, increased birth weight and environmental pollutants may all have contributed to this phenomenon.

5. Ovarian torsion occurs when an ovary and its fallopian tube twist around their pedicle, occluding the ovarian artery and/or vein. The ovarian vessels are the major blood supply to the ovary so occlusion causes ischaemia and severe pain. Torsion occurs commonly in enlarged ovaries containing cysts or tumours; any delay in diagnosis can lead to the loss of the ovary.

6. Removing one ovary does not affect the length of the menstrual cycle because the remaining ovary compensates by releasing an egg every cycle. Although removing an ovary reduces the number of eggs, women go in to the menopause only slightly earlier than women with two functioning ovaries because a smaller proportion of developing follicles degenerate each month.

7. One per cent of all pregnancies are ectopic and over 90% of these occur in the fallopian tubes. The majority occur as a result of scarring from pelvic infections that lead to the formation of adhesions and damage to the tubal cilia. Scarring impedes efficient transport of the fertilised egg into the uterus. Progesterone-based contraceptives, cigarette smoking and chromosomal abnormalities of the embryo are all risk factors for ectopic pregnancies.

8. During pregnancy the uterus grows from approximately 50 g to over 1kg. This growth is a combination of uterine smooth muscle hypertrophy and hyperplasia. At labour the uterus becomes contractile: uterine smooth muscle fibres shorten with each contraction rather than returning to their fully-stretched length.

Answers *continued*

After delivery these contractions continue and falling oestrogen levels reduce size further by signalling for excess muscle cells to be broken down. By 6 weeks after birth the uterus has returned to its pre-pregnancy weight.

9. Cervical cancer is caused by the human papillomavirus (HPV), which is transmitted through skin-to-skin contact during sexual activity. HPV infection interferes with the production and function of proteins involved in proliferation and DNA repair, meaning cells can divide in an uncontrolled manner and become cancerous. Cells in the cervical transformation zone are particularly vulnerable to these changes, making cervical cancer more common than other HPV-associated cancers.

10. Probiotic supplements that contain strains of *Lactobacillus* (which normally colonise the vagina) can be given either orally or vaginally to treat and prevent the overgrowth of pathogenic bacteria (bacterial vaginosis). To date only a handful of small studies have been conducted and therefore the optimal type of probiotic, doseage and route of administration has yet to be established.

11. The hymen is a thin fold of mucous membrane separating the vaginal vestibule from the vaginal canal. In the perinatal period, it ruptures and allows the flow of menstrual blood after menarche. In some cultures, there is a misconception that the presence of a hymen that completely encircles the vaginal orifice is an indication of a woman's virginity. In such cultures, a woman with an incomplete hymen is thought to have engaged in premarital intercourse. 'Virginity testing' is still used in some countries: the practice is degrading and has no scientific validity.

12. Eighty-five per cent of women experience a perineal injury during vaginal birth. Some factors such as ethnicity, parity and infant birthweight cannot be addressed. Perineal massage in the third trimester of pregnancy and the application of warm compresses to the perineum during the second stage can reduce the rate of perineal trauma. Episiotomies (a surgical incision in the perineum) are not used routinely because they do not prevent spontaneous injury.

13. Women are more prone to urinary tract infections than men due to their shorter urethra. Twenty-five per cent of women experience a urinary tract infection at least once in their lifetime. The relative proximity of the anal canal means that pathogenic bacteria from the gastrointestinal tract have a shorter distance to travel to reach the bladder.

14. The theory of menstrual synchrony is based on the observation that the periods of women living in close proximity became closer together. It is thought this is due to the secretion of pheromones that could affect LH production in other women. Many researchers have criticised this observation, suggesting that due to the variation in the length of women's menstrual cycles there are inevitably times when these might converge or diverge simply by chance.

Answers *continued*

15. Conception only occurs around the time of ovulation due to the finite lifespan of both sperm and ovum within the genital tract. Women have a fertile window of approximately 6 days. If a woman has intercourse on the day of ovulation she has a 1 in 3 chance of conceiving. This falls to less than 10% if she has intercourse 5 days before she ovulates. Many women's menstrual cycles vary in length so the day of ovulation is difficult to predict accurately.

16. Fetuses hiccup from 9 weeks gestation and they increase in frequency in the second and third trimesters. In the third trimester they accompany fetal breathing movements. It is thought that these movements prepare the fetus for breathing postnatally.

17. At term, 97% of babies are in the cephalic (head down) position; they change position through a combination of kicks, stretches and rolls. It is unclear what triggers such a high proportion of babies to adopt this position, but it is thought it happens as a result of the development of the nervous system, a progressive increase in muscle tone and response to gravity.

18. Seventy-five per cent of women experience breathlessness in the third trimester. Physiological breathlessness is caused by the increased drive to breathe and the increased work of breathing caused by the enlarging uterus. Other factors that contribute include increased pulmonary blood volume, nasal congestion and anaemia.

19. Food cravings are a common phenomenon in pregnancy. The aetiology is not fully understood, but it is thought that hormonal influences, nutritional deficits, alleviation of nausea by certain ingredients in craved foods and complex psychological and cultural influences contribute to cravings.

20. Many women describe childbirth as the most painful experience of their lives. It is suggested that three factors affect the intensity of the pain felt: the amount of activity in pain fibres, the amount of activity in other touch fibres and the influence of messages from the brain as a result of stress or anxiety. Pain relief works by modifying any one of these pathways, e.g. continuous one-to-one support reduces anxiety, therefore improving the experience of labour and reducing the need for pharmacological intervention.

21. Women are often told that spicy food, pineapple and herbal remedies such as raspberry leaf tea trigger labour. Although there is anecdotal evidence that they cause abdominal cramps, there is very little evidence to suggest that they trigger labour. The onset of labour is a cascade of physiological events that are interrupted by high levels of stress. Self-help techniques to bring on labour make women feel more empowered and therefore reduce stress levels, allowing spontaneous labour to occur.

22. Women's fertility decline with age and by the time the average woman goes through the menopause at 51 years old, conception is very unlikely. However, ovulation can occur sporadically in the transition period so women are advised to continue using contraception for 1–2 years after their last period. Post-menopausal women can become pregnant with the assistance of in vitro fertilisation of donor eggs. Although the quality of eggs falls with age, the uterus can be primed using oestrogen and progesterone to carry a pregnancy after menopause.

Answers *continued*

23. Over half of postmenopausal women will experience sexual dysfunction. The decline in oestrogen causes vaginal dryness, pain with penetration and reduced sexual desire. These symptoms have a significant impact on a woman's quality of life, affecting her self-esteem and the relationship with her partner.

Chapter 2
Clinical essentials: gynaecology

Introduction

In gynaecology, as in other medical specialties, 90% of diagnoses are made on the basis of history alone. Targeted examinations and investigations are then carried out to confirm or refute this diagnosis. However, gynaecology differs from other medical specialties in that the history includes questions, particularly those about menstruation and sexual function, that are potentially embarrassing and necessitate a sensitive approach, with the patient's answers treated in confidence and accepted without judgement.

Establishment of a rapport makes gynaecological history taking easier for both physician and patient. It also enables exploration of the effects of the disease on the patient's life, and her expectations from treatment. Many gynaecological conditions are managed to improve quality of life, such as treatment of heavy menstrual bleeding, rather than to prolong it. Patients' satisfaction is increased when their wishes, particularly with regards to future fertility, are taken into account through shared decision making.

Common symptoms and how to take a history

Starter questions

Answers to the following questions are on page 117.

1. Can sinister causes of abnormal bleeding be distinguished from benign causes from the history?
2. Why does treating a cystocele make symptoms of stress incontinence worse?

Gynaecology patients may present acutely, to an accident and emergency department, a dedicated gynaecology assessment unit or an early pregnancy assessment unit, or they may present with chronic symptoms to an outpatient department.

A history is taken at presentation, with the aim of finding out a patient's main symptoms. Using this information, doctors create a list of potential diagnoses, ranked in order of likelihood. These are known as differential diagnoses. The essential components of a gynaecological history are the same in any setting, but it is truncated and carried out simultaneously with resuscitation if the patient is compromised.

> **Remember to introduce yourself and the purpose of your questioning.** For example, 'My name is Alex Lewis, and I'm a fifth-year medical student. Would you mind if I ask you some questions about why you have come to the hospital today, as I'm learning how to take a history?'

> **Asking intimate questions about menstruation and sexual intercourse becomes easier with practice.** Signpost these questions, for example by asking for permission: 'Is it all right if I ask you some personal questions?' Also try to hide your own embarrassment at the situation. Women will answer freely if they have been made to feel comfortable.

History taking

History taking is approached in a problem-solving manner; it should not be viewed simply as a list of questions to ask. Symptoms are explored to confirm or exclude differential diagnoses based on a thorough understanding of their underlying causes. For example, if a woman presents with heavy menstrual bleeding it is essential to ask about the nature of the bleeding,

its frequency and any associated pain. If a postmenopausal woman attends clinic with urinary incontinence these questions are inappropriate; instead, focus on the causes of incontinence and its impact on her life. A gynaecological history follows the same basic format as those taken in other specialties, but with some additional questions. The following are the key areas to explore:

- presenting complaint
- history of presenting complaint
- menstrual history
- obstetric history
- cervical screening and contraception history
- medical history
- surgical history
- drug history, including allergies and any use of hormone replacement therapy (HRT)
- family history
- social history
- systems review
- ideas, concerns and expectations

> **The order in which questions are asked is not important, but consultants and examiners expect cases to be presented using the format given above.** Develop a style of questioning that suits you, and use these headings to ensure that crucial questions are not forgotten.

Presenting complaint

The presenting complaint is the reason for the patient's visit. Open questions are used, such as 'What has brought you to clinic today?'. Signpost more sensitive questions, for example by asking 'May I ask you some personal questions?' Avoid interrupting the patient, because most information is gathered from the patient's responses to these opening questions.

Examples of presenting complaints are heavy and painful periods, urinary incontinence and subfertility (see page 83).

Usually a woman presents with more than one complaint. Ask her to prioritise her complaints in order of severity, because different treatment recommendations are based on the most troublesome symptom. For example, endometrial ablation treats heavy periods but is ineffective at relieving painful periods, whereas the levonorgestrel-releasing intrauterine system (Mirena coil) is an effective treatment for both symptoms.

History of presenting complaint

Further detailed information about the presenting symptoms are discussed in the history of the presenting complaint. This includes their duration, severity, pattern, exacerbating and relieving factors, and associated symptoms. The main questions to ask are:

- 'How long have you had this problem?'
- 'Does it change with your menstrual cycle?' and if the answer is positive, 'When is it better or worse?'
- 'Is there anything that makes it better or worse?'
- 'Do you have any other symptoms with it?'

Summarise what the patient has told you so far. This allows you to check your understanding of what you have been told, and gives the patient the opportunity to correct any inaccuracies. It also shows her that you have been listening. Use this as an opportunity to signpost areas that still need to be covered.

Menstrual history

This includes questions about the onset of the patient's periods, the date of her last period, the regularity and duration of bleeding, and any abnormal bleeding or pain.

- 'How old were you when you had your first period?'
- 'When was the first day of your last period?' or 'When did your periods stop?' (if the patient is post-menopausal)

- 'Are your periods regular, for example every 28 days?'
- 'How long do you usually bleed for?'
- 'Do you bleed between periods or after sex?'
- 'Are your periods painful?'
- 'Is this something you want treatment for?'

A 'normal' cycle differs between women; find out what the patient's usual cycle is like and whether she has any menstrual symptoms with a negative effect on her life.

Early menarche and late menopause increase the length of time a woman is exposed to oestrogen, and thereby increase her risk of endometrial and breast cancer. Abnormal bleeding patterns are 'red flag' symptoms warranting urgent investigation (see page 293).

If a woman says that she has missed her period, arrange a urinary pregnancy test. She may not have considered the possibility of being pregnant.

Obstetric history

In the obstetric history, questions are asked to obtain information about previous pregnancies and deliveries.

- 'Do you have any children?'
- 'Were there any problems in the pregnancy?'
- 'How was the baby delivered?'
- 'Have you had any other pregnancies, for example miscarriages, terminations, ectopic pregnancies?'

Gravidity (G) is the number of pregnancies a woman has had, regardless of outcome. Parity (P) is the number of livebirths or stillbirths after 24 weeks' gestation plus the number of losses before 24 weeks. For example, if a woman has had two children born at 37 weeks' gestation and one miscarriage, this information is recorded as 'G3 P2+1 (miscarriage)'.

Amenorrhoea after surgical management of miscarriage or termination is investigated for intrauterine adhesions (Asherman's syndrome), i.e. scarring and potential obliteration of the uterine cavity as a result of trauma to the endometrium. Intra-abdominal adhesions are expected after abdominal surgery, including previous caesarean section, and increase the risk of bowel and bladder damage in future operations.

Cervical screening and contraception history

A history of normal test results from up-to-date cervical screening (see page 375) substantially reduces the likelihood that abnormal bleeding is a consequence of cervical cancer. Cervical cancer is considerably more likely if a woman's screening test is overdue or if she has had abnormal results.

Abnormal vaginal bleeding can be related to contraception use. The progestogen implant (Nexplanon) causes irregular or prolonged bleeding in 50% of users, and missing either combined oral or progestogen-only contraceptive pills leads to intermenstrual bleeding.

Questions to ask in this part of the history are:

- 'When was your last cervical smear?'
- 'Have you had any abnormal smears?' and if the answer is positive, 'What treatment did you have?'
- 'What contraceptive are you currently using?'

The gathering of this information is also an opportunity to promote screening and sexual health. Cervical smears are carried out opportunistically in clinic for women who have failed to attend routine screening appointments. Advice on contraception is given to those at risk of unwanted pregnancy.

> Ask specifically about whether a woman has undergone sterilisation or if her partner has had a vasectomy. Many women forget to mention these procedures, especially if they were carried out some time ago.

Medical history and surgical history

The medical and surgical histories include questions about any current or previous medical conditions and any operations.

- 'Do you have any other health problems?'
- 'In particular, do you have asthma, diabetes, epilepsy or high blood pressure?' and 'Have you had a heart attack or stroke?'
- 'Have you had an operation before?' and if the answer is positive, 'What operation did you have?' and 'Were there any complications?'

The presence of comorbidities influences likely diagnoses and treatment options. A woman with glaucoma is not given anticholinergic drugs to treat urge incontinence, because they increase intraocular pressure. Similarly, an ovarian cyst with benign appearances on scan is managed conservatively in a woman who has had two previous heart attacks and coronary artery stenting, and who is, therefore, at high risk of anaesthetic complications.

Drug history

A complete drug history is taken, and includes questions about HRT and allergies.

- 'Are you taking any medications at the moment?'
- 'Have you ever taken HRT?'
- 'Are you allergic to anything?'

Drug interactions are checked before new medication is prescribed. Women may have already tried several different treatments for their presenting complaint before being referred to secondary care; acknowledging this avoids repetition of ineffective treatment and subsequent frustration.

> Hormone replacement therapy and over-the-counter preparations are often not considered medication by patients, so ask specifically about these.

Family history

A minority of women are at increased risk of gynaecological malignancies from the inheritance of specific genetic mutations. The breast cancer susceptibility genes BRCA1 and BRCA2 are associated with an increased risk of ovarian and breast cancer, whereas mutations in one of the mismatch repair genes, in patients with Lynch syndrome, predispose to endometrial and colorectal cancer. Questions to ask are:

- 'Are there any conditions that run in your family?'
- 'Has anyone in your family had breast, ovary, womb or bowel cancer?'

Understanding a woman's family history often puts her anxieties into context; acknowledging and addressing these fears is vital.

> **Verbal and non-verbal communication are equally important.** Pick up on cues and explore these areas as they arise rather than sticking to the above schema rigidly. Women will talk if they are given the space and opportunity to do so.

Social history

The social history includes questions about smoking, alcohol consumption, recreational drug use and occupation.

- 'Do you smoke?' and if the answer is positive, 'How many a day?'
- 'How much alcohol do you drink in a week?'
- 'Do you use any recreational drugs?'

As well as promoting general health, this information is also used to identify modifiable risk factors for gynaecological conditions. Smoking reduces fertility in both men and women. Alcohol irritates the bladder mucosa and exacerbates urge incontinence (see page 340).

Systems review

This is a brief screen for symptoms in other body systems. Specific questions relevant to a gynaecological history include:

- 'Any bowel or urinary tract symptoms?' (causes of pelvic pain)
- 'Shortness of breath, tiredness, swollen ankles?' (anaemia)
- 'Excess hair, spots, weight gain?' (polycystic ovary syndrome and androgen excess)

- 'Skin changes, rashes?' (generalised skin conditions causing vulval itching)
- 'Loss of appetite and weight?' (malignancy)

Ideas, concerns and expectations

Asking about a patient's ideas, concerns and expectations increases her satisfaction with the consultation, adherence to treatment and improves the physician–patient relationship. Ask the following questions:

- 'What are your thoughts about your symptoms?'
- 'What are you concerned about?'
- 'What do you hope to achieve from the consultation today?'

> **Do not rush this part of the consultation or leave it until the last minute in objective structured clinical examinations.** Several marks are available for exploring a patient's ideas, concerns and expectations.

Gynaecological symptoms

The following symptoms are common reasons for referral to a gynaecologist. The underlying causes are described, along with specific questions used to discriminate between disease processes.

Describing pain

Specific types of pain reported by gynaecology patients are lower abdominal and pelvic pain, dysmenorrhoea and dyspareunia. Pain is described in the same way as for other parts of the body, by using the acronym SOCRATES (**Table 2.1**).

Lower abdominal pain and pelvic pain

This is pain located below the level of the umbilicus. It can be on one side (unilateral) or both sides (bilateral) and varies in character depending on the underlying cause, from

SOCRATES: mnemonic for taking a history of pain		
Letter	Meaning	Example question(s)
S	Site	'Where does it hurt?'
O	Onset	'When did the pain start?'
C	Character	'What sort of pain is it?'
R	Radiation	'Does the pain move to other areas?'
A	Alleviating factors	'Is there anything that makes the pain better?'
T	Timing	'How long does the pain last?'
		'Does it change depending on where you are in your cycle?'
E	Exacerbating factors	'What makes the pain worse?'
S	Severity	'How severe is the pain on a scale of 1 to 10, with 10 being the worst pain you have ever felt?'

Table 2.1 The SOCRATES mnemonic for taking a history of pain

crampy pain associated with endometriosis to acute onset, severe stabbing pain in cases of torsion or rupture of a ovarian cyst (**Table 2.2**). Visceral pain from the reproductive tract radiates to the back and upper thighs, and is difficult to localise because of the low density of sensory nerve fibres in these areas.

Chronic pelvic pain is intermittent or constant lower abdominal or pelvic pain, lasting for ≥ 6 months, which is not associated exclusively with menstruation, sexual intercourse or pregnancy. It is a symptom, not a diagnosis, and affects one in six women. Common causes are:

- endometriosis
- adhesions
- irritable bowel syndrome
- musculoskeletal pain or nerve entrapment

Women often have coexisting depression and sleep disorders, either as a cause or a consequence of living with chronic pain.

Lower abdominal and pelvic pain: causes		
Category	Cause	Discriminating feature(s)
Pregnancy related	Miscarriage	Crampy, suprapubic pain; associated bleeding (may be heavy)
	Ectopic pregnancy	Unilateral pain, minimal bleeding and vaginal discharge, possible collapse
	Rupture of corpus luteal cyst	Unilateral pain, no bleeding, known intrauterine pregnancy
Gynaecological	Ovulation (mittelschmerz)	Mid-cycle unilateral pain that recurs each month
	Pelvic inflammatory disease	Bilateral pain, associated fever, offensive discharge, new sexual partner
	Rupture or torsion of ovarian cyst	Unilateral pain, acute onset, associated vomiting in cases of torsion, unwell
	Fibroid degeneration	Acute onset; low-grade temperature; history of heavy, painful periods; palpable pelvic mass
	Endometriosis	Cyclical pain that is worse leading up to menstruation and eases afterwards; may become chronic pelvic pain
	Pelvic tumour	Constant pain, associated urinary and bowel symptoms as a result of compression
Non-gynaecological	Irritable bowel syndrome	Alternating diarrhoea and constipation, exacerbated by certain foods
	Constipation	Irregular bowel habit
	Adhesions	Constant and usually chronic pain, previous abdominal surgery
	Urinary tract infection or kidney stone	Suprapubic pain with or without loin pain, haematuria, dysuria, urinary frequency
	Appendicitis	Umbilical to right iliac fossa pain, vomiting, fever, anorexia (loss of appetite)

Table 2.2 Causes of lower abdominal and pelvic pain

Dysmenorrhoea

Dysmenorrhoea is pain during menstruation. It affects 90% of women. Symptoms begin about the time bleeding starts. The pain is crampy, and a significant number of women have associated back pain, nausea and vomiting.

- Primary dysmenorrhoea occurs from menarche, is not associated with underlying conditions and improves with age and after childbirth
- New onset dysmenorrhoea in later life requires investigation for secondary causes, such as adenomyosis and leiomyomas (fibroids)

Common causes of dysmenorrhoea are listed in **Table 2.3**.

Dyspareunia

Dyspareunia is painful intercourse. It is felt either superficially at the entrance of the vagina on initial penetration or deep within the pelvis. The distinction is clinically helpful, because different conditions cause superficial or deep dyspareunia.

> **Dyspareunia is not a term commonly used by the lay public.** Instead of asking the patient if she has 'experienced dyspareunia', ask if sexual intercourse is painful for her. If the answer is positive, ask whether the pain is at the entrance of the vagina or deeper, and if it is relieved by a change in position. Pain that occurs only in certain positions is generally benign, but pain unaffected by position is a more worrying feature.

Dyspareunia has both physical causes and psychological risk factors (**Table 2.4**). Once dyspareunia is experienced, fear of future pain leads to loss of vaginal lubrication and dilation, making penetration more painful. A vicious circle is established of anticipated pain and avoidance of sexual intercourse, which has adverse effects on the woman's relationship with her partner. Explore this area:

Dysmenorrhoea: causes	
Cause	Discriminating features
Endometriosis	Pain persists when not menstruating, associated dyspareunia
Adenomyosis	As for endometriosis *
Leiomyoma (benign smooth muscle mass arising from the myometrium)	Heavy periods, palpable pelvic mass
Pelvic inflammatory disease	Offensive discharge, new sexual partner

Table 2.3 Causes of dysmenorrhoea. *Adenomyosis is diagnosed by pathological examination of the uterus after a hysterectomy. A diagnosis can be suspected when a thickened, bright myometrium is visualised by ultrasound or MRI.

- 'What effect is the pain having on your life?'
- 'Is it affecting your relationship with your partner?'

Referral for psychosexual counselling is helpful but requires both partners to want to seek help.

Bleeding

Bleeding is a normal part of the menstrual cycle. Quantification of the volume of blood lost each month is difficult and unnecessary. A woman's perception of her bleeding pattern is the most important factor; what is perceived as normal for one woman is regarded as unacceptably heavy by another. Key points to establish are:

'Are your periods heavy?'

On average, women lose 30–40 mL of blood during their period. Loss of >80 mL constitutes heavy menstrual bleeding. Ask:

- 'Do you have to change tampons or pads more than every 2 h?'
- 'Do you flood the bed at night?'
- 'Do you have to use both pads and tampons? (double protection)'

Positive answers provide more information about the effects of heavy menstrual bleeding on the patient's life than measuring volume of blood lost.

Dyspareunia: causes		
Category	**Cause or risk factors**	**Discriminating features**
Superficial	Anatomical anomalies (e.g. vaginal septum, imperforate hymen)	Pain on initial penetration, confirmation of anomaly by physical examination
	Painful episiotomy scar	New onset dyspareunia after childbirth
	Skin conditions (e.g. lichen sclerosus, lichen planus)	Vulval itching, skin changes
	Vulval and vaginal infections (e.g. herpes, candidiasis, chlamydia)	Vaginal discharge, bleeding, ulcers, itching
	Vestibulodynia	Pain on light touch (e.g. during tampon insertion as well as sexual intercourse); localised or generalised pain; contrasts with vulvodynia, in which pain is continuous and unprovoked by penetration
	Oestrogen deficiency	Vaginal dryness, itching, post-menopausal status
	Vaginismus	Inability to insert tampons or tolerate speculum examination because of involuntary contraction of pubococcygeal muscles
	Psychological factors	History of sexual abuse, relationship difficulties
Deep	Endometriosis	Cyclical dyspareunia, pelvic pain, dysmenorrhoea
	Pelvic inflammatory disease	Fever, offensive discharge, new sexual partner
	Pelvic mass (e.g. ovarian cyst, fibroid)	Pelvic pain unrelated to intercourse, heavy periods, bloating
	Retroverted uterus	Pain relieved by changing position
	Irritable bowel syndrome	Alternating diarrhoea and constipation, passage of mucus
	Interstitial cystitis	Dysuria but no infection, urinary frequency

Table 2.4 Causes of dyspareunia

Heavy periods since menarche are unlikely to have an underlying cause. However, new onset heavy menstrual bleeding prompts investigation for fibroids, endometrial polyps and cancer.

Periods become heavier after starting anticoagulant medication. Blood loss is also greater after insertion of an intrauterine device (copper coil). In contrast, the levonorgestrel-releasing intrauterine system (Mirena coil) reduces blood loss in 90% of women. Excess bleeding after a period of amenorrhoea occurs in women with polycystic ovary syndrome. It is a result of the delay in shedding an endometrial lining that has become abnormally thick during the long interval between periods.

'Do you get bleeding in between your periods?'

Intermenstrual bleeding is bleeding between periods. Breakthrough bleeding is irregular blood loss associated with the use of hormonal contraception. Most cases of intermenstrual bleeding have a benign aetiology. However, gynaecological malignancies, i.e. vaginal, cervical and endometrial cancers, also present this way, so all women are investigated, regardless of age.

Specific questions to elicit the cause of the intermenstrual bleeding include:

- 'What contraception are you using?' and 'Have you missed any pills (or injections)?'
- 'Do you have any unusual vaginal discharge?'
- 'Do you bleed after sexual intercourse as well?'

Missed combined oral and progestogen-only contraceptive pills are a common cause of breakthrough bleeding. Over-the-counter preparations, including St John's wort, gingko and ginseng, interfere with the effectiveness of the pill and can also cause intermittent bleeding. A thorough drug history

chronic conditions such as fibroids or lichen sclerosus, however, usually look well.

Does she look pale or jaundiced?

Anaemia causes pallor, particularly of the conjunctiva. Women with sickle cell anaemia and increased breakdown of red blood cells appear jaundiced and may present to a gynaecologist with acute lower abdominal pain during a sickle cell crisis (blockage of blood vessels by sickle-shaped cells). Liver metastases from a gynaecological malignancy and hepatic dysfunction secondary to pelvic abscess can also cause jaundice.

Is she over- or underweight?

Significant weight loss suggests an underlying neoplastic process. Increased BMI is a significant risk factor for endometrial cancer and contributes to irregular periods, urinary incontinence and subfertility.

Does she have nicotine-stained fingers?

Smoking weakens the immune system, thereby delaying clearance of human papillomavirus and increasing the risk of developing cervical cancer. In the UK, couples may be ineligible for IVF funded by the National Health Service if either partner smokes.

Does she have any gait abnormalities or use walking aids?

Neurological conditions, such as spinal cord injuries, multiple sclerosis and Parkinson's disease, affect the bladder causing incontinence, retention and recurrent urinary tract infections. Difficulties with mobility may affect positioning for vaginal examination. Arthritis affecting the hand joints can make women unable to carry out intermittent self-catheterisation.

What are her observations?

A full set of observations, including blood pressure, pulse, respiratory rate and temperature, are required for patients who present acutely unwell. These measurements are used to guide resuscitation and monitor response to treatment. In the outpatient setting, they are recorded as part of preoperative assessment for patients due to undergo surgery. Control of new onset hypertension and cardiac arrhythmias needs to be optimised before anaesthesia.

Abdominal examination

After the general examination comes the abdominal examination, which follows the usual format of inspection before palpation. It is an opportunity to locate the source of pain and characterise abdominal and large pelvic masses.

Abdominal examination is carried out from the right-hand side of the bed, with the patient supine, her hands at her sides and her head at a comfortable height on a pillow. The abdomen is exposed from just below the breasts to the symphysis pubis; sheets are used to cover the genitalia until this examination is complete.

Inspection

Systematically examine all quadrants of the abdomen for scars or distension.

Scars

Evidence of previous surgery is provided by the location and number of scars (**Figure 2.1**). Midline incisions have a higher rate of adhesion formation than transverse ones; adhesions are associated with chronic lower abdominal pain and a greater chance of organ damage in subsequent surgical procedures. Keloid scars are overgrowths of granulation tissue at sites of injury, and are more common in women with pigmented skin. The cosmetic appearance of these scars can dissuade women from undergoing further surgery.

> **Remember to look specifically inside the umbilicus for any scars.** Gynaecologists carry out laparoscopies through an intraumbilical incision rather than a subumbilical incision, as used by surgeons. The scar from an intraumbilical incision is difficult to see if it has healed well.

Distension

This is an outward expansion beyond the normal girth of the abdomen. The presence of distension is best appreciated by

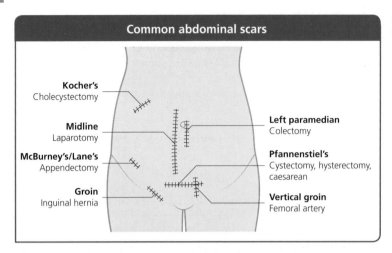

Figure 2.1 Common abdominal scars.

inspecting the abdomen from its level; the clinician crouches down so that their eye-line is at the level of the bed. Distension can be localised, as in cases of a discrete mass, or generalised, because of the presence of ascites or pregnancy.

Palpation

Palpation is the touching of a patient with the fingers to determine the size, consistency, tenderness and location of body parts. Ask the patient to relax before palpation begins; it is difficult to palpate masses accurately if the abdomen is tense. Check if the woman has any pain and where it is located; examine this area last. Carry out the palpation systemically so that all areas of the abdomen are covered, and observe the patient's face to detect any signs of discomfort during the examination.

Tenderness

This can be localised or generalised, and is felt on superficial as well as deep palpation. Ovarian cyst haemorrhage causes unilateral pelvic pain, whereas peritoneal inflammation caused by pelvic inflammatory disease or endometriosis is felt as a more diffuse pain. Guarding (tensing of the abdominal wall muscles) and rebound tenderness, i.e. pain induced by the quick release of pressure, is found in cases of peritonitis, ruptured ovarian cyst and ectopic pregnancy.

Palpable masses

A mass is arising from the pelvis if it is not possible to feel below it. It is further characterised by its consistency – soft, hard, irregular or smooth – and whether it feels mobile or fixed to adjacent structures.

- Malignant masses are hard, irregular and fixed
- Benign ovarian cysts are regular in shape and mobile

The size of a mass is equated to that of the gravid uterus in number of weeks' gestation, for example 20 weeks if it extends to the umbilicus and 36 weeks if it reaches the xiphisternum.

The location of a mass is described in terms of the quadrant of the abdomen in which it is found (**Figure 2.2**).

The finding of a pelvic mass prompts assessment for lymph nodes enlarged by metastatic disease in the groin and left supraclavicular region (Virchow's node). The abdomen is also palpated for hepatosplenomegaly.

Ascites

This is accumulation of fluid in the peritoneal cavity. The presence of ascites is confirmed by demonstration of a fluid thrill; place the patient's hand along the midline of her abdomen and gently flick one side of the abdomen while feeling for transmission of an impulse to the other flank (**Figure 2.3**). Ascites can

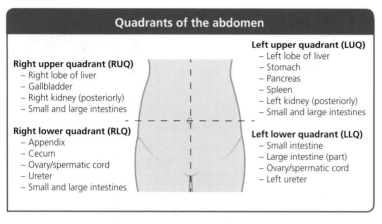

Quadrants of the abdomen

Right upper quadrant (RUQ)
– Right lobe of liver
– Gallbladder
– Right kidney (posteriorly)
– Small and large intestines

Right lower quadrant (RLQ)
– Appendix
– Cecum
– Ovary/spermatic cord
– Ureter
– Small and large intestines

Left upper quadrant (LUQ)
– Left lobe of liver
– Stomach
– Pancreas
– Spleen
– Left kidney (posteriorly)
– Small and large intestines

Left lower quadrant (LLQ)
– Small intestine
– Large intestine (part)
– Ovary/spermatic cord
– Left ureter

Figure 2.2 Division of abdomen into quadrants.

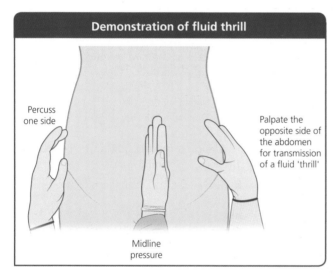

Demonstration of fluid thrill

Percuss one side

Palpate the opposite side of the abdomen for transmission of a fluid 'thrill'

Midline pressure

Figure 2.3 Demonstration of fluid thrill indicating the presence of ascites.

also be shown by shifting dullness; percuss the abdomen until the sound becomes dull, mark the spot while rotating the patient away, and then repeat percussion at that site, where the sound will now be resonant.

Vaginal examination

The vaginal examination is a key part of the gynaecological examination, but it is also the most intrusive. The aim of the examination is to assess the internal and external genitalia for abnormalities.

Talking to the patient during the examination distracts her from what is happening and helps her to relax, thereby making the procedure less uncomfortable. Position the woman on her back on the couch, with her ankles together, and ask her to let her knees fall as far apart as possible. If a colposcopy couch is available, place the woman's feet in the stirrups, with her legs relaxed open and her bottom at the end of the bed.

> **Wash your hands and put on gloves before a vaginal examination.** Check whether the woman has an allergy to latex before proceeding.

External genitalia

Inspect the external genitalia first. In particular, look for any:

- swelling
- skin changes
- ulceration
- signs of infection
- scarring
- anatomical abnormalities
- unusual distribution of hair

Normal external genitalia are shown in Figure 1.2. A Bartholin's abscess (localised infection within the Bartholin's gland) presents with a red, hot swelling in the lower vagina, which can be considerable in size. In lichen sclerosus (a dermatological condition of unknown aetiology), there is labial atrophy, white discoloration of the perineal skin and excoriation or ulceration as a result of scratching. In the most severe form of female genital mutilation, type 3, the labia minora, labia majora or both are sewn together to narrow the vaginal opening, and the clitoris may also have been removed (see Chapter 15). The presence and distribution of pubic hair is assessed in girls with primary amenorrhoea and in women with suspected polycystic ovary syndrome; in the latter condition, excess androgen secretion causes hair growth on the lower abdomen, back and inner thighs.

Ask the woman to cough. Stress incontinence is shown by the leakage of urine, and pelvic organ prolapse becomes more evident with increased intra-abdominal pressure.

Speculum examination

Two types of speculum are used in gynaecological examinations (**Figure 2.4**).

- A Cusco speculum is used for examination of the cervix
- A Sims speculum allows assessment of vaginal prolapse

Examination with a Cusco speculum

Lubricate the speculum with water or water-based lubricant. Part the labia with the left hand and use the right hand to insert the speculum with the blades closed and parallel to the labia. Direct the speculum posteriorly and stop once it is flush with the vagina.

Once the speculum is inserted, rotate it 90° and then open it. The handle should point

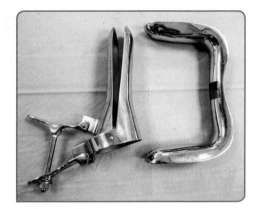

Figure 2.4 Speculums used in gynaecological examinations. Cusco speculum (left) and Sims speculum (right).

upwards if a standard examination couch is used, and downwards if the woman is on a colposcopy couch or theatre bed from which the lower half has been removed. Fix the speculum in position by tightening the ratchet to free the hands to carry out any required procedures.

A normal cervix is shown in Figure 15.6. The cervix is examined for:

- discharge
- bleeding
- cysts
- the presence or absence of threads from an intrauterine device
- polyps (fleshy overgrowths of tissue)
- ulceration or masses

While removing the speculum, examine the vaginal walls for discharge, ulcers and foreign bodies. Withdraw the speculum with the blades slightly open, ensuring that the vaginal walls and cervix are not trapped within it as it closes. The cervix may not be visualized for a number of reasons:

- It is not present. Check with the woman that she has had a hysterectomy and forgotten to tell you about it
- The cervix is very anterior or posterior due to the position of the uterus. Remove the speculum and adjust the position, aiming more anteriorly or posteriorly. If still struggling, perform a bimanual examination (see below) to find the cervix and then re-insert the speculum in that direction

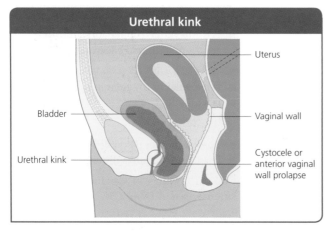

Figure 2.5 Urethral kink caused by cystocele. The prolapsed anterior vaginal wall distorts the usual anatomy of the urethra, causing a kink to form and a reduction in the flow of urine.

- The vaginal walls are obstructing the view. This is a problem particularly in obese women who have had several children or if a prolapse is present. Changing the size of the speculum or cutting a finger off a glove and placing it over the speculum blades can help push the vaginal walls away

> When choosing a speculum, consider the individual patient. A 90-year-old woman who has not been sexually active for 30 years will require a smaller speculum than a premenopausal woman.

Examination with a Sims speculum

This examination is carried out in the left lateral position, with the hips and knees flexed and the top leg elevated. The blade is inserted first along the anterior vaginal wall to allow assessment of the cervix and detection of a rectocele or enterocele, and then along the posterior vaginal wall to enable visualisation of a cystocele (anterior vaginal wall prolapse) (**Figure 2.5**). Ask the woman to strain as though opening her bowels to make any prolapse more evident.

> Most speculums are plastic and disposable. Metal speculums are cold and need to be warmed by placing them under warm running water before insertion; they are sent for sterilisation before reuse.

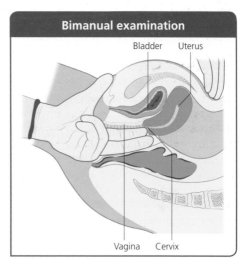

Figure 2.6 Bimanual examination.

Bimanual examination

In this examination, the lubricated index and middle finger of the right hand are inserted into the vagina to assess the vagina, cervix, uterus and adnexa, while the left hand simultaneously palpates the abdomen (**Figure 2.6**).

During assessment of the vagina, ask the following questions:

- Are there any masses?
- Is there good vaginal tone? (This is assessed by asking the patient to squeeze the clinician's inserted fingers during the examination)
- Are the vaginal walls well supported?

During assessment of the cervix, ask the following:

■ Is it smooth or hard?
■ Are any masses palpable?
■ Does movement of the cervix cause pain?
■ Is the cervical os open or closed? It is not important whether the external os is open or not (after a woman has had children vaginally the external os never closes completely). Whether the internal os is open or closed is more important, an open internal os in a woman in the first trimester of pregnancy means an inevitable miscarriage and in the third trimester is indicative of labour

During assessment of the uterus, ask:

■ Is it anteverted (tipped forwards) or retroverted (tipped backwards)?
■ What size is it?
■ Is it regular or irregular in shape?
■ Is it mobile?

For the adnexa, ask:

■ Are any masses palpable?
■ Does examination of the adnexa cause pain?

Clinical findings in specific conditions are summarised in **Table 2.5**.

Bimanual examination: clinical findings and associated conditions		
Organ	Finding	Associated condition(s)
Vagina	Irregular, firm, fixed mass	Vaginal cancer
	Weak or no vaginal tone	Vaginal prolapse (pelvic floor exercises required)
	Loss of vaginal wall support	Vaginal prolapse Anteriorly: cystocele Posteriorly: rectocele
Cervix	Smooth, firm (like the tip of the nose), internal os closed, no pain on movement	Normal
	Soft cervix (similar consistency to lips)	Normal in latter stages of pregnancy
	Internal os open	Inevitable miscarriage (in multiparous women, external os is normally open but internal os is closed)
	Hard, irregular, palpable mass	Cervical cancer
	Pain on sideways movement of the cervix (cervical excitation)	Pelvic inflammation (e.g. pelvic inflammatory disease, ectopic pregnancy)
Uterus	Uterus palpated between two hands when fingers of one hand are in anterior fornix of vagina	Anteverted uterus (85% of women)
	Uterus palpated when fingers of one hand are in posterior fornix of vagina	Retroverted uterus (15% of women)
	Firm, smooth, smaller than a lemon	Normal in non-pregnant women
	Size of a small orange	Enlarged uterus: pregnancy of 6 weeks' gestation (in a molar pregnancy, uterus is larger than expected for dates), fibroids, malignancy
	Size of a large orange	Pregnancy of 8 weeks' gestation
	Size of a grapefruit	Pregnancy of 10 weeks' gestation
	Size of a cantaloupe	Pregnancy of 12 weeks' gestation
	Hard, irregular	Fibroids
	Non-mobile, fixed	Endometriosis, adhesions

Continued...

Bimanual examination: clinical findings and associated conditions		
Fallopian tubes and ovaries	Nothing palpable between two hands when fingers of one hand are in right or left lateral fornices and the hand on the abdomen is pressing down on the same side just above the symphysis pubis	Normal
	Smooth, mobile mass	Benign ovarian cyst or tubal mass (e.g. hydrosalpinx)
	Irregular, hard, fixed mass	Tubal or ovarian malignancy
	Bilateral adnexal tenderness; may have firm, fixed mass	Endometriosis, pelvic inflammatory disease or abscess
	Unilateral adnexal tenderness, mass, positive pregnancy test	Ectopic pregnancy

Table 2.5 Clinical findings on bimanual examination and associated conditions

Investigations

Starter questions

Answers to the following questions are on page 117.

5. Does the CA125 protein rise in all cases of ovarian cancer?
6. Why is cervical cytology not performed in women with suspected cervical cancer?
7. When is a CT preferable to a MRI scan during investigation of suspected gynaecological malignancy?

Investigations are carried out to answer specific questions raised by the history and examination. The results are used to:

- confirm a suspected diagnosis
- exclude differential diagnoses
- establish the extent of disease
- monitor disease progression

Not all patients require investigation. Women with regular, heavy periods or primary dysmenorrhoea are treated empirically with non-steroidal medication or hormonal contraceptives, and investigations are carried out only to exclude other diagnoses if symptoms do not settle.

Always ask 'Why is this test being done?' If the result is not going to affect management, then it is unnecessary.

Blood tests

Blood tests are done to investigate a number of gynaecological conditions. They include:

- full blood count
- renal and liver function tests
- measurement of inflammatory markers
- hormonal profiles
- measurement of tumour markers

The indications for blood tests in gynaecology and the interpretation of their results are shown in **Table 2.6**.

Urine tests

Urine testing is done for several indications:

- confirmation of pregnancy, by urinary pregnancy test

Blood tests in gynaecology		
Test	When required	Purpose
Full blood count (FBC)	Heavy or chronic bleeding	Normal MCV identifies anaemia caused by acute blood loss Low MCV identifies anaemia caused by iron deficiency in chronic bleeding
	Suspected infection	Increased white cell count confirms infection
	Preoperatively	Crossmatched blood is required for surgery in anaemia Bleeding is exacerbated if platelet count low
Group and save (G+S)	Preoperatively; in heavy bleeding	Ensure blood for transfusion is compatible
Coagulation tests: prothrombin time (PT), activated partial thromboplastin time (APTT), international normalised ratio (INR)	Preoperatively	Prolonged PT and APTT and high INR demonstrates clotting factor deficiency
	Acute haemorrhage	Diagnose disseminated intravascular coagulation
	Menorrhagia from menarche	Low von Willebrand's protein confirms von Willebrand's disease (a cause of heavy periods)
Urea and electrolytes (U+E) – assessment of renal function	Systemic infection Hypovolaemia	Sepsis and hypovolaemia cause hypoperfusion and acute kidney injury
	Large pelvic mass causing ureteric compression Overflow incontinence	Pressure on the kidneys causes loss of renal function
	Recurrent urinary tract infections	Scarring of the kidneys reduces renal function
Liver function tests (LFTs)	Hyperemesis	Abnormal LFT results reflect: ■ cause of chronic vomiting (e.g. gallstones) ■ consequences of chronic vomiting (alanine transaminase is increased)
	Suspected metastatic gynaecological malignancy	Abnormal LFT results suggest liver metastases
C-reactive protein (CRP)	Suspected infection Monitoring treatment response	↑CRP suggests inflammation or infection Serial measurements monitor treatment response
Oestradiol	Investigating amenorrhoea	Low oestradiol + high FSH + high LH: ovarian failure Low oestradiol + low FSH + low LH: hypothalamic or pituitary conditions (e.g. stress, anorexia, , see Chapter 8)
Progesterone (at day 21 of cycle)	Investigating subfertility	Day 21 progesterone > 30 nmol/L: ovulation has occurred

Continued....

Blood tests in gynaecology *continued*		
Total and free testosterone, sex hormone-binding globulin	Suspected polycystic ovary syndrome or hirsutism due to this	↑free testosterone and low sex hormone-binding globulin (cause the hirsutism and acne)
	Suspected Sertoli–Leydig cell tumour	Androgen secretion suggests Sertoli–Leydig tumour; serial testosterone detects recurrence
Prolactin	Investigating amenorrhoea	Significantly increased prolactin confirms prolactinoma
	Investigating subfertility if periods irregular	
Human chorionic gonadotrophin (hCG)	Confirming pregnancy if high clinical suspicion but negative urine test	hCG confirms pregnancy (secreted by placenta to maintain pregnancy)
	Investigating pregnancy of unknown location	Suboptimal hCG increase suggests miscarriage or ectopic pregnancy (hCG increases ≥ 66% per 48 h in normal early pregnancy)
	Follow-up of gestational trophoblastic disease and choriocarcinoma	Increasing hCG measurements suggests disease recurrence
Luteinising hormone (LH) and follicle-stimulating hormone (FSH)	Investigating subfertility if periods irregular	High day 2 or 3 LH and FSH: ovarian failure Low LH and FSH: hypothalamic or pituitary disease (AMH has superseded FSH as marker of ovarian reserve; see below)
	Confirming menopausal status if history unclear	↑LH and ↑FSH on 2 occasions 6 weeks apart confirm menopause Used when amenorrhoea is due to other causes, e.g. previous hysterectomy with ovarian conservation, levonorgesterol-releasing intrauterine system (Mirena coil) in situ. Not valid if patient uses other hormonal contraceptives
Antimüllerian hormone (AMH)	Work-up for IVF	Low AMH indicates poor ovarian reserve and need to adjust drug doses to increase egg availability
Cancer antigens 125, 19-9 and 15-3 (CA 125, 19-9 and 15-3) and carcinoembryonic antigen (CEA)	Investigating adnexal mass	CA125 + ultrasound score + menopausal status give risk of malignancy index which guides management Ovarian metastases from other cancers (Krukenberg's tumours) suspected if: ■ ↑CEA in bowel cancer ■ ↑CA19-9 in upper GI cancers and mucinous ovarian tumours ■ ↑CA15-3 in breast cancer
	Monitoring ovarian cancer	Detect disease recurrence if elevated at baseline
α-Fetoprotein (AFP) and lactate dehydrogenase (LDH)	Investigating complex adnexal mass in patient aged < 45 years	hCG secreted by germ cell tumours AFP secreted by yolk sac tumours Increased LDH levels in dysgerminomas

AKI, acute kidney injury; MCV, mean corpuscular volume.

Table 2.6 Blood tests in gynaecology

- detection of infection, by dipstick urinalysis and microscopy and culture
- screening for malignancy, by cytological investigation

A midstream sample of urine is needed for detection of infection, because urine passed at the start of urination is likely to be contaminated with bacteria from the skin. To collect midstream urine, the clean catch method is used. After washing her hands, the patient passes a small amount of urine before stopping. She then urinates into a container held away from the body. Once the container is half full and sealed, she may empty her bladder as normal.

Urinary pregnancy test

A urinary pregnancy test is carried out on all women of childbearing age before gynaecological surgery and during investigation of amenorrhoea. A woman is asked to perform a midstream urine sample into a sterile container. A few drops of urine are then added onto a test strip with a pipette and the strip is read after 2–3 minutes (**Figure 2.7**). The strip contains anti-hCG antibodies bound to an enzyme; hCG in the urine binds to the antibody and the enzyme causes a colour change of the coating on the strip. The presence of a single lines means a negative test, two lines indicate a positive pregnancy test. If no lines appear then the test has not worked. It is either repeated or a blood hCG

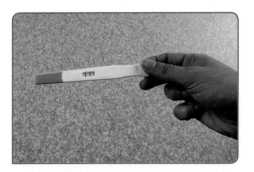

Figure 2.7 The home pregnancy test. The two lines are a control line and a positive test line. If both are visible this indicates a positive pregnancy test result. The test is negative if only one line is present and not valid if no lines appear.

test is performed. A urine pregnancy test is positive when the hCG level is >25 mIU/mL, 12–14 days after conception. False negative results occur if the test is performed too soon after conception, false positive results occur with hCG secreting tumours and some medications, such as chlorpromazine and fertility drugs containing hCG.

> Urine pregnancy tests used in hospitals and general practice surgeries work in the same way as those bought in shops by patients and done at home.

Culture and cytology

Urine is sent for culture and cytology if a woman has macroscopic or microscopic haematuria or recurrent urinary tract infections. A midstream urine sample is required to perform these tests. For culturing, urine is kept under conditions to allow bacteria and fungi to grow. If no organisms grow after 48 hours then the test is negative. If organisms grow in large numbers the test is positive and sensitivity to commonly prescribed antibiotics is tested.

Cytology is the examination of urine under the microscope by specially trained pathologists. Abnormal cells are found in bladder cancer and infection and warrant further investigation with cystoscopy (camera examination of the bladder) and biopsy.

Imaging

Imaging in gynecology is used to confirm diagnoses and to assess disease severity. Ultrasound does not involve radiation and is used first line, with CT and MRI reserved for cases where more detailed information is required.

Ultrasound

In ultrasound, high-frequency soundwaves emitted from a probe are used to generate a picture of an area of the body. Waves pass through soft tissue and fluid but are reflected by denser structures such as bone, and the reflected waves are detected by the same probe. A computer converts the soundwaves into images; fluid appears black and solid structures appear white.

Ultrasound is a first-line investigation for many signs and symptoms, because it is easily available and inexpensive and involves no exposure to radiation. This last advantage of ultrasound makes it a particularly suitable imaging modality for women who are pregnant or are trying to become pregnant.

Scans can be carried out transabdominally or transvaginally (see **Figure 2.8**); each type of scan has its advantages and disadvantages (**Table 2.7**). Frequently, both techniques are used to maximise diagnostic accuracy (**Figure 2.8**).

When women are referred for an ultrasound scan, they are made aware that it may include both abdominal and internal scans and that they need to attend with a full bladder. This prepares them for the examination and avoids the sonographer having to send them away to drink more if their bladder is empty.

The use of ultrasound in pregnancy is described in Chapter 3. It is also particularly useful for characterising ovarian masses and fibroids and assessing endometrial thickness (**Table 2.8** and **Figures 2.9–2.11**). It is used to guide biopsies of pelvic masses and the omentum. The soundwaves are disrupted

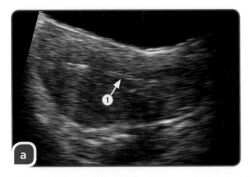 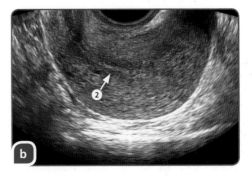

Figure 2.8 Endometrial stripe shown on a (a) transabdominal ultrasound scan and (b) transvaginal ultrasound scan.

Transabdominal and transvaginal ultrasound: advantages and disadvantages		
Technique	Advantages	Disadvantages
Transabdominal	Non-invasive Allows full assessment of large pelvic masses Other abdominal organs (e.g. liver, spleen) can be examined simultaneously	Full bladder required to improve image quality; it pushes the bowel away and provides a window to allow transmission of soundwaves to internal pelvic organs Image quality adversely affected by bowel gas Poorer image resolution, because low-frequency soundwaves emitted
Transvaginal	Better image resolution, because higher frequency soundwaves used Unaffected by bowel gas and body fat Gestational sac seen from 5 weeks' gestation (compared with 7 weeks with transabdominal scan)	Invasive Cannot visualise mid and upper abdomen

Table 2.7 Advantages and disadvantages of transabdominal and transvaginal ultrasound

Ultrasound findings in gynaecological conditions		
Finding	Questions to ask	Interpretation
Adnexal mass	Where does it arise from?	Not all adnexal masses are ovarian cysts; hydrosalpinx (fluid-filled fallopian tube), tubo-ovarian abscess and appendiceal or diverticular abscess can all present as an adnexal mass
	How big is it?	Cysts ≤ 3 cm in size in premenopausal women are normal and are not reported
		Cysts of < 7 cm are usually benign and can be monitored
		Cysts > 7 cm need further characterisation with MRI with or without surgery, because ultrasound alone is insufficient
	Is it unilateral or bilateral?	Unilateral masses are more likely to be benign
		Bilateral masses are found in endometriosis and malignancy, including metastatic disease from elsewhere in the body
	Is it cystic or solid, and does it have internal septations?	Simple cystic masses without septations are functional or benign
		Solid areas increase suspicion for malignancy
	Is ascites present?	Ascites increases the likelihood of malignancy
	Does it contain diffuse low-level echoes?	This is consistent with blood products and is found in haemorrhagic cysts and endometriomas
Fibroid	How big is it?	Fibroids < 3 cm in size are managed medically with non-steroidal medication and hormonal contraceptives, if symptomatic
		Fibroids > 3 cm in size require surgical management if symptomatic
		A fibroid that is rapidly increasing in size is concerning because it suggests a leiomyosarcoma (malignant smooth muscle tumour)
	Where are the fibroids?	Ultrasound is used to determine if the fibroids are under the lining of the uterus (submucous), in the uterine wall (intramural) or on the outer wall of the uterus (subserosal)
		Submucous fibroids prevent implantation and are removed hysteroscopically
		Subserosal fibroids press on adjacent organs, thereby causing urinary frequency and constipation
	How many fibroids are there?	More than one is usual; a single large fibroid responds better to uterine artery embolisation than multiple smaller ones
Endometrium	How thick is it?	In premenopausal women, endometrial thickness varies widely depending on the stage of the menstrual cycle
		In post-menopausal women:
		the risk of endometrial cancer with endometrial thickness < 5 mm is very low, so biopsy is not required
		endometrial thickness ≥ 5 mm warrants histological sampling
		Localised thickening suggests a polyp
	Is it cystic in appearance?	Endometrium with a cystic appearance is found in endometrial hyperplasia and with tamoxifen use

Table 2.8 Ultrasound findings in common gynaecological conditions

by air and fat, making imaging difficult if bowel obscures the pelvic organs or if the patient is obese. MRI is more useful in these situations.

Intrauterine contraceptive devices are visible on ultrasound (**Figure 2.12**); this is performed to confirm intrauterine placement if the coil threads can not be seen or felt.

Radiography

An X-ray is a high energy electromagnetic wave. In radiography, an image is created

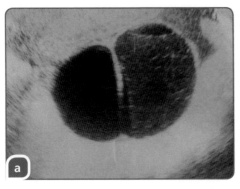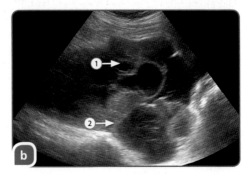

Figure 2.9 Ultrasound scans showing (a) benign and (b) malignant ovarian cysts. The benign cyst is fluid filled with a thin septation. The malignant cyst is multicystic with ① hypoechoic and ② solid echogenic areas.

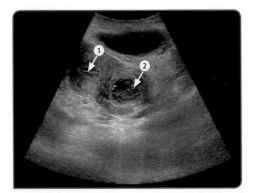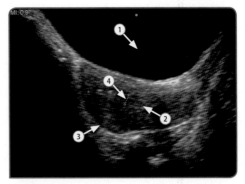

Figure 2.10 Transabdominal ultrasound scan of the left ovary showing an ovarian cyst containing echogenic debris, consistent with an abscess (pelvic inflammatory disease (PID). ① Uterus showing endometrial stripe, ② ovarian abscess.

Figure 2.11 Assessment of endometrial thickness on ultrasound. The echo bright area is measured at its widest point (shown here between the two crosses). ① Bladder, ② endometrium, ③ uterus, ④ calipers to assess endometrial thickness.

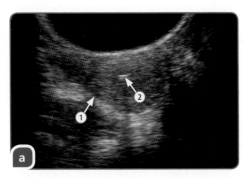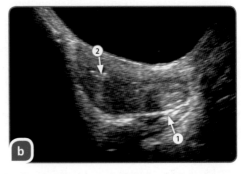

Figure 2.12 Ultrasound scans of a levonorgestrel-releasing intrauterine system (coil) in situ. (a) Transverse image. (b) Longitudinal image. ① Uterus, ② Mirena coil.

by the differential absorption of X-rays by tissues of varying density as the radiation passes through the body.

- Bone, which is dense, readily absorbs X-rays so appears white
- Pelvic organs and fat, which are less dense, do not impede the passage of X-rays so appear as darker areas

Radiography is useful in the diagnosis of bony abnormalities but of limited value in gynae-cology, because the tissues of interest are of similar density and, therefore, poorly differen-tiated. Its use is avoided in pregnant women, because of the potential harmful effects of ion-ising radiation on the developing fetus, includ-ing miscarriage and birth defects.

Abdominal and pelvic radiography are used to locate missing intrauterine devices, which are clearly visualised because of their metal-lic components, as well as in investigations of postoperative abdominal distension to distin-guish bowel obstruction from paralytic ileus (paralysis of intestinal muscles causing a func-tional blockage of the intestine).

Computerised tomography

Computerised tomography (CT) is an advanced radiographic technique. In CT a narrow beam of X-rays are aimed at and rotated around the body. X-rays that pass through the body are recorded by detectors, and a computer uses the data to create cross-sectional images. Contrast agents are given intravenously or orally to highlight blood ves-sels or the gastrointestinal tract, respective-ly. CT images are more detailed than those obtained using conventional radiography.

Computerised tomography is used in the staging of ovarian cancer (**Figure 2.13**) and other advanced malignancies of the female genital tract, as well as the detection of disease recurrence. Systematic examination of the chest, abdomen and pelvis is carried out to identify the involvement of other organs and lymph nodes. The use of CT in pregnancy is avoided because of the risks of radiation exposure.

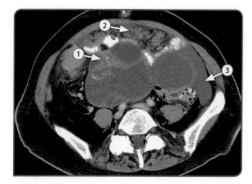

Figure 2.13 CT scan showing ovarian cancer seen as a multicystic pelvic mass with ① solid enhancing areas, ② omental caking and ③ ascites. Courtesy of Rishi Sethi.

Magnetic resonance imaging

In MRI, a strong magnetic field and radio-frequency waves are used to produce images of the body. A magnet within the MRI scan-ner forces protons within hydrogen atoms to line up. Short bursts of radiofrequency waves are then applied, which knock the protons out of alignment. Once the waves are turned off, the protons realign, and in the process emit radio signals that are detected by receivers. The protons in dif-ferent tissues realign at varying speeds, and therefore emit distinct signals that are used to create detailed images of the body. Gadolinium is used as a contrast agent to aid identification of blood vessels, inflam-mation and tumours.

Magnetic resonance imaging has several advantages over ultrasound and CT. It is bet-ter at discriminating between types of tissue, particularly in the assessment of soft tissues. It is used to help stage cervical cancers and to determine depth of myometrial invasion in endometrial cancer (**Figure 2.14**). It is also used to establish the extent of endometriosis, further characterise complex adnexal masses and plan reconstructive surgery in girls with müllerian anomalies (abnormal development

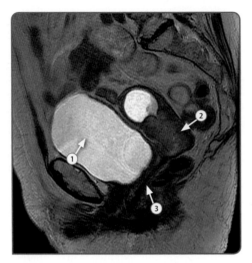

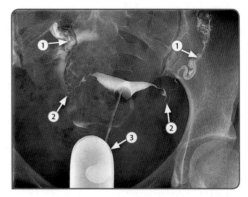

Figure 2.15 Hysterosalpingogram showing bilateral patent fallopian tubes. ① Free spill of contrast from fallopian tubes, ② contrast within fallopian tube, ③ cannula. Courtesy of Roy Craven.

Figure 2.14 Sagittal T2-weighted MRI scan showing a large cervical mass infiltrating the corpus of the uterus causing haematometra and debris in the uterine cavity. ① Bladder, ② cervical tumour, ③ vagina. Courtesy of Rishi Sethi.

of internal reproductive organs). It is safe for use in pregnancy, because there is no radiation exposure; however, contrast is not used because of its potential teratogenicity.

The space within the MRI scanner is narrow and can provoke claustrophobia. It is also noisy and women have to lie still for up to an hour and a half while the images are collected. MRI cannot be used if the patient's body contains metallic implants, including a pacemaker, cerebral artery clips or cochlear implants. Furthermore, all jewellery must be removed.

Tubal patency testing

Tubal patency testing is used to check for blockages in the fallopian tubes that might prevent a fertilised egg from reaching the uterus. It can be carried out using hysterosalpingography, hysterosalpingo-contrast sonography or laparoscopy and dye test. All involve the injection of dye or contrast through the cervix, and visualisation of its spill from the ends of the fallopian tubes.

Hysterosalpingography

In hysterosalpingography, radio-opaque dye is injected into the uterus and fallopian tubes through a cannula inserted into the cervical canal. The distribution of the dye in the uterus and tubes is then visualised by radiography. Tubal patency is confirmed by spillage of the dye from the ends of the fallopian tubes (**Figure 2.15**).

The investigation is used in women at low risk of having tubal disease and avoids the need for general anaesthesia. A false positive diagnosis of tubal blockage can be caused by tubal spasm, so a laparoscopy and dye test is carried out to confirm the result.

Hysterosalpingo-contrast sonography

This investigation is similar to hysterosalpingography in that contrast is injected through a cannula inserted into the cervix. However, in hysterosalpingo-contrast sonography the passage of contrast through the fallopian tubes is monitored with ultrasound rather than radiography. Thus radiation exposure is avoided, and the uterus and ovaries can be evaluated simultaneously.

Endoscopy

In endoscopy (Greek, 'to look inside'), an endoscope, a thin tube with a light source and camera at the end, is inserted into the body and images from the camera are transmitted to a screen. The following endoscopic procedures are used in gynaecology:

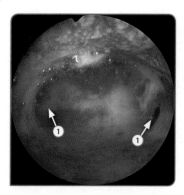

Figure 2.16 Hysteroscopic visualisation of the uterine cavity. ① Tubal ostia.

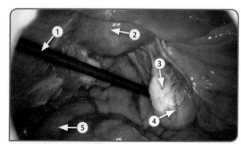

Figure 2.17 Laparoscopic appearance of a simple right ovarian cyst. ① Laparoscopic instrument, ② uterus, ③ right ovary, ④ right ovarian cyst, ⑤ loops of small intestine.

- hysteroscopy to visualise the uterine cavity
- laparoscopy to visualise the abdominal cavity
- colposcopy to visualise the cervix

Hysteroscopy

In hysteroscopy, a hysteroscope (the endoscope used in this procedure) is passed through the cervix to visualise the uterine cavity and endometrium (**Figure 2.16**). It is used in the investigation of various symptoms:

- abnormal bleeding, including intermenstrual and postmenopausal bleeding
- dysmenorrhoea
- subfertility
- suspected uterine anomalies

Fibroids, endometrial polyps, cancers and uterine septa can be assessed by hysteroscopy, and directed biopsy done to make a histological diagnosis. This can be carried out using local anaesthesia in the outpatient setting or under general anaesthesia as a day-case procedure. Therapeutic procedures, including resection of submucous fibroids and sterilisation, can also be carried out with hysteroscopy.

Potential complications are bleeding, infection, perforation of the uterus, and creation of a false passage when the hysteroscope is not inserted through the cervical canal but is inserted into the cervical tissues.

Laparoscopy

In laparoscopy, the abdomen is first inflated with carbon dioxide using a Veress needle inserted through a small skin incision in the umbilicus. Once the abdomen is adequately distended, the laparoscope is inserted through the same incision. The distension of the abdomen allows better visualisation of the internal organs (**Figure 2.17**). Further incisions along the 'bikini line' are made if other instruments are needed during the procedure. General anaesthesia is required.

Indications for carrying out a diagnostic laparoscopy include:

- investigation of subfertility (when combined with dye test to assess tubal patency)
- investigation of pelvic pain
- suspected endometriosis
- suspected ovarian or primary peritoneal cancer, to obtain a biopsy sample for diagnosis and to assess surgical resectability

Laparoscopy is also used to treat a wide range of gynaecological conditions, such as resection of endometriosis and removal of fibroids (myomectomy).

Complications include bleeding and infection, as well as damage to bowel, bladder and ureters (1 in 1000 cases; higher in therapeutic procedures).

If all the carbon dioxide is not allowed to escape from the abdomen at the end of the procedure, it irritates the diaphragm and causes referred pain to the shoulder tip. Warn women having a laparoscopy that this may happen, otherwise they are confused if they wake up and find that their shoulders hurt.

Colposcopy

This investigation is classified as a form of endoscopy. However, the colposcope does not enter the body; it is placed at the entrance to the vagina. Colposcopy is used to assess the cervix in women with an abnormal smear test result or symptoms suggesting cervical cancer (see Chapter 15).

Urodynamics

Urodynamic testing is used to study bladder and urethral function. It is carried out in women with urinary incontinence that has not responded to conservative management, and those who are due to undergo surgical treatment. A number of specific tests are done to assess different lower urinary tract functions (Table 2.9).

Women are asked to stop anticholinergic medication 5 days before the test to prevent masking of signs, and to attend the appointment with a full bladder. They first pass urine on a special commode containing a flowmeter to measure the volume and flow of urine. Catheters are then placed in the rectum and bladder to measure the pressure both inside and outside the bladder. The bladder is slowly filled with fluid through the catheter, and the woman is asked to report when she starts to feel the urge to pass urine and when this urge becomes unbearable. She is also asked to stand up, cough and listen to running water in case these provoke leakage. Once the bladder is full, she is allowed to fully void the fluid while on the commode with the tubes in place to monitor detrusor pressure during urination.

Urodynamic testing is done selectively, because it takes 30 min and is invasive. The results, combined with the information in a bladder diary, are used to guide surgical treatment.

Urodynamic testing		
Test	What it involves	What it shows
Post-void residual volume	Catheter inserted into the bladder after voiding to measure residual volume	Residual volume < 50 mL is normal Larger amounts cause overflow incontinence and occur in neurogenic bladder (e.g. in Parkinson's disease) and infection
Uroflowmetry	Rate of urine flow measured as patient voids urine on a special commode at the start of the procedure; pressure of flow measured at the end, when voiding with the catheter in situ	High pressure and low flow rate in lower urinary tract obstruction Low pressure and low flow rate caused by detrusor weakness (e.g. in multiple sclerosis, diabetes)
Cystometry	Detrusor pressure = vesical pressure (bladder catheter) − abdominal pressure (rectal catheter)	A normal bladder is compliant; there is no increase in detrusor pressure with filling An overactive bladder contracts inappropriately during filling, causing leakage In stress incontinence, there is leakage of urine during coughing and increases in intra-abdominal pressure without corresponding increases in detrusor pressure

Table 2.9 Components of urodynamic testing

Management options

Starter questions

Answers to the following questions are on pages 117–118.

8. What are the principles of obtaining informed consent?
9. Why has use of hormone replacement therapy decreased for the treatment of menopausal symptoms?
10. When is a hysterectomy indicated for the treatment of heavy menstrual bleeding?

The aims of management in gynaecology are to:

- provide a cure
- prevent disease progression
- reduce or alleviate symptoms
- improve quality of life
- improve fertility

Most gynaecological conditions are treated to reduce symptoms and improve quality of life. Early stage malignancies are managed with a view to curing the disease. However, ovarian cancer generally presents at an advanced stage, when this is no longer an option; the aim then becomes prolongation of survival.

Therapeutic interventions are:

- non-pharmacological interventions
- pharmacological treatment
- radiological procedures
- surgical procedures

Patients use the Internet to research symptoms and treatment options. Ask patients what they have found out. This provides an opportunity to gauge their level of understanding and engages them in joint decision making.

A combined approach using several different treatment modalities is usually required. Multiple options for managing a particular condition are frequently available; selecting the right treatment for an individual woman depends on several factors, including the presence of comorbidities and fertility intentions. Therefore patient education to promote understanding of their condition is critical. This allows women to make informed choices about their treatment, as well as improving adherence to therapy and satisfaction with their care.

Observe other health professionals providing information to patients, and learn from their technique. Avoid using medical jargon; instead, use simple terms supplemented with pictures. Patient information leaflets for many conditions are available from organisations such as the Royal College of Obstetricians and Gynaecologists.

Non-pharmacological interventions

Many gynaecological symptoms are relieved by simple, non-pharmacological interventions. They can be used to treat a range of symptoms, including urinary incontinence, pelvic organ prolapse and subfertility. They are often used alongside pharmacological treatments, but also improve general health. Non-pharmacological interventions are cheap, non-invasive and have no side effects, but are frequently less effective in the short and long term than other treatments; and compliance is a problem.

Conservative management refers to situations where a 'watch and wait' approach is employed to see if a condition improves with time. It differs from medical management, in which pharmacological interventions are used to improve symptoms.

Weight reduction

As well as being a risk factor for many health problems generally, obesity contributes to and exacerbates several gynaecological conditions, including stress incontinence, prolapse and subfertility. It also makes surgical procedures technically more difficult to carry out and increases the risk of postoperative wound infection and thromboembolism.

Advice about healthy eating and exercise, through individual patient advice and leaflets, is given to women with BMI > 25 kg/m², and referral to a dietitian offered. Weight loss drugs or bariatric surgery is suitable for a minority of patients.

When discussing the impact of obesity on reproductive health with a patient avoid blaming her for her condition; instead explore her understanding of how her weight influences her symptoms and management options. Most women have good insight and will appreciate an open discussion.

Smoking cessation

Smoking has a negative effect on many aspects of reproductive and gynaecological health. For example, it:

- reduces fertility
- impairs wound healing
- increases the risk of cervical cancer
- can cause chronic coughing, which exacerbates stress incontinence

Advice on smoking cessation is given to all women, supplemented with information leaflets, highlighting the harmful effects of smoking on health in both the short and long term. Women who are motivated to quit are referred to smoking cessation services for further advice and counselling in combination with nicotine replacement.

Physiotherapy

Pelvic floor physiotherapy is the first-line treatment for prolapse and urinary incontinence. It also improves dyspareunia caused by vaginismus. Pelvic floor exercises are used to improve muscle tone. Exercises supervised by a health professional are proven to be effective; exercises learned from leaflets without supervision are often unsuccessful as they are performed incorrectly.

Regimens for pelvic floor exercises vary but follow the same basic pattern. When starting these exercises, the woman learns to identify the correct set of muscles by trying to stop the flow during urination. She holds these muscles in a contraction for 3 s before relaxing them for 3 s, and repeats these actions 10 times, three times every day. As the muscles strengthen, she gradually works up to 10-s contractions with 10-s intervals of relaxation, again with 10 repetitions three times daily.

Other techniques for strengthening the pelvic floor muscles are:

- electrical stimulation
- biofeedback, i.e. provision of information about muscle contraction from electrical sensors
- the use of vaginal cones, a set of progressively heavier weights, inserted into the vagina, that the pelvic floor muscles must contract around to hold in place, thus providing 'weight training' for these muscles

Exercises need to be carried out regularly for several months to be effective, which requires commitment from the patient. If the symptoms do not improve after 3 months, further medical or surgical treatment is warranted.

Pharmacological treatment

The main drugs used in gynaecology are non-steroidal anti-inflammatory drugs (NSAIDs), hormonal medication, fertility drugs and anticholinergic agents.

Non-steroidal anti-inflammatory drugs

These drugs provide analgesia (pain relief) and also act as antipyretics, i.e. reducing temperature, and anti-inflammatories. They act by inhibiting cyclo-oxygenases 1 and 2, thereby reducing the synthesis of prostaglandins and thromboxanes, which mediate transmission of pain signals to the brain and have roles in the inflammatory response. Examples of NSAIDs are ibuprofen, diclofenac and mefenamic acid; most NSAIDs are available over the counter.

Non-steroidal anti-inflammatory drugs are used as first-line treatment for pelvic pain, endometriosis and dysmenorrhoea, conditions in which the release of prostaglandins stimulates an inflammatory response and activation of pain. They are contraindicated in pregnancy, because:

- exposure to NSAIDs in the first trimester is associated with miscarriage and cardiac, abdominal wall and cleft defects
- NSAID use in the third trimester causes oligohydramnios and pulmonary hypertension

NSAIDs are used with caution in women with asthma, because they can cause bronchospasm. Adverse effects with long-term use include stomach ulcers, gastrointestinal bleeding and anaemia.

Hormonal medication

A broad range of hormonal medications are available, including oestrogen and progestogen (a synthetic form of progesterone), either alone or in combination and in various formulations. They are used to replace hormonal deficiencies and, in higher doses, to inhibit the hypothalamic-pituitary-ovarian axis, preventing pregnancy and alleviating symptoms from hormonally-responsive conditions, such as endometriosis.

Hormone replacement therapy

Low-dose oestrogen, with or without progestogen, is given as HRT to peri- and post-menopausal women to treat symptoms of the menopause, such as hot flushes, night sweats and vaginal dryness. The different types of HRT are described in **Table 2.10**.

Long-term use of HRT, i.e. for >5 years, is associated with an increased risk of breast cancer, venous thromboembolism and cardiovascular disease. Therefore HRT is used at the lowest dose for the shortest period of time.

> **Additional contraception is required if a woman is premenopausal and using HRT for the treatment of menopausal symptoms.** The doses of the hormones used are too low for it to be relied on to prevent pregnancy.

Progestogen-only preparations

These are used mainly for contraception. They are available in many forms to suit an individual's needs and preferences:

- tablets, e.g. Cerazette
- subdermal implants, e.g. Nexplanon
- intramuscular injections, e.g. Depo-Provera
- intrauterine systems, e.g. Mirena coil
- pessaries, e.g. Cyclogest

In women who are menstruating, the exogenous progesterone supplied via each of these methods causes cervical mucus to thicken, thereby preventing sperm from reaching the uterus and fallopian tubes, where fertilisation can take place. It also inhibits ovulation in up to 99% of cycles, depending on the dose and type of progestogen given.

Progestogen-only preparations are used in many circumstances when oestrogen is contraindicated, including in women who are breastfeeding or who have venous thromboembolism, migraine with aura and cardiovascular disease. Irregular bleeding is the commonest adverse effect, but this usually settles with time. Breast tenderness, mood swings and heavy bleeding also occur.

Hormone replacement therapy				
Type	Description	Who uses it?	Methods of administration	Contraindications
Oestrogen only	Continuous administration of oestrogen only	Women without a uterus or with only local vaginal symptoms	Either systemic (via tablet, patch or implant) or local (to the vagina as a cream or pessary)	Increased risk of endometrial cancer if uterus present
Sequential combined	Continuous administration of oestrogen, with 14 days of progestogen every 1–3 months	Women who are still menstruating regularly but have menopausal symptoms	Oral or patches	Oestrogen receptor–positive breast or endometrial cancer, deep vein thrombosis or pulmonary embolism, acute myocardial infarction, liver disease
Continuous combined	Continuous administration of oestrogen and progestogen	Post-menopausal women (bleed-free)	Oral, patch; the progestogen component can be delivered via the levonorgestrel-releasing intrauterine system (Mirena coil)	Oestrogen receptor–positive breast or endometrial cancer, deep vein thrombosis or pulmonary organism, acute myocardial infarction, liver disease

Table 2.10 The different types of hormone replacement therapy

Non-contraceptive indications for exogenous progesterones include:

- prevention of miscarriage after embryo transfer in IVF, because progesterone helps maintain early pregnancy by thickening the endometrium
- endometriosis
- menstrual disorders
- endometrial hyperplasia
- endometrial protection from unregulated proliferation and the risk of hyperplasia and endometrial cancer when oestrogen-only HRT is used.

Combined preparations

These contain both oestrogen and progesterone. Combined hormonal contraceptives act by suppressing ovulation. They are available as tablets (the combined oral contraceptive pill), patches and vaginal rings, and are taken or worn for 3 weeks followed by a 1-week break in which a withdrawal bleed occurs. Combined preparations are also used to treat endometriosis and menstrual problems.

> Hormone tablets are taken at the same time every day to maximise contraceptive effect; there are free apps available to remind patients. Ensure patients are aware that the package insert contains instructions on what to do if they miss a pill; different formulations have different margins of error (e.g. 3 hours for a POP, 12 hours for cerazette, 24 hours for a COCP).

Contraindications to its use include migraine with aura, BMI >35 kg/m^2, smokers aged >35 years and current or previous breast cancer. Adverse effects, which include breast tenderness and headaches, are unusual. However, combined preparations increase the risk of venous thromboembolism and breast cancer.

Fertility drugs

Drugs are used in the treatment of subfertility to stimulate ovulation. In IVF, they are also used to temporarily suppress production of reproductive hormones, essentially shutting down natural menstrual cycles in preparation for a treatment cycle, in which the timing of ovulation is controlled.

Clomifene citrate

By a process of negative feedback, oestrogen inhibits gonadotrophin-releasing hormone (GnRH) production by the hypothalamus. This prevents the release of follicle stimulating hormone (FSH) and luteinising hormone (LH) by the anterior pituitary and prevents further oestrogen production. Clomifene, a selective oestrogen receptor modulator, blocks the effect of oestrogen on the hypothalamus and thus causes a surge in FSH and LH. This stimulates increased production and release of eggs from the ovaries.

Clomifene is used to treat women with anovulatory subfertility. However, it increases the risk of multiple pregnancies and ovarian hyperstimulation syndrome. Ultrasound monitoring is performed in at least the first cycle to monitor for these risks.

Gonadotrophins

Exogenous LH and FSH are used to stimulate ovulation:

- in women who have low levels of these gonadotrophins as a result of pituitary disease
- as part of an IVF cycle
- when clomifene treatment has been unsuccessful

They are given as daily injections.

Gonadotrophin-releasing hormone analogues

These initially stimulate gonadotrophin production but prolonged use causes down-regulation of LH and FSH secretion. They are used in the short protocol of IVF treatment to stop the natural cycle in older women and women who have had a poor ovarian response under the long protocol. They are administered as a nasal spray several times a day or by daily or monthly injection.

Gonadotrophin-releasing hormone antagonists

Like gonadotrophin-releasing hormone analogues, these drugs inhibit gonadotrophin production; however, there is no initial increase. They are given as daily or monthly injections:

- in the long protocol of IVF treatment, to prevent natural menstrual cycles and to delay ovulation until the optimal time for egg collection
- to remove hormonal stimulation of fibroids and endometriosis

Induction of a menopausal state with low oestrogen levels causes hot flushes and night sweats, and increases the risk of osteoporosis and cardiovascular disease if used long term. To counteract these effects, add-back HRT is required if gonadotrophin-releasing hormone antagonists are used for > 6 months.

Anticholinergic medication

Anticholinergic drugs block acetylcholine transmission in the central and peripheral nervous systems. They are used to treat urge incontinence, because they inhibit parasympathetic stimulation of the bladder detrusor muscle. Many different preparations are available, all with similar efficacy and adverse effect profiles. Examples of commonly used anticholinergic drugs are oxybutynin, tolterodine and solifenacin.

> **Intolerable side effects is the most common reason for discontinuing anticholingeric medication.** Mirabegron, a β-3-adrenoreceptor agonist, is used second-line in such cases. Its efficacy for treating overactive bladder symptoms is similar, but it has fewer anticholinergic side effects. It is contraindicated in severe renal and liver disease and uncontrolled hypertension.

Adverse effects are caused by the reduction in cholinergic neurotransmission; dry eyes, dry mouth, blurred vision, constipation and confusion are the most common. Anticholinergic drugs are contraindicated in myasthenia gravis and acute angle closure glaucoma, because they worsen symptoms.

Interventional radiology

In interventional radiology, minimally invasive, image-guided procedures are used to treat various conditions. In gynaecology, uterine artery embolisation is an interventional radiology procedure for the treatment of fibroids. A catheter is inserted through the femoral or radial artery and directed to the uterine artery by using real-time imaging (**Figure 2.18**). Once in position, tiny particles or coils are fed through the catheter to occlude blood supply to the fibroid, thereby causing it to necrose (die) and shrink.

Uterine artery embolisation is used for women who do not wish to have a hysterectomy but who do not wish to have children or have completed their family, because subsequent pregnancy outcomes are adversely affected. The procedure takes an hour to perform but the maximal effect is only apparent after 6–12 months.

Surgery

Surgery is used when conservative or medical management is inappropriate, or when less invasive options have been unsuccessful. The type of operation to be carried out depends on the condition in question, whether the woman has had previous surgery, her fertility intentions and the skill of the surgeon. The most common gynaecological procedures are listed in **Table 2.11**.

Minimally invasive surgery

Minimal access surgery in gynaecology is carried out either hysteroscopically through a hysteroscope or laparoscopically (through a laparoscope; **Figure 2.17**). The benefits include quicker recovery and lower risk of wound infection. The disadvantages are longer operating time, particularly while the surgeon is learning, and the requirement for more advanced surgical skills.

Radiotherapy

Radiotherapy is used to treat cancers of the female genital tract. It can be given as primary treatment or in addition to surgery, chemotherapy or both. High-energy X-rays are used to kill cancer cells. Radiotherapy is delivered in specialist hospitals in radiotherapy departments. It is given as multiple doses and the majority of patients go home between treatments.

External beam radiotherapy

In this technique, radiotherapy is delivered externally; a machine is used to target precisely the area to be treated. It is used to treat abdominal or pelvic disease or to reduce the risk of recurrence.

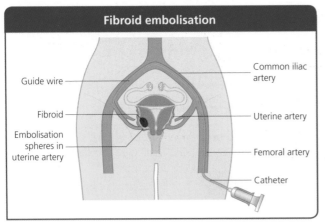

Fibroid embolisation

Guide wire

Fibroid

Embolisation spheres in uterine artery

Common iliac artery

Uterine artery

Femoral artery

Catheter

Figure 2.18 Fibroid embolisation via the uterine vasculature. Uterine vessels are accessed via the femoral arteries.

Gynaecological operations				
Name	When is it carried out?	How is it carried out?	Type of anaesthesia	Risks*
Evacuation of retained products of conception	To treat miscarriages or terminate pregnancies	A wide-bore catheter is inserted through the cervix into the uterus and suction used to remove tissue	Local or general	Uterine perforation Injury to the cervix Incomplete procedure Intrauterine adhesions (Asherman's syndrome)
Endometrial ablation	To treat heavy periods in women who do not want children or who have completed their family	Hysteroscopy is carried out to assess uterine size and shape; this is followed by ablation of the endometrium by heated water (balloon ablation) or high-energy radiofrequencies (NovoSure)	Local or general	Uterine perforation Injury to the cervix Ineffective treatment (10% of cases)
Diagnostic laparoscopy	To investigate abdominal or pelvic pain, suspected ectopic pregnancy	The abdomen is inflated with carbon dioxide through a Veress needle before the laparoscope is inserted via an umbilical incision	General	Injury to bowel, bladder or ureters (1 in 1000 procedures)
Laparoscopy and dye	To investigate subfertility	Laparoscopy is carried out and dye is injected through the cervical canal while simultaneously looking for spill abdominally through the fallopian tubes	General	Injury to bowel, bladder or ureters Uterine perforation
Salpingectomy	To treat ectopic pregnancy, or to improve IVF outcomes if a hydrosalpinx is present	Removal of tube by cauterising and dividing mesosalpinx (part of the broad ligament between the ovary and fallopian tube) and proximal tubal; carried out laparoscopically or by laparotomy (open surgery)	General	Injury to bowel, bladder or ureters
Salpingostomy	To treat ectopic pregnancy if the other fallopian tube is abnormal or absent	An incision is made in the tube over the site of the ectopic pregnancy, and suction used to remove the products of conception	General	Injury to bowel, bladder or ureters Retained placental tissue (8 in 100 procedures) Repeat ectopic pregnancy (18 versus 8 in 100 procedures after salpingectomy)

Continued....

Gynaecological operations *continued*				
Name	When is it carried out?	How is it carried out?	Type of anaesthesia	Risks*
Sterilisation	To provide permanent contraception	Either laparoscopically, when Filshie clips are applied to both fallopian tubes, or hysteroscopically, when coils are inserted into the tubal ostia (openings)	General or local (local possible for hysteroscopic procedure only)	Laparoscopy ■ Injury to bowel, bladder or ureters ■ Uterine perforation ■ Failed procedure (1 in 200) ■ Increased risk of ectopic pregnancy, if pregnancy occurs Hysteroscopy ■ Uterine perforation ■ Failed procedure (<1 in 100) ■ Need to use contraception for 3 months until hysterosalpingography to confirm correct placement of coils
Ovarian cystectomy	To treat benign ovarian cysts	Ovarian capsule incised and cyst dissected from remaining normal ovary; carried out either laparoscopically or at laparotomy	General	Injury to abdominal organs Need for further surgery if cyst is borderline or malignant on histology
Salpingo-oophrectomy	To treat large ovarian cysts if the ovary cannot be conserved, as part of cancer treatment, and prophylactically in women with BRCA mutations	Removal of tube and ovary by opening broad ligament and dividing infundibular pelvic ligament, mesosalpinx and proximal end of tube	General	Injury to bowel, bladder or ureters Hot flushes and osteoporosis if patients is premenopausal and procedure is carried out bilaterally
Hysterectomy	To treat heavy periods, prolapse or gynaecological cancer	Uterus, with or without cervix, removed by dividing round, cardinal and uterosacral ligaments and tying off the uterine arteries; carried out laparoscopically, vaginally or as an open procedure and combined with bilateral salpingo-oophorectomy	General or spinal	Injury to bowel, bladder or ureters Recurrent prolapse

BRCA, breast cancer susceptibility gene.

*Excluding general risks of bleeding, infection and thrombosis.

Table 2.11 Common gynaecological operations

Internal radiotherapy (brachytherapy)

In brachytherapy, radioactive material is placed within the vagina. Placement of the radioactive material at the site of the tumour allows a lower dose of radiation to be used. Consequently, there is less damage to surrounding organs, though the effectiveness is similar to that of external beam radiotherapy. Brachytherapy is used to treat pelvic disease and to reduce the risk of local recurrence.

Chemotherapy

In chemotherapy, anticancer drugs are used to kill malignant cells. Because the drugs target all dividing cells, they also affect normal tissues to varying degrees; this causes hair loss, nausea and immunosuppression.

Carboplatin, paclitaxel and methotrexate are the chemotherapy drugs most commonly used to treat gynaecological malignancies. They are either given alone or in combination with surgery and radiotherapy. Chemotherapy is particularly effective for germ cell tumours of the ovary and gestational trophoblastic disease. These conditions are described as being chemosensitive.

Answers to starter questions

1. Although most cases of abnormal bleeding have a benign aetiology, history alone is inadequate at excluding an underlying malignancy and investigations are required for any woman who presents with red flag symptoms. Heavy, but regular, periods, are rarely associated with female genital tract cancers and are treated symptomatically, with investigations only used when first-line medical management is unsuccessful.

2. A cystocele causes kinking of the urethra, slowing down the flow of urine and acting like a sphincter to prevent leaking in association with increases in intra-abdominal pressure. When it is treated, this kink is removed and any deficiencies in the actual urethral sphincter are exposed.

3. Cervical excitation is significant pain on sideways movement of the cervix during a bimanual examination. It indicates pelvic inflammation and is caused by pelvic inflammatory disease, endometriosis or an ectopic pregnancy. It is distinguished from the normal uncomfortable sensation caused by the examination by looking at the woman's face for sign of substantial discomfort.

4. The patient being a virgin is not a contraindication to a vaginal examination, but it might influence the decision as to whether the examination is necessary or not. A speculum does not affect the hymen, but is more uncomfortable for people who have not had sexual intercourse before. If the cervix needs to be visualised to diagnose or exclude abnormalities then a speculum is the only means by which this can be achieved. A general anaesthetic is used in the rare instances where examination in clinic is not acceptable to the patient.

5. Although CA125 is a useful marker of ovarian cancer and is raised in advanced disease, only 50% of stage 1 (early) ovarian cancer cases are associated with a raised CA125. It is also not specific and is raised in other conditions, including endometriosis, fibroids, pelvic inflammatory disease and pregnancy.

6. Cervical cytology is used during the cervical screening programme to detect asymptomatic precancerous cervical lesions (CIN). It provides a cytological, but not a histological diagnosis. If cervical cancer is suspected, a definitive histological diagnosis is required: this is obtained by taking a biopsy of the mass either from the edge as a wedge biopsy or by performing a loop excision of the cervix if the lesion is small.

7. CT scans are used to stage malignancies when distant metastases are suspected, e.g. high grade endometrial or ovarian cancers, because it provides better definition of the lungs and bone than an MRI scan. A CT of the chest, abdomen and pelvis is requested to perform complete staging. It is also used in patients with cardiac pacemakers and other metallic implants who are not able to have a MRI scan.

8. For consent to be valid it must be voluntarily given, made on an informed basis and be given by a person with capacity to make decisions. This means the patient should be free from coercion and be able to make up their own mind about proceeding with investigations or treatment. They should receive sufficient information about the risks and benefits, alternative options and what would happen if they did not proceed. They should be able to understand this information, weigh it up and covey their answer to a medical professional.

Answers *continued*

9. Studies performed into hormone replacement therapy (HRT) have shown that while the benefit of short-term use outweighs any risks, longer term exposure (>10 years) is associated with an increased risk of breast, endometrial (oestrogen-only HRT) and ovarian cancer, thromboembolism and stroke.

10. The number of hysterectomies performed for heavy menstrual bleeding has significantly decreased with the introduction of levonorgestrel-releasing intrauterine systems (Mirena coils) and endometrial ablation, both of which reduce bleeding by 90% and avoid the risks of surgery. A hysterectomy is indicated if:

    *   medical and non-surgical treatments fail
    *   the patient desires no periods at all (this cannot be promised with other treatment options)
    *   the uterus contains fibroids >3 cm in size
    *   the bleeding is related to endometrial abnormalities, e.g. hyperplasia or cancer

Chapter 3
Clinical essentials: obstetrics

Introduction

Obstetrics differs from other specialities in that there are two patients – the mother and the baby – to consider simultaneously, and they have potentially conflicting needs. Also, the mothers are generally young and healthy; they may be seeing a health professional other than their general practitioner for the first time in years. In obstetrics, symptoms and signs develop late and quickly, making history taking and examination as much about identifying asymptomatic disease as about diagnosing the cause of symptoms.

Obstetrics is an emotionally charged speciality, with frequent high points and, fortunately rarer, heartbreaking moments. It is necessary to acknowledge how each woman feels about being pregnant, because not all pregnancies are planned. Furthermore, not all mothers are able to take home a healthy baby; those who lose a baby to miscarriage or stillbirth, or whose baby is unwell, need particular support. Eliciting background information before taking a history prevents entering into conversations based on incorrect assumptions about an individual patient's situation.

> **Gestational age** is documented as the number of weeks gestation (X) plus the number of days (Y), written in superscript (X^{+Y}).

> **'Booking visit'** is the term used in the UK, Australia and various other countries for the first antenatal visit.

Common symptoms and how to take a history

Starter questions

Answers to the following questions are on pages 145–146.

1. What are Braxton Hicks contractions?
2. Why is it important to find out if the pregnancy was planned?
3. How many fetal movements should a woman feel during the third trimester of pregnancy?

Pregnant women present either acutely to an assessment unit or delivery suite or routinely to an outpatient antenatal clinic. History taking follows the same format in each situation, but in an emergency focuses on the presenting complaint and obstetric history to guide immediate management. In the outpatient setting, adequate time is available to explore all topics in greater detail.

History taking

The format of the obstetric history follows that used in other specialities, but also includes a summary of antenatal care in the current and any previous pregnancies, as well as their outcomes. The key areas to cover are:

- presenting complaint
- history of presenting complaint
- pregnancy history
- obstetric history
- gynaecological history
- medical and surgical history
- drug history, including allergies
- family history
- social history
- systems review
- ideas, concerns and expectations

As in gynaecology, the order in which these areas are covered is not critical. The most important tasks are to ensure that all the information is gathered and to develop a style that works for the individual and promotes trust between the patient and those responsible for her care.

Introduce yourself and explain the purpose of the interview. Ask the patient how they would like to be addressed; 'What would you like me to call you?' makes them feel comfortable and puts them in charge of the consultation. Most women will reply with their first name, but others prefer to be addressed by their title and surname.

Presenting complaint

The presenting complaint is the reason for the patient's visit. Use open questions to gather as much information as possible; 'What has brought you in today?' and 'Tell me about your symptoms' are suitable opening questions. Avoiding interrupting the patient, and allow time for her to answer, because most information is provided at this stage of the consultation. Examples of presenting complaints include headache, abdominal pain and reduced fetal movements.

In obstetrics, women often present with concerns about their baby rather than about their own health. Acknowledging this and providing reassurance about fetal well-being, for example by listening to the fetal heartbeat, relieves these anxieties and thereby improves the quality of the history subsequently obtained.

History of presenting complaint

Further details about the presenting complaint are explored, including their duration, exacerbating and relieving features, severity and associated symptoms. Questions to ask include:

- 'How long have you had this problem?'
- 'Did anything provoke it?'
- 'Have you found anything that makes it better or worse?'
- 'Have you noticed any other symptoms?'

Summarise the information gathered to check that you have understood the patient correctly, and ask if anything has been missed. Signpost the topics that remain to be covered, for example by stating, 'Next, I would like to discuss how this pregnancy has been'.

> A significant minority of patients visiting the antenatal clinic have been referred because they have been identified by their midwife as being at risk of future pregnancy complications rather than because of a current problem. However, this information may not have not been relayed to the patient. Check the handheld notes to see if the reason for referral has been documented.

Pregnancy history

The pregnancy history is a summary of the current pregnancy and includes the estimated date of delivery. The frequency and content of antenatal visits are determined by the risk of pregnancy complications; women having only routine blood tests and scans and who are in the care of a community midwife, have pregnancies considered low risk, whereas those seeing a consultant for growth scans every 2 weeks have been identified as having high-risk pregnancies. Chapter 4 and Chapter 6 detail normal antenatal care and care in high-risk pregnancies, respectively.

Questions to ask in the pregnancy history are:

- 'When was the first day of your last period?'
- 'When did you stop using contraception?'
- 'Were your cycles regular before you became pregnant?'
- 'Was it a planned pregnancy?'
- 'Did you take folic acid?'
- 'Did you have an early pregnancy scan?' and if the answer is positive, 'What is your due date?'
- 'Were any problems detected on your dating and 20-week scans?' and 'Have you had any scans apart from these?'
- 'What other tests have you had?'
- 'Did you have screening for Down's syndrome?' and if the answer is positive, 'What was the estimated risk?'

Estimated date of delivery is initially based on the date of the woman's last menstrual period. However, this can be unreliable if her periods are irregular or if she conceived while using contraception. Gestational age, calculated at the dating scan from the crown–rump length, is more exact and is used as the working estimated date of delivery.

An unplanned pregnancy can be a source of anxiety, generating confusing feelings, including guilt, about whether or not to continue with the pregnancy. Offer additional support and referral to counselling services to these women.

> Show sensitivity when asking whether the pregnancy was planned, and respond with compassion if the answer is 'No'. 'It must have been a shock for you. How do you feel about things now?' helps identify women who remain ambivalent about being pregnant.

Cases of domestic abuse may only become known when the victim fails to engage with obstetric services. All women are asked whether they are experiencing domestic abuse (see page 123).

Obstetric history

The obstetric history summarises any previous pregnancies and their outcomes. It helps guide management of the current pregnancy by providing information that is used to identify conditions that can recur, make decisions about mode of delivery and put the woman's emotions surrounding the pregnancy into context. The following questions are asked:

- 'Is this your first pregnancy?'
- 'How old are your children now? and 'Are they well?'
- 'How were they delivered?'
- 'What did they weigh?'
- 'Were they born at the right time, or early?'
- 'Were there any complications in your previous pregnancies?'
- 'Have you had any other pregnancies apart from these?'

The risk of preterm birth or having a small-for-gestational-age fetus is increased for women for whom either has occurred in previous pregnancies. The greater the number of children affected, the higher the risk for the current pregnancy.

Miscarriages, terminations and stillbirths need to be handled sensitively. A woman who has been pregnant before but who has no live children is likely to be highly anxious.

Gynaecological history

In obstetrics, the gynaecological history is not as detailed as that for a gynaecology patient, but it needs to include the following questions.

- 'What was the date of your last cervical cytology test?'
- 'Have you had any treatment for abnormal cervical cytology?'

Overdue cervical screening tests are done 12 weeks after delivery. The greater the number of previous loop excisions of the cervix, the higher the risk of preterm birth. A previous trachelectomy, i.e. surgical removal of the cervix, for cervical cancer means that vaginal delivery is not possible.

Medical and surgical history

The medical history includes any previous or current medical problems. To elicit this information, ask open questions such as 'How would you describe your general health?'. In particular, diabetes, epilepsy, previous venous thromboembolism, hypertension and thyroid problems affect pregnancy, and

control of these disorders is affected by the physiological changes of pregnancy.

Ask about previous operations, particularly those involving the abdomen and pelvis. Abdominal surgery increases the risk of adhesion formation and injury to the bowel and bladder if a caesarean section is required for delivery. It occasionally contraindicates vaginal delivery, for example in cases of previous myomectomy, i.e. surgical removal of uterine fibroids.

Drug history, including allergies

The following questions need to be asked.

- 'Do you take any medication?'
- 'Did you take folic acid at the start of the pregnancy?'
- 'Are you taking iron tablets or vitamins or any other supplements?'
- 'Have you ever taken any illegal drugs?'
- 'Do you have any allergies?'

Many drugs cross the placenta and can affect the developing fetus. Therefore women may stop taking vital medication on discovering that they are pregnant, for fear of possible effects on the baby. If this has not been done on the advice of a physician, this can result in deterioration of disease control. A thorough history of previous and current medications is taken to evaluate any risks.

Women may be taking tablets that they do not consider to be drugs, often because they have been bought 'over the counter.' These include folic acid, iron and vitamin supplements.

The use of recreational drugs poses a number of risks to the pregnancy. For example, cocaine use causes placental abruption, and heroin use leads to withdrawal symptoms in the newborn baby. Ask questions about recreational drug use in an open, non-judgemental manner. Women need to know that they will not face recrimination for their actions, and that your interest is purely to minimise the risk of harm to them and their baby.

Family history

A family history is useful to assess a woman's risk of developing a particular condition during pregnancy. It includes information on diseases that have occurred both during and outside pregnancy in close family members. For example, if a first-degree relative has diabetes, the woman is screened for gestational diabetes. Similarly, if there is a family history of venous thromboembolism, depending on the circumstances in which it occurred and other risk factors for the disease, prophylactic anticoagulation is given. For women with a sister or mother who has been affected by pre-eclampsia, the prescription of low-dose aspirin is considered to reduce the risk of developing this disorder. Examples of suitable questions are:

- 'Are there any conditions that run in your family?'
- 'In particular, has anyone got diabetes, or has anyone had a blood clot in the legs or lungs, or pre-eclampsia?'

A growing number of inherited conditions, including major cardiac abnormalities (half of all cases), haemophilia and cystic fibrosis, can be diagnosed antenatally. They are detected by ultrasound in combination with amniocentesis. The specific genetic mutation needs to be known for testing to be possible.

If screening is not possible, information about the inherited condition is registered on a paediatric alert form, for paediatricians to use to guide postnatal examination and investigation.

Social history

The social history covers a number of topics, with questions such as:

- 'Do you smoke?' and if the answer is positive, 'How many a day?' and 'Do you want to give up?'
- 'Do you drink alcohol?' and if the answer is positive, 'How much in an average week?'
- 'How are you coping with the pregnancy?' and 'Do you have support at home?'
- 'Domestic abuse is common, and we ask all women about it. Is this something that has ever affected you?'

Smoking increases the risk of many pregnancy complications, including placental abruption, fetal growth restriction and stillbirth. All women who smoke are asked if they are willing to give up, and a referral is made to the smoking cessation team for those wishing to engage with their services.

Alcohol should be avoided throughout pregnancy; because alcohol is harmful to the fetus at any stage of its development, and no safe limit has been established. Frequent intake of alcohol and binge drinking are particularly damaging and significantly increase the risk of fetal alcohol syndrome.

Social support is essential in pregnancy, particularly if a previous pregnancy resulted in an adverse outcome such as stillbirth. For women who have lost a baby at any stage, the emotions triggered by another pregnancy are difficult to manage.

Women are more likely to experience domestic abuse in pregnancy than at other times in their life, and attacks may become more severe or frequent at this time. Abuse during pregnancy threatens the well-being of both mother and baby.

Questions about domestic abuse are phrased in a way that encourages disclosure by avoiding judgement and reassuring any woman experiencing such abuse that she is not alone. A positive response is investigated further by asking about the type of abuse, whether children are affected and if it is safe to return home (see Chapter 15, page 370).

Systems review

The systems review includes a brief screen of symptoms in other organs. In obstetrics, questions about the fetus are also included here if not asked previously.

- 'Do you have a headache, blurred vision or pain at the top of the abdomen?' (These are symptoms of pre-eclampsia)
- 'Any pain on passing urine?' (A sign of infection)
- 'Is the baby moving normally?' (To check for reduced fetal movements)
- 'Any leaking or unusual discharge from the vagina?' (Signs of ruptured membranes or vaginal infection)

Ideas, concerns and expectations

Asking about the patient's ideas, concerns and expectations shows a willingness to listen and to acknowledge her role in managing her health. It improves the physician–patient relationship and is more likely to result in adherence to treatment.

- 'What do you think might be causing your symptoms?'
- What are your concerns?'
- 'What did you hope for from the consultation today?'

Obstetric symptoms

During pregnancy, a woman's body undergoes significant physiological changes. Differentiating normal symptoms of pregnancy from those caused by underlying disease can be difficult. The following are common symptoms causing women to present to the obstetric department. The questions listed narrow down the differential diagnosis and focus the examination and subsequent investigations.

Abdominal pain

Discomfort is a common feature of pregnancy, especially in the latter stages, but abdominal pain is not. It is described in the same way as pain in other parts of the body by using the SOCRATES acronym (see page 84).

Common causes of abdominal pain and their specific features are shown in **Table 3.1**. They are divided into obstetric, gynaecological, surgical, medical and musculoskeletal causes. Benign causes of pain settle with time, whereas pathological conditions worsen.

Vaginal bleeding

Any vaginal bleeding in pregnancy is abnormal and requires assessment. There are several underlying causes, which can be distinguished by asking:

- 'How much blood have you lost? A spot, a teaspoon, a tablespoon, a cup, a pint?'
- 'Did anything provoke the bleeding?'

- 'Do you have any associated pain?'
- 'Is this the first time you have had bleeding in this pregnancy, or has it happened before?'
- 'Is the baby moving normally?'

Small-volume bleeds after sexual intercourse occur in women with cervical ectopy. This type of bleed is the result of trauma from contact between the penis and the cervix.

Placental abruption is associated with sudden, severe, constant abdominal pain and a degree of maternal collapse which does not match the evident blood loss. This is because further blood is trapped behind the placenta (concealed haemorrhage). The fetus is at risk of hypoxia and stillbirth, and its movements are reduced to conserve energy.

In cases of bleeding, the patient's handheld notes are consulted to check the placental site. Painless bleeding occurs as a result of placenta praevia and vasa praevia.

> **In the UK, all pregnant women receive a set of maternity notes in which their antenatal care is recorded.** They are asked to bring these handheld notes to all appointments with health care professionals, as well as to carry them at all other times in case emergency care is required. The use of handheld notes increases women's involvement in their care. It also enables partners to be better informed and feel more involved in the pregnancy.

A single unexplained, small antepartum haemorrhage, i.e. bleeding after 24 weeks' gestation, is not associated with increased risk to the pregnancy. However, repeated unexplained bleeding is a symptom of placental insufficiency, which is a cause of fetal growth restriction; regular monitoring of fetal well-being with ultrasound is warranted, and delivery is in an obstetric-led unit.

> **The woman's blood group is always checked after any episode of bleeding.** Rhesus-negative women need anti-D prophylaxis within 72 h to prevent development of rhesus autoantibodies.

	Abdominal pain in pregnancy: common causes	
Category	Causes	Discriminating features
Obstetric	Labour, either term or preterm	Intermittent, generalised pain, initially crampy then increasing in frequency and severity; tightening of the abdomen; may have loss of mucus plug and waters
	Pre-eclampsia	Right upper quadrant pain caused by liver capsule distension, associated headache, blurred vision
	Placental abruption	Sudden, severe, constant pain; bleeding (may not be a large amount); reduced fetal movements
	Uterine rupture	Previous caesarean section; intermittent contractions followed by constant, severe pain, bleeding and collapse
	Chorioamnionitis	Previous rupture of membranes, foul-smelling fluid, temperature
	Acute fatty liver of pregnancy	Upper abdominal pain, vomiting, jaundice, headache, unwell
Gynaecological	Ectopic pregnancy	Early pregnancy, unilateral pelvic pain, minimal bleeding, collapse
	Miscarriage	Crampy, suprapubic pain; associated bleeding (may be heavy)
	Rupture or torsion of ovarian cyst	Unilateral pain, acute onset, associated vomiting in cases of torsion, unwell
	Fibroids (red degeneration) i.e. blockage in the blood supply to the fibroid causing it to turn red and die	Acute onset; low-grade temperature; history of heavy, painful periods; palpable pelvic mass
	Ovarian hyperstimulation syndrome	Early pregnancy, infertility treatment, generalised abdominal pain and bloating, shortness of breath, vomiting, thirst
Surgical	Appendicitis	Umbilical to right iliac fossa pain, vomiting, fever, anorexia
	Cholecystitis	Right upper quadrant pain, exacerbated by consumption of fatty foods; vomiting; jaundice
	Intestinal obstruction	Generalised, colicky pain; vomiting; constipation; previous abdominal surgery
Medical	Constipation	Colicky pain, irregular bowel habit
	Urinary tract infection or stone	Suprapubic pain with or without loin pain, haematuria, dysuria, frequency of micturition
	Venous thromboembolism (pelvic deep vein thrombosis)	Constant lower abdominal pain; may also have swollen, red, hot, painful calf
Musculoskeletal	Round ligament pain	Sudden, sharp pain in lower abdomen, which radiates to groin; short lasting; exacerbated by movement or exercise
	Pelvic girdle pain or symphysis pubis dysfunction	Gnawing pain over pubis and lower back, exacerbated by movement; audible clicking or popping of pelvic joints

Table 3.1 Common causes of abdominal pain in pregnancy

Vaginal discharge

Blood flow to the uterus increases during pregnancy, and the cervix softens in response to high levels of progesterone. These changes increase the amount of physiological vaginal discharge. However, a change in discharge may be a sign of infection. Genital tract infections are more common during pregnancy, because of suppression of the immune system to prevent rejection of the fetus.

Vaginal discharge is determined to be normal or abnormal by asking:

- 'What colour is the discharge?'

- 'Do you have any itching with the discharge?'
- 'Is there any blood in the discharge?'

Normal discharge is milky white and odourless. Thick, curdy discharge with itching signifies candidiasis (thrush). Grey, fishy-smelling discharge indicates bacterial vaginosis, which is caused by an imbalance in the normal vaginal flora. Yellow, frothy discharge is the result of *Trichomonas* infection.

A 'show' is a bloody, mucous discharge that may be noticed several days or weeks before the start of labour. This represents the loss of the mucus plug, a protective seal within the cervical canal, as a consequence of the softening and stretching of the cervix as it dilates in preparation for birth.

Chlamydia and gonorrhoea infections are usually asymptomatic. However, they can present with a change in vaginal discharge and bleeding after sex.

Headache

This symptom is a manifestation of many different conditions. However, appropriate questioning can help differentiate between disease processes (**Table 3.2**):

- 'Where is the headache?'
- 'Did it come on suddenly or gradually?'
- 'Have you ever had a headache like this before?'
- 'Have you noticed anything else, for example blurred vision or vomiting?'
- 'Have you taken any painkillers?' and if the answer is positive, 'Did they work?'

Women are reluctant to take analgesics in pregnancy, because of fears of teratogenicity; they need reassurance that paracetamol (acetaminophen), and in small and infrequent doses codeine, are safe to use. Benign types of headache, such as tension headache and migraine, ease with simple analgesia, whereas headaches with more sinister causes do not. 'Red flag' symptoms and signs are:

- sudden onset headache
- fever
- change in consciousness
- focal symptoms and signs

Headaches with these features warrant immediate investigation.

Headache in pregnancy: causes	
Type of headache or cause	Specific clinical features
Tension headache	Related to stress, no features of migraine, no 'red flag' symptoms and signs*
Migraine	Throbbing, unilateral pain; vomiting; difficulty looking at lights or hearing loud sounds; aura (i.e. visual symptoms, flashing lights, partial loss of vision); loss of sensation or movement in hemiplegic migraine; symptoms resolve with time
Drug-related headache	Headache occurs when starting a drug, for example a calcium channel blocker such as nifedipine
Epidural-related headache	Occurs after epidural or spinal anaesthesia, frontal headache, worse when standing and relieved by lying down
Pre-eclampsia	Frontal headache, associated flashing lights, oedema, upper abdominal pain
Idiopathic intracranial hypertension	Symptoms pre-date pregnancy, retro-orbital pain, double vision, obesity
Subarachnoid haemorrhage	Sudden onset, severe pain, occipital, vomiting, neck stiffness, loss of consciousness
Cerebral vein thrombosis	Post-partum, vomiting, photophobia, seizures, impaired consciousness
Meningitis	Fever, photophobia, vomiting, neck stiffness, rash
Space-occupying lesion	Gradual onset, seizures, focal symptoms depending on area of brain affected
*Sudden onset headache, fever, changes in consciousness, and focal symptoms and signs.	

Table 3.2 Causes of headache in pregnancy

Oedema (swelling)

Oedema of the lower limbs is common in pregnancy, particularly in the third trimester. The enlarging uterus compresses the vena cava, thereby reducing the return of blood to the heart; as a result, blood pools in the feet and ankles. The swelling is more marked at the end of the day and after standing for prolonged periods. It disappears overnight when the woman is lying flat. Pathological causes of oedema include pre-eclampsia and venous thromboembolism, and can be distinguished by asking:

- 'Where have you noticed the swelling?'
- 'Has it come on suddenly or been present for some time?'
- 'Does the swelling disappear overnight in bed?'
- 'Have you noticed any other symptoms?'

In pre-eclampsia, oedema affects the face and hands, i.e. non-dependent areas, rather than the lower limbs. It is also associated with headaches and visual disturbances.

Deep vein thrombosis (DVT) causes oedema in one leg rather than both legs, develops suddenly and is not relieved by lying down. The leg is also red, hot and tender to the touch.

> **Anticoagulation (low molecular weight heparin) is started while unilateral leg oedema in pregnancy is being investigated.** It poses no harm to the fetus and potentially prevents fatal pulmonary embolism. Anticoagulation is stopped if the results of investigations for a DVT are negative.

Urinary symptoms

In pregnancy, as blood volume increases and the enlarging uterus presses on the bladder, women need to pass urine more frequently. Although urinary frequency is a normal feature of pregnancy, pain on passing urine is not; it is a symptom of infection. Infections of the lower and upper urinary tract are more common in pregnant women, because of the short length of the female urethra, immunosuppression, incomplete emptying of the bladder as a consequence of its compression by the uterus, and progesterone-induced relaxation of the ureters.

Pyelonephritis (kidney infection) can have potentially serious consequences: sepsis, preterm labour and, if untreated, kidney damage. Questions to ask are:

- 'Have you needed to go to the toilet to pass urine more frequently than usual?'
- 'Does it hurt to pass urine?'
- 'Have you had a temperature or been vomiting?'

Pyelonephritis presents with loin pain, fever and systemic symptoms of vomiting and loss of appetite. If a woman is vomiting, oral antibiotics will be ineffective so need to be given intravenously instead.

Itching

Mild itching is common in pregnancy, affecting almost a quarter of women, but it disappears after delivery. It is caused by hormonal changes, increased blood flow and stretching of the skin. The abdomen and breasts are preferentially affected. There is no rash, but evidence of excoriation from scratching is present. Itching can also be a symptom of underlying skin and systemic diseases (**Table 3.3**). Pathological itching is identified by asking:

- 'When did the itching start?'
- 'Have you noticed a rash?'
- 'Have you changed soaps, washing powder or shampoo?'
- 'Have you had a temperature or felt generally unwell?'
- 'Have you noticed a change in the colour of your urine or stools?'

The history, combined with inspection of the skin, is sufficient to make a diagnosis.

Itching in pregnancy: causes			
Cause	Time of onset	Features of rash	Characteristics
Underlying skin condition (e.g. eczema, psoriasis)	Before pregnancy	Eczema: dry, thickened skin Psoriasis: red, scaly plaques (**Figure 3.1**)	Symptoms improve in pregnancy because of immunosuppression
Pruritic urticated papules and plaques of pregnancy (**Figure 3.2**)	Third trimester	Plaques (raised areas > 1 cm in size) and papules (raised areas < 1 cm in size) Start in stretch marks then spread across the abdomen and on to the thighs	Resolves quickly after delivery
Prurigo of pregnancy	Any time in pregnancy	Papules all over the body	Systemically well
Pemphigoid gestationis (**Figure 3.3**)	Second and third trimester or after delivery	Blisters, which start around the umbilicus then spread over entire body	Risk of preterm labour and fetal growth restriction Recurs in future pregnancies
Allergic or contact dermatitis	Any time in pregnancy	Erythema papules, blisters at site of contact ('hives')	Occurs after change in soap, washing powder, shampoo, etc. Disappears when contact with causative agent stops
Parasitosis (e.g. scabies, head lice infestation)	Any time in pregnancy	Scabies: itching under armpits, between fingers, under buttocks or breast creases; tiny red spots and burrow marks Lice: itching of scalp; lice identified on inspection of hair	Close contacts also affected
Chickenpox	Any time in pregnancy	Red spots and blisters in dermatomal distribution	Fever, pneumonia, hepatitis and encephalitis more common in adults with chickenpox Contact with others with similar symptoms
Obstetric cholestasis	Third trimester	No rash but signs of excoriation	Fetal risks debatable (see Chapter 6) Pale stools and dark urine as a result of cholestasis

Table 3.3 Causes of itching in pregnancy

Rupture of membranes

Rupture of the amniotic sac is called rupture of membranes, also referred to as 'waters breaking'. It occurs either before or during labour and presents with fluid leaking vaginally. Women frequently attend assessment units with suspected rupture of membranes, which is easily confused with vaginal discharge and urine. The following questions are asked to confirm rupture of membranes.

- 'Have your waters broken?'
- 'Was there a sudden gush of fluid?'
- 'Have you needed to wear a pad since?'
- 'What colour is the fluid?'

Rupture of membranes results in a sudden gush of fluid followed by constant trickling, so that pads need to be changed every 2–4 hours. Amniotic fluid is clear or straw-coloured and has a sweet smell. Cloudy or offensive-smelling fluid suggests infection, green or brown fluid indicates meconium. Increased maternal and fetal monitoring and expediated delivery (either following induction of labour or caesarean section) is warranted in these circumstances. Coughing exacerbates leakage of both amniotic fluid and urine, but the latter is yellow and has a characteristic smell.

Reduced fetal movements

Each baby has its own pattern of movements. Reduced fetal movements is the term for the maternal perception of a decrease in the usual frequency of movements.

As pregnancy progresses, the magnitude of movements decreases because the fetus has less room to move in; the movements become more rolls than kicks, but their number stays the same. Ask 'Is your baby moving normally?'

Reduced fetal movements is a consequence of placental dysfunction and growth restriction,

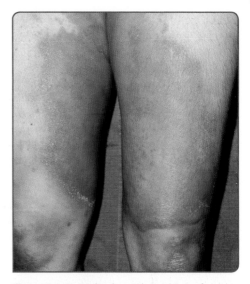

Figure 3.1 Generalised pustular psoriasis of pregnancy in 23-year-old woman. It cleared rapidly after parturition. Courtesy of Robert Chalmers.

and can warn of impending stillbirth. If a woman is concerned about her baby's movements, she is seen immediately and the fetal heart is listened to.

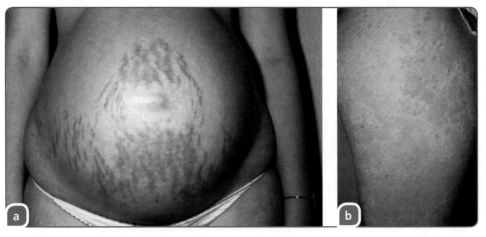

Figure 3.2 Pruritic urticated papules and plaques of pregnancy (a) on the abdomen, and (b) on the left leg. Courtesy of Robert Chalmers.

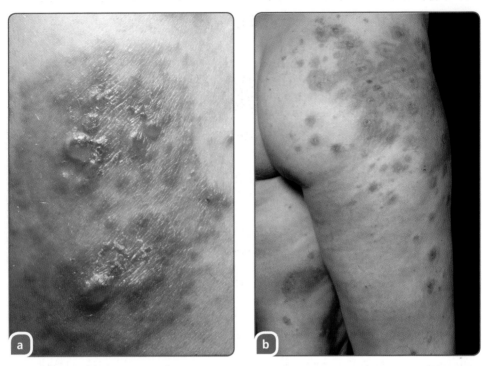

Figure 3.3 Pemphigoid gestationis showing characteristic (a) blistering and (b) target lesions. Courtesy of Robert Chalmers.

Common signs and how to examine a patient

Starter questions

Answers to the following questions are on page 146.

4. From when can a fetal heart be heard?
5. Are digital vaginal examinations performed during pregnancy?
6. How much blood does a pregnant woman need to lose before her heart rate increases and her blood pressure falls?

The examination is an opportunity to exclude differential diagnoses generated from the history and thereby identify the most likely underlying cause. A systematic approach is required to ensure that significant signs are not missed. It includes general and abdominal examinations, and assessment of fetal well-being, supplemented with vaginal examination, if appropriate.

Setting

Obstetric examination includes all the components detailed above but they are applied selectively depending on the clinical situation.

- In an acute situation on the labour ward, the immediate priority is maternal well-being: simultaneous resuscitation and examination are required to identify the cause of collapse; fetal assessment is delayed until the mother's condition has been stabilised
- In the antenatal clinic, vaginal examination is unnecessary if the woman has no symptoms of vaginal bleeding or discharge; abdominal examination to establish fetal well-being is more important in this situation

Maintain the patient's dignity at all times. Provide privacy when women undress, and use a sheet to cover areas not currently being examined. For patient reassurance, arrange to have a chaperone present for all vaginal examinations.

When examining any pregnant woman, position her as flat as she is able to lie but at a slight incline to avoid compression of the inferior vena cava, particularly in late pregnancy.

General examination

The general examination begins from the moment the clinician or patient walks into the room. It includes a rapid inspection and assessment of maternal well-being as well as more detailed review for systemic signs of disease.

Consent is obtained from the patient before the examination begins. It is explained that the consultation will include a general and an abdominal examination, as well as a vaginal examination, if necessary. The woman is asked if she needs to empty her bladder first, otherwise palpation can be uncomfortable.

Does the patient look acutely unwell?
Women attending antenatal clinic usually look well. Those who present to the labour ward with severe abdominal pain or bleeding will be pale and appear anxious. Blood running down the legs is a sign of a significant haemorrhage. A woman with sepsis is flushed.

Does she look pale or jaundiced?
Anaemia causes pallor, particularly conjunctival pallor. Jaundice, caused by obstetric

cholestasis or acute fatty liver of pregnancy, presents with yellow sclera.

Does she have any oedema?

Bilateral lower limb oedema is normal in pregnancy, especially after prolonged periods of standing. However, swelling of non-dependent areas (face and hands), or of one leg only, is pathological and needs investigation.

Is she over- or underweight?

Body mass index is recorded at the first antenatal visit; it is weight in kilograms divided by height in metres squared. Obesity increases the risk of miscarriage, fetal anomaly, pre-eclampsia, gestational diabetes and delivery complications. Eating disorders worsen during pregnancy as affected women struggle to cope with changes to their body. Malnutrition causes fetal growth restriction.

Is she able to get on to the couch easily?

Most pregnant women are fit and healthy. Symphysis pubis dysfunction is the result of excess movement between the two pubic bones as a consequence of progesterone-mediated softening of the pelvic ligaments. Pain limits leg abduction, making walking and getting on to couches difficult.

Does she have nicotine-stained fingers?

Smoking increases the risk of many pregnancy complications, including growth restriction, placental dysfunction and stillbirth.

What are her observations?

A full set of observations, including blood pressure, heart rate, respiratory rate and temperature, is required for a patient presenting acutely unwell. These measurements are used to guide resuscitation and response to treatment. In the antenatal clinic, blood pressure is checked at each visit to screen for pre-eclampsia.

> **Always record the respiratory rate.** Healthy women are able to compensate for significant blood loss or infection, maintaining a normal heart rate and blood pressure until they are moribund. Tachypnoea is the first sign of an unwell woman.

> **An appropriately sized cuff must be used to measure blood pressure.** If the cuff is too small, the blood pressure is overestimated. If the cuff is too large, blood pressure is underestimated.

Abdominal examination

An abdominal examination is performed to determine the site and cause of abdominal pain and to assess fetal well-being. For full assessment, the woman's abdomen is exposed from the ribcage to the pubis. Areas not currently being examined are covered to maintain her dignity.

Inspection

Inspection of the abdomen begins from the foot of the bed. More close inspection is done while standing on the patient's right-hand side.

Symmetry

The abdomen is assessed to determine if it is symmetrically distended, consistent with normal pregnancy. Asymmetry is a sign of fetal malposition, commonly transverse lie.

Surgical scars

The abdomen is examined closely for surgical scars. Particular scars to note are Pfannenstiel's or Joel Cohen incisions from previous caesarean sections (see page 92) and any midline laparotomy scars.

Cutaneous signs of pregnancy

Skin changes in normal pregnancy include stretch marks (striae gravidarum), spider naevi (**Figure 3.4**) and linea nigra. The latter is a dark line down the centre of the abdomen, and is caused by increased secretion of melanocyte-stimulating hormone.

Fetal movements

These are visible on inspection of the abdomen from 24 weeks' gestation. Identification of fetal movements is a sign of fetal well-being.

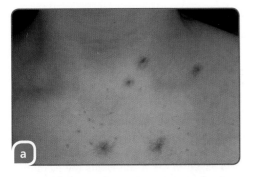
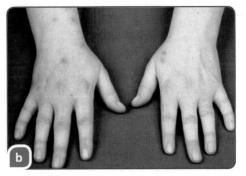

Figure 3.4 Eruptive spider telangiectasias arising during pregnancy (a) on the neck, and (b) on the hands. Courtesy of Robert Chalmers.

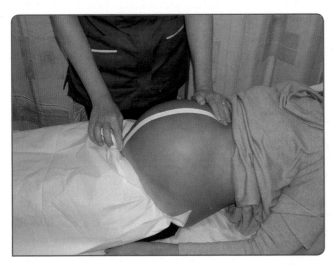

Figure 3.5 Measurement of symphysis–fundal height.

Palpation

The abdomen is palpated to determine the symphysis–fundal height, number of fetal poles, fetal lie and presentation, as well as to assess the amniotic fluid volume.

> **Before palpation begins, the woman is asked if she has any abdominal pain.** The painful area is assessed last.

Symphysis–fundal height

This is measured from 24 weeks' gestation as a screening test for abnormalities of fetal growth. In particular, it is used to identify small-for-gestational-age babies in women with low-risk pregnancies.

To determine symphysis–fundal height, a tape measure is used to measure from the fundus to the pubic symphysis. The result is recorded in centimetres, with the height equating to the number of weeks' gestation (plus or minus 2 cm).

1. Identify the top of the uterus (fundus) by palpating from the ribcage down the abdomen, using the inner aspect of the left hand (**Figure 3.5**); the uterus feels firm
2. Mark this spot with the tape measure, placing it face down to hide the numbers and thereby avoid bias
3. Locate the upper border of the symphysis pubis with the right hand, and mark this with the other end of the tape measure
4. Now turn the tape measure over and document the measurement

Causes of a deviation in symphysis–fundal height from that expected for the gestation are described in Chapter 6 (see page 195).

Fetal lie

This is the relation between the long axis of the fetus and the long axis of the mother. Fetal lie is normally longitudinal but can be transverse, i.e. across the abdomen, or oblique, i.e. diagonal. It is assessed from 36 weeks' gestation, because non-longitudinal lies are incompatible with vaginal delivery. External cephalic version or caesarean section is offered in these cases.

Fetal lie is assessed by placing the hands on either side of the woman's uterus (**Figure 3.6**).

The number of poles, i.e. heads and buttocks, that can be felt is checked. In a singleton pregnancy, two poles are palpable; in multiple pregnancies, there are four or more poles.

> When palpating the maternal abdomen, a fullness on one side indicates the location of the fetal back. Limbs are occasionally palpable on the other side. When presenting, include the side of the maternal abdomen on which the back was felt. It is a useful guide to the position of the fetal head, and influences how an external cephalic version is carried out.

Fetal presentation

The presentation of the fetus is the part closest to the pelvis:

- the head in a cephalic presentation
- the bottom in a breech presentation
- the shoulder in a transverse lie

This part of the examination is carried out with the clinician facing the woman's feet. She is warned that it may be uncomfortable, and asked to say if she wants the examination to stop. The palms of the hand are placed on either side of the lower abdomen, with fingers facing towards the pelvis, and the presenting part is moved between the hands (**Figure 3.7**). A head feels round and hard, whereas a bottom is softer and is not ballotable. In Pawlick's grip, the presenting part is grasped between the thumb and index finger of the right hand while facing the mother's head; it is more uncomfortable for the woman and is used only by trained professionals and should not be replicated in exam situations.

Assessment of engagement

If the fetus is presenting cephalically (head first) then engagement is determined. The head is engaged when the widest part has descended into the pelvis in preparation for labour. This occurs several weeks before contractions begin in a first pregnancy, but may

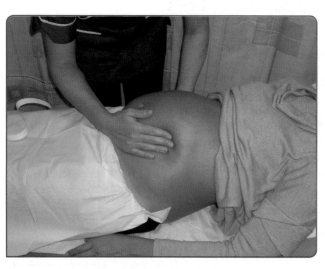

Figure 3.6 Assessment of fetal lie. The hands are placed on either side of the woman's uterus, facing towards her, in order to check for any discomfort. Gentle pressure is applied to the sides of the uterus, balloting (moving) the fetus between the hands. The fetal back feels firm and on the other side the limbs can be identified.

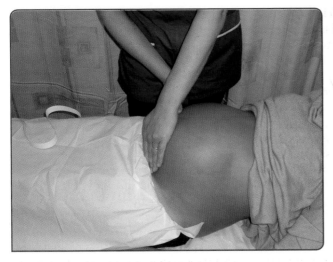

Figure 3.7 Assessment of fetal presentation.

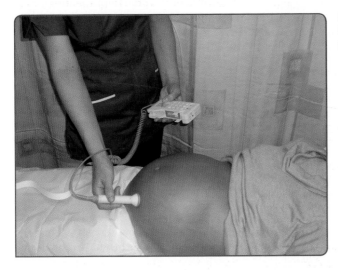

Figure 3.8 Auscultating the fetal heart using a handheld Doppler monitor (sonicaid).

happen only during labour in subsequent pregnancies.

Engagement is assessed by determining the proportion of the head that can be felt. It is expressed in fifths: the head is 5/5ths palpable if it can all be felt abdominally, and 0/5ths palpable if none of the head can be felt. The head is engaged when 2/5ths or fewer of the head are palpable.

Assessment of liquor volume

The amount of amniotic fluid is assessed during abdominal palpation.

- In oligohydramnios, the uterus is small and the parts of the fetus are easily felt

- In polyhydramnios, the uterus is tense and larger than expected, the skin of the abdomen is stretched and shiny, and the fetus is difficult to palpate

Auscultation

In this part of the examination, a stethoscope is used to listen to the fetal heart, thereby providing maternal reassurance. Auscultation is carried out by feeling for the fetal back and listening with a Pinard stethoscope or Doppler ultrasound over the anterior shoulder, halfway between the umbilicus and the superior iliac spine on the same side as the back (**Figure 3.8**).

Auscultation is done for 1 min. A normal fetal heart rate is 110–160 beats/min and is differentiated from the maternal pulse by feeling and counting her radial pulse at the same time.

Vaginal examination

Vaginal examination is carried out selectively in obstetrics in response to particular symptoms, such as vaginal bleeding or abdominal pain. Speculum examination, with a Cusco speculum, is done to assess bleeding and discharge. Cervical dilation and effacement (thinning) are determined by digital examination before or during labour.

External genitalia

The first part of a vaginal examination is inspection of the external genitalia (see page 94 and Figure 2.6). Evidence of blood, discharge or amniotic fluid secondary to ruptured membranes is looked for. Women who have experienced female genital mutilation are seen in special obstetric clinics to plan their antenatal and intrapartum care, including consideration of whether defibulation is necessary (see Chapter 15, page 372).

Vulval varicosities

These are dilated veins caused by increased blood flow during pregnancy, progesterone induced relaxation of vessel walls and compression of the inferior vena cava by the enlarging uterus (**Figure 3.9**). They are frequently asymptomatic but can cause itching or discomfort, particularly after prolonged standing. They do not affect mode of delivery and disappear post-partum.

Ulcers

Genital herpes causes multiple painful ulcers on the external genitalia. Primary infection requires treatment with the antiviral aciclovir. Delivery is by caesarean section if lesions are present in the 6 weeks prior to delivery, to reduce the risk of neonatal transmission.

Speculum examination

A Cusco speculum (see Figure 2.7) is used to assess the vagina and cervix in the antenatal and postnatal period. It is of limited use intrapartum, because a dilated cervix is not easily visualised and the procedure is more uncomfortable. Speculum examination is carried out in the same way as for gynaecological patients (see page 94).

In cases of bleeding, the volume of blood loss and obvious causes are assessed. Cervical polyps or cancers are visible on speculum examination.

Differentiation of normal from infective discharge is possible on visual inspection alone. Swab samples are taken for confirmation and to determine susceptibility to antimicrobial drugs. A cotton-tipped swab is rotated inside the cervix (endocervical), in the posterior vaginal fornix (high vaginal) or in the lower half of the vagina (low vaginal) and inserted into tubes containing charcoal or chlamydia-specific media. They are sent to the lab to be

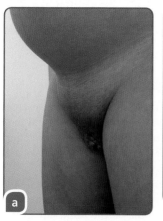 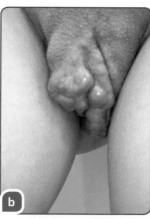

Figure 3.9 (a and b) Vulval varicosities in pregnancy. Prominent vulval varicose veins at 30 weeks.

processed under conditions compatible with bacterial and fungal growth. Growth of a large number of organisms indicates a positive result and no growth a negative result.

Amniotic fluid is a straw-coloured liquid pooling in the posterior fornix of the vagina and leaking through the cervix on coughing. The Actim Prom (see Chapter 7) test is used to detect insulin-like growth factor–binding protein-1, which is found only in amniotic fluid. It is taken by rotating the given swab in the vagina for 10–15 seconds before placing it in the test tube. It is used if the history strongly suggests membrane rupture but no amniotic fluid is visible at the time of speculum examination. After 5 minutes incubation, the presence of two lines (positive result) confirms rupture of membranes, one line (negative result) indicates the membranes are intact.

> The external cervical os never completely closes once a woman has had a vaginal delivery; it is always 1–2 cm dilated. This makes it difficult to distinguish whether or not a woman is in labour in subsequent pregnancies. A non-labouring cervix is long and thick; this is a multips os. Labour is diagnosed when the cervix starts to thin as well as dilate.

Cervical assessment

The cervix is assessed by inserting lubricated index and middle fingers of the right hand into the vagina until they reach the cervix. Cervical assessment is done before labour to assess the likelihood of successful induction of labour and to carry out a sweep (see Chapter 4, page 166), and during labour to determine progress. The following features are noted.

- Position of cervix: the cervix moves from a posterior to an anterior position as labour approaches
- cervical consistency, length and effacement: the cervix becomes softer, shorter and thinner as it effaces, until it becomes paper thin in labour
- dilation: this ranges from closed to 10 cm, i.e. fully dilated
- fetal station: the position of the fetal head or bottom relative to the ischial spines
- position of presenting part: the position of the presenting part is determined by locating the posterior fontanelle if it is a head, or the sacrum if it is a bottom
- presence or absence of membranes: intact membranes are felt as a tense balloon of fluid in front of the presenting part; once the membranes have ruptured, the fontanelles are easier to identify.

> Once the membranes have ruptured, digital cervical assessments are carried out only when necessary. The risk of infection increases with the number of examinations done, so extra care if needed to maintain a sterile technique.

> The placental site must be reviewed before a digital cervical assessment is performed. If the placenta is reaching up to or covering the internal os (placenta praevia) a vaginal examination is not performed as it causes significant bleeding.

Investigations

Starter questions

Answers to the following questions are on page 146.

7. Should X-rays be avoided in pregnancy?
8. Why is excess sugar in the urine frequently seen in pregnancy?

In obstetrics, investigations are carried out to screen for asymptomatic disease and to answer specific clinical questions, such as is a woman's shortness of breath caused by anaemia or is her urinary frequency due to a urinary tract infection. They are selected based on the differential diagnoses being considered and are used to rule out certain conditions and confirm others.

Blood tests

Blood tests are carried out in pregnancy for screening and to narrow down the list of differential diagnoses. They include:

- full blood count
- identification of blood group and antibody profile (group and save)
- acid elution test (Kleihauer test)
- renal and liver function tests
- coagulation tests
- measurement of inflammatory markers
- serological tests

Table 3.4 summarises the situations in which these tests are required, as well as the interpretation of test results.

Kleihauer's test is used to assess the amount of fetal blood in the maternal bloodstream. Maternal blood samples are exposed to acid, which causes fetal blood cells to stain pink and maternal blood cells to turn pale. The number of fetal blood cells is used to estimate the volume of a fetomaternal haemorrhage.

Urine tests

Urine is tested to screen for infection and pre-eclampsia. In the UK, cultures are done (see page 100) on samples from all women at their first antenatal visit to detect asymptomatic bacteriuria, which increases the risk of pyelonephritis and possibly preterm labour.

Dipstick urinalysis (see page 100) is carried out at each antenatal visit to screen for proteinuria. The greater renal blood flow in pregnancy causes proteinuria, which is exacerbated by increased glomerular basement membrane permeability. Levels greater than 300 mg/24 hours are, however, abnormal and can indicate infection, pre-eclampsia or underlying renal disease. Differentiation between these diagnoses is achieved by quantifying protein excretion using a protein: creatinine ratio (30 mg/mol is equivalent to 300 mg/24 hours), urine culture, blood pressure measurement and renal ultrasound and autoantibody screen. Persistent proteinuria in the first trimester or after delivery signifies renal disease.

Monitoring of fetal heart rate

Fetal heart rate is monitored to assess fetal well-being:

- a Pinard stethoscope or Doppler ultrasound monitor is used intermittently during labour in women with a low-risk pregnancy
- cardiotocography is used continuously in women with a high-risk pregnancy

Blood tests in pregnancy

Test	When required	Reason for test, interpretation of results and further action
Full blood count (FBC)	As a screening test at booking and 28 weeks' gestation Bleeding Suspected infection Pre-eclampsia	Hb < 110 g/L in 1st trimester and < 105 g/L in 3rd trimester: anaemia Normal MCV: acute blood loss Low MCV: chronic anaemia caused by iron deficiency Increased white cell count: infection Low platelets: HELLP syndrome or disseminated intravascular coagulopathy caused by consumption of platelets
Group and save (identification of blood group and antibody profile) (G+S)	As a screening test at booking and 28 weeks' gestation Heavy bleeding	Ensure group-compatible blood is transfused in heavy bleeding Identify risk of haemolytic disease of the newborn (HDN), caused by atypical alloantibodies detected during the group and save process; (see page 205): ■ Use of serial titre measurements, cerebral US and intrauterine transfusion depends on type and levels of antibody detected ■ Rhesus-negative women: give prophylactic anti-D at 28 weeks and after potentially sensitising effects, to prevent HDN
Acid elution test (Kleihauer test)	In rhesus-negative women: ■ After surgical management of miscarriage or ectopic pregnancy ■ Antepartum haemorrhage ■ Abdominal trauma ■ After delivery In all women after stillbirth	To measure volume of fetal blood that has come into contact with maternal blood; the result determines the dose of anti-D required to prevent sensitisation
Urea and electrolytes (U+E)	Systemic infection Hypovolaemia Pre-eclampsia	To assess renal function: ■ Sepsis and hypovolaemia cause hypoperfusion and AKI ■ Pre-eclampsia increases blood vessel permeability, causing redistribution of fluid into third spaces (unusual accumulation of fluid in tissues, e.g. in peritoneal cavity [ascites] or pleural space [pleural effusion]). Also causes under-perfusion of the kidneys
Liver function tests, (LFTs) including measurement of bile acids (BA)	Itching without a rash Pre-eclampsia Severe abdominal pain and vomiting	Increased BA with or without increased alanine transaminase: obstetric cholestasis Abnormal LFTs: hepatic oedema in pre-eclampsia or HELLP syndrome; gallstones, infective hepatitis or acute fatty liver of pregnancy ■ Alanine transaminase is significantly higher in acute fatty liver of pregnancy ■ Ultrasound and viral immunology distinguish between the other causes of abnormal LFT results
Coagulation tests: prothrombin time, activated partial thromboplastin time, international normalised ratio	Acute haemorrhage Abnormal LFT results	Prolonged PT and APTT and high INR: clotting factor deficiency ■ Diagnose disseminated intravascular coagulation ■ Assess bleeding risk in patients with liver damage (hepatocytes produce some clotting factors)
C-reactive protein (CRP)	Suspected infection	Increased CRP: inflammation or infection Result is non-specific but serial measurements are used to monitor response to treatment

Continued..

Blood tests in pregnancy *Continued...*		
Serological tests (HIV, hepatitis N, syphilis and rubella)	At first antenatal visit	Positive result: test repeated to ensure genuine result. Follow up: ■ HIV: implement antiretroviral treatment to reduce maternal–fetal transmission depending on stage of pregnancy and viral load ■ Chronic hepatitis B: plan neonatal vaccination and immunoglobulin after delivery ■ Syphilis: immediate antibiotic treatment; ultrasound screening for congenital infection ■ Rubella non-immune: postnatal maternal vaccination

HELLP, haemolysis, elevated liver enzymes and low platelets.

Table 3.4 Blood tests in pregnancy: when they are required and interpretation of results

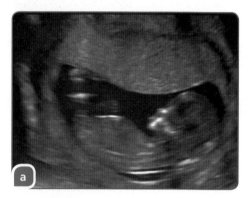 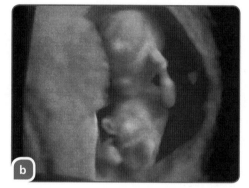

Figure 3.10 2D Ultrasound scan (a) and 4D scan (b) at 12 weeks' gestation. Courtesy of Katherine and Jacob Nadarajah.

Chapter 4 describes the techniques as well as normal and abnormal findings (see page 163).

Imaging

Ultrasound is the predominant imaging method used in obstetrics, because it is easily available and there is no exposure to radiation. It is supplemented with MRI or ventilation–perfusion (V/Q) scanning in cases of suspected placenta accreta and PE, respectively.

Ultrasound

The way in which ultrasound works is described in Chapter 2 (see Chapter 2, page 100). After the first trimester, it is done transabdominally because the fetus is too large to assess completely using a transvaginal probe.

Ultrasound is used to investigate maternal symptoms as well as to assess the fetus. It is done to:

■ investigate causes of abdominal pain
■ diagnose DVT
■ date pregnancies (**Figure 3.10**)
■ screen for fetal anomalies
■ assess fetal growth and well-being
■ locate placental site
■ determine fetal lie, presentation and position, if abdominal palpation is unhelpful

Hydronephrosis

Hydronephrosis refers to a dilated renal pelvis. It is more common in pregnancy, particularly on the right-hand side, because of ureteric compression by the enlarged uterus, which is naturally rotated to the right (dextrorotated). It increases the risk of urinary tract infection and kidney stones as a result of urinary stasis.

Appendicitis

Appendicitis is diagnosed by finding a dilated, oedematous appendix on ultrasound.

Doppler ultrasound

In cases of suspected venous thromboembolism, Doppler ultrasound of the lower limbs is carried out. Soundwaves are emitted from the probe and, because of the Doppler effect, reflected back at a different pitch when they come into contact with moving blood cells. In cases of DVT, blood flow is static because of the presence of a clot within the vessel, so no change in pitch is detected.

Doppler ultrasound is also the first-line investigation for suspected pulmonary embolus. Most cases arise from DVTs and are similarly managed with anticoagulation. Detection of a DVT in one or both limbs avoids the need for further radiological procedures and the associated exposure to radiation. If the result is negative, a ventilation–perfusion (V/Q) scan is the next investigation of choice.

V/Q scan

A V/Q scan is a nuclear medicine investigation in which gamma cameras are used to detect emitted radiation from radioisotopes inserted into the body. It is composed of two phases.

- In the ventilation (V) phase, the gaseous radionucleotide technetium-99m is inhaled and images are recorded to study airflow in the lungs

- In the perfusion (Q) phase, technetium-99m macroaggregated albumin is injected into the veins and images recorded to study blood flow to the lungs

Pulmonary embolism is diagnosed if there is a mismatch between the areas of the lungs being ventilated and those being perfused.

A V/Q scan exposes the maternal breasts to a lower dose of radiation than a CT pulmonary angiogram, but it is associated with a higher fetal radiation dose (see Figure 7.7). The ventilation phase is frequently omitted to reduce radiation exposure, with ventilation assumed to be normal. A V/Q scan is not helpful if any abnormalities have been identified on chest radiograph, because they prevent accurate interpretation of the results.

Magnetic resonance imaging

The physics underlying MRI are described in Chapter 2 (see page 104). It is used in obstetrics to characterise fetal anomalies, particularly those of the head, neck and spine, in greater detail than can be achieved with ultrasound.

MRI is also used in women with a low-lying anterior placenta who have had a previous caesarean section when it is not possible to conclusively diagnose placenta accreta by ultrasound. It aids subsequent management of delivery by enabling accurate identification of the depth of invasion and bladder involvement.

Management options

Starter questions

Answers to the following questions are on page 146.

9. Why is it important to keep the caesarean section rate low?
10. When maternal and fetal interests conflict, which patient takes precedence?

In obstetrics, the aim of management is to ensure a healthy mother and a healthy baby. To achieve this:

- maternal medical conditions are optimised before pregnancy
- teratogenic medications are replaced with safer alternatives
- delivery is timed to optimise maternal and fetal well-being
- prompt intervention is used to prevent complications in cases of asymptomatic disease detected by screening
- in utero treatment of fetal disease is carried out in selected cases, and preparations made for postnatal management

Therapeutic interventions include:

- non-pharmacological interventions
- pharmacological treatment
- in utero procedures
- delivery

The best interests of the mother and fetus are occasionally in conflict. For example, drugs required to treat maternal medical conditions may have adverse effects on the developing fetus, and early delivery required in cases of pre-eclampsia puts the fetus at risk of prematurity. The pros and cons of intervention from the perspective of both mother and baby are discussed to try to reach a compromise. However, many women are willing to put their own health at risk to give their baby the best possible start in life.

Non-pharmacological interventions

Non-pharmacological interventions increase the chance of a successful pregnancy outcome. They are used to treat urinary incontinence, symphysis pubis dysfunction and to improve general health, with the aim of minimising the risk of pregnancy complications. They are used alongside pharmacological treatments, which are frequently more effective, but avoid potentially harmful side effects for the mother and fetus. For non-pharmacological interventions to be effective, patient compliance is necessary, which is often difficult to achieve.

Weight reduction

Obesity is associated with multiple pregnancy complications affecting both mother and baby (see page 200). Active weight loss is not advisable in pregnancy, because it results in fetal growth restriction, but weight gain should be avoided. Advice on healthy eating and encouragement of light exercise is provided (see Chapter 2, page 109). Women who are overweight or obese are advised to reduce their weight to achieve a body mass index within the normal range before pregnancy.

Smoking cessation

Exposure to cigarette smoke during pregnancy increases the risk of fetal growth restriction and placental abruption, as well as causing maternal respiratory disease. Smoking cessation is discussed at each antenatal visit, and women who want to stop smoking are referred to support services (see Chapter 2, page 109). Nicotine replacement is safe in pregnancy. There is insufficient information on the effects of the use of electronic cigarettes during pregnancy to allow them to be suggested as alternatives.

Physiotherapy

Pressure from the weight of the gravid uterus on the maternal pelvis and pelvic floor can cause prolapse, stress incontinence, lower back pain and symphysis pubis dysfunction. Pelvic floor exercises (see page 109) and musculoskeletal physiotherapy relieve symptoms by improving muscle tone and by educating women about movements that will exacerbate the pain. Exercising in water is particularly beneficial as the water provides buoyancy, reducing weight and burden on the spine and limbs.

Musculoskeletal physiotherapy focuses specifically on the assessment and treatment of lower back and pelvic girdle pain, whereas pelvic floor exercises are taught to manage prolapse and urinary tract symptoms.

Pharmacological treatment

Unlike in other specialities, drugs are actively avoided in obstetrics. Clinical trials to determine drug safety and effectiveness exclude pregnant and breastfeeding women therefore guidelines on the use of drugs during pregnancy are based on anecdotal evidence. Therefore it is difficult to be precise about levels of risk when discussing pharmacological treatment with patients. However, many drugs have been used in pregnant women over many years without adverse effect.

The main drugs used in obstetrics are heparin, corticosteroids, prostaglandins and uterotonics. The use of antihypertensives and tocolytics (uterine relaxants, commonly used to stop preterm labour) are discussed in Chapter 6 (see page 192) and Chapter 7 (see page 222), respectively.

Low-molecular-weight heparin

Heparin inactivates thrombin and other proteases responsible for blood clotting by activating the enzyme inhibitor antithrombin III. It is used to both prevent and treat established blood clots by inhibiting further thrombus formation. The body is able to break down existing clots by using its own natural lysis system.

Low-molecular-weight heparin is a separated component of unfractionated heparin. It is more pharmacodynamically stable than its parent compound, so is administered once or twice daily without the need for monitoring. The dose is adjusted according to body weight.

The main adverse effects are:

- increased risk of bleeding
- osteoporosis, because of the associated decrease in bone formation
- thrombocytopenia, because of the generation of antiplatelet antibodies

Fewer adverse events are experienced with short-term use of low-molecular-weight heparin than with longer term use of unfractionated heparin.

Corticosteroids

Corticosteroids stimulate the expression of genes encoding an enzyme needed to mature the fetal lungs in preparation for breathing, in particular, they increase production of surfactant by type 2 pneumocytes. These cells line the alveolar sacs in the lungs and are the site of storage of surfactant, a rich lipid and protein mixture, which spreads across the lung tissue-air interface. By doing so, it prevents the alveoli from collapsing during expiration and allows them to open easily with the next inspiration. Type 2 pneumocytes only begin to differentiate between 24 and 34 weeks' gestation, meaing babies born preterm are at risk of respiratory distress syndrome. Corticosteroid administration reduces this risk and increases survival rates. These drugs also help prevent necrotising enterocolitis, intraventricular haemorrhage and sepsis, although the mechanisms underlying these effects are unclear.

They are administered antenatally to mothers whose babies are:

- at risk of preterm birth before 35 weeks' gestation, or 36 weeks in cases of growth restriction
- to be delivered by elective caesarean section before 39 weeks

The latter group are at higher risk of transient tachypnoea of the newborn. This is because fluid is not expelled from their lungs to the same extent as from the lungs of babies born by vaginal delivery.

Betamethasone is preferred over dexamethasone, because it is more effective. It is given as two intramuscular injections 24 h apart. The clinical benefit is evident 24 h after the second dose. Corticosteroids negatively affect glucose control in diabetic patients, so additional insulin on a sliding scale is sometimes required to cover administration. Repeated courses impair brain development in sheep and are not recommended.

Prostaglandins

Two prostaglandin analogues commonly used in obstetrics are misoprostol (prostaglandin E$_1$) and dinoprostone (prostaglandin E$_2$). They soften the cervix and stimulate uterine contractions.

Dinoprostone is licensed for induction of labour, but it is expensive and needs to be stored in the cold. It is available as tablets, gel or pessaries. Misoprostol has not been licensed for this indication, because of concerns about the risk of uterine rupture caused by hyperstimulation.

In the UK, misoprostol is used off-label after stillbirth, because it is more effective than dinoprostone at inducing labour. It is also used to treat post-partum haemorrhage caused by poor uterine tone. In low- and medium-income countries without cold storage facilities, misoprostol is used as the primary method of inducing labour in all pregnancies. The uterus becomes increasingly sensitive to prostaglandins with gestation, so lower doses are needed to induce labour as pregnancy progresses.

Common adverse effects of prostaglandins include bronchospasm and diarrhoea secondary to relaxation of smooth muscle in the gastrointestinal tract. They are used with caution in patients who have had a previous caesarean section, because of the risk of scar rupture.

Uterotonics

Uterotonics are a group of drugs that cause uterine contraction. They include oxytocin, ergometrine, misoprostol and carboprost.

Synthetic oxytocin

Syntocinon is a synthetic version of the natural hormone oxytocin. It activates oxytocin receptors to stimulate rhythmic uterine contractions. It is given as an intravenous infusion to initiate or augment contractions; the dose is titrated according to response. It is also used to both prevent and treat post-partum haemorrhage; it is administered as:

- a single 5- to 10-IU intramuscular bolus for prevention
- a 40-IU infusion for treatment. Syntocinon has a short duration of action as it is promptly broken down by the enzyme oxytocinase, produced by the syncitiotrophoblast. When persistent uterine contraction is required, it is delivered by infusion rather than a bolus to ensure continuous oxytocin receptor activation.

All uterotonics can cause hyperstimulation of the uterus and fetal distress if used intrapartum. Oxytocin has an antidiuretic effect because of its molecular similarity to antidiuretic hormone; excessive use leads to water intoxication, hyponatraemia and seizures. Therefore it is used with caution in women with pre-eclampsia. Cardiac arrhythmias can be precipitated by oxytocin use.

Ergometrine

Ergometrine is an ergot alkaloid that is chemically similar to LSD (lysergic acid diethylamide). It acts on unknown receptors in the uterus to stimulate tonic contractions. It is given either intramuscularly or intravenously to prevent or treat post-partum haemorrhage.

Its activation of α-adrenergic, dopaminergic and serotonergic receptors commonly causes vomiting and increased blood pressure after administration. Therefore it is relatively contraindicated in women with hypertension.

Carboprost

Carboprost (trade name, Hemabate) is a synthetic analogue of prostaglandin F2α. It causes uterine contraction via activation of prostaglandin receptors, and it also has oxytocin-like properties. It is administered either intramuscularly or directly into the myometrium as a bolus every 15 min to treat post-partum haemorrhage if other drugs have failed to reduce the bleeding.

It has similar adverse effects to those of other prostaglandin analogues but causes more severe bronchospasm than misoprostol. Therefore it is used cautiously in women with asthma.

In utero procedures

Fetal surgery is required in a small number of highly selected cases to prolong life in utero until the fetus is sufficiently mature to survive being born. Procedures are carried out in specialist fetal medicine units and include:

- laser surgery on connecting vessels in twin-to-twin transfusion syndrome
- insertion of pleural–amniotic shunts to treat pleural effusions
- repair of some neural tube defects
- vesicoamniotic shunting for urinary tract obstruction
- in utero transfusion to treat anaemia, commonly caused by haemolytic disease of the newborn

In utero procedures are not without risk. They can trigger preterm labour and cause fetal death.

Delivery

The ultimate management of many conditions in obstetrics is delivery of the fetus. This has the benefit of:

- relieving maternal physiology of the demands of the fetus
- allowing the administration of medication contraindicated in pregnancy
- allowing surgical procedures to be carried out without concerns about the effects on the fetus
- allowing postnatal treatment of neonatal conditions

The timing of delivery is a complicated balance between prematurity and the risks of continuing with the pregnancy. Induction of labour is possible in many cases after 34 weeks' gestation, depending on the urgency and indication for delivery. If delivery needs to occur at an earlier gestation, induction is unlikely to be successful because of the lower numbers of oxytocin receptors, so a caesarean section is carried out.

Answers to starter questions

1. Braxton Hicks contractions are tightenings of the uterine muscle and are a sign of the body preparing itself for the delivery of a baby. They are felt from the second to third trimester of pregnancy and are infrequent and irregular, lasting 1–2 minutes. Not all mothers feel Braxton Hicks contractions and they vary in severity from mild, crampy discomfort to causing significant pain, when they need to be distinguished from the symptoms of labour. Braxton Hicks do not cause any change to the cervix and they settle spontaneously.

2. If a pregnancy is planned this allows the mother to take folic acid prior to, and following, conception to prevent neural tube defects. Women with unplanned pregnancies are vulnerable because of financial and social problems, lack supportive relationships and are at increased risk of postnatal depression. They may also fail to attend routine antenatal appointments and feel ambivalent or even negatively about their unborn baby. Extra support is provided to help these women through pregnancy.

3. There is no set number of fetal movements that a woman should feel during the third trimester of pregnancy. Every baby is different and will develop its own waking and

Answers *continued*

sleep pattern. Women are advised to report any deviation from their normal pattern so that fetal CTG monitoring can be performed.

4. The fetal heart can be heard with a Pinnard or sonicaid through the abdominal wall from 12 weeks' gestation, when the uterus has risen out of the pelvis. It can be heard from 5 weeks on ultrasound scan using a Doppler, but this is not performed routinely because of the teratogenic risk due to excess heat generation.

5. Digital vaginal examinations are contraindicated when a woman has a placenta praevia because it can provoke significant bleeding. It is also contraindicated following the rupture of the membranes, particularly if this occurs prematurely, due to the risk of infection. However, if labour is suspected then cervical assessment is warranted.

6. Young, healthy women are able to compensate for a significant loss of blood before developing signs of shock. Between 15–30% of blood volume (approximately 1.8 L) needs to be lost before they become tachycardiac. Systolic blood pressure decreases when 40% (approximately 2.4 L) of blood is lost; the woman will lose consciousness once the loss exceeds this.

7. All imaging investigations involving radiation are avoided in pregnancy, due to the risks of teratogenicity and childhood cancers. There are circumstances, however, where the benefits of performing a chest X-ray outweigh the risks, such as investigating a suspected pulmonary embolus or pneumonia. Fetal radiation exposure is very low after a single chest X-ray and the abdomen is shielded to reduce the exposure further.

8. During pregnancy, the increased blood flow to the kidneys overwhelms the ability of the proximal renal tubules to reabsorb glucose resulting in its increased excretion. Glycosuria (excess glucose in the urine) can be a normal sign of pregnancy, but is also seen in gestational diabetes. Persistent glycosuria therefore warrants an oral glucose tolerance test.

9. Caesarean sections carry risks, including bleeding, infection and damage to the bowel, bladder and ureters. It is also associated with adverse outcomes in future pregnancies, such as scar rupture during labour and placenta accreta, and the incidence of these rises with the number of procedures performed. The most common indication for an elective caesarean section is a previous caesarean section, therefore reducing the number of first-time operations and encouraging vaginal delivery reduces health care costs and complications in the long term.

10. The mother always takes precedence over the fetus when conflicts in interest arise. A fetus would not be able to survive in utero if the mother were to die and does not have any legal rights until it is born in the UK. If the mother has a cardiac arrest, a caesarean section is performed within 4 minutes of an unsuccessful resuscitation. This is not done for any fetal benefit, but to remove the physiological burden of the fetus and to improve the effectiveness of maternal resuscitation and, hence, her chance of survival.

Chapter 4
Normal delivery and antenatal and postnatal care

Starter questions

Answers to the following questions are on page 169.

1. Where is the safest place for a woman to deliver her baby?
2. What triggers labour?
3. Do epidurals slow down labour?

Introduction

Pregnancy is an exciting time for a woman and the people who are close to her. Complications can arise, but for most women this is a normal physiological event resulting in the birth of a healthy baby.

In many countries, care during pregnancy and childbirth is routinely provided by midwives, with support from obstetricians in high-risk cases. Many pregnant women will not require a physician. However, it is essential for all physicians to have an understanding of normal pregnancy and delivery, so that they are able to reassure patients, when appropriate, and recognise any deviation from normality.

Case 1 Booking visit

Presentation

Sally Brookes, aged 25 years, attends her local general practitioner (GP) surgery for her booking appointment (first antenatal visit) with her midwife. This is her first pregnancy.

Initial interpretation

Women are able to book an appointment directly with a midwife or their GP as soon as they know they are pregnant. This enables referral to appropriate obstetric services to be arranged as soon as possible for high-risk cases.

At the booking visit, the midwife takes a detailed medical, surgical, drug, obstetric, family and social history to determine the likelihood of the woman or her baby experiencing difficulties during pregnancy or after the birth. If the pregnancy is deemed low risk, antenatal care is provided solely by the midwife or a team of midwives in the community. Women whose pregnancy is high risk are cared for by a named obstetrician at the hospital as well as by their community midwife.

Further history

Sally is fit and well and has no medical history of note such as hypertension, diabetes or epilepsy. She has been taking folic acid for the past 3 months, but no other medication. She is a non-smoker and stopped drinking alcohol when she started trying for a baby. Her husband, Tom, appears supportive and has accompanied her to the appointment. The first day of Sally's last period was 8 weeks ago.

Examination

Sally's body mass index is 24 kg/m^2, and her blood pressure is 110/70 mmHg. She is well-kept and interacts appropriately with her partner and the midwife. No abdominal or pelvic examination is carried out.

Interpretation of findings

Sally is a primigravida with a planned pregnancy of 8 weeks' gestation by dates. She is neither a teenager nor over 40, putting her in a low-risk age category for pregnancy. By taking folic acid since before conception, she has reduced the risk of the baby developing a neural tube defect. She has no medical comorbidities that could have an adverse effect on the pregnancy, and her body mass index and blood pressure are normal. She appears to have good social support. However, her midwife will try to speak to Sally on her own to enquire about any previous pregnancies that Sally may not have disclosed to her husband and to ask whether she is experiencing domestic abuse.

Abdominal and pelvic examinations are not routine at the booking visit. Assessment of gestational age by uterine palpation is inaccurate at this stage of pregnancy and has been superseded by ultrasound scanning.

Investigations

A urine test confirms that Sally is pregnant. No abnormalities are detected on dipstick urinalysis. A sample of urine is sent for microscopy and culture, as is routine; the results are negative. Blood is taken for a full blood count, blood grouping and antibody screening, and haemoglobinopathy screening, as well as tests for HIV, hepatitis B, syphilis and rubella immunity. An ultrasound scan is arranged for 4 weeks later.

Diagnosis

The ultrasound scan shows a singleton pregnancy of 12 weeks' gestation. Sally continues to attend antenatal visits with her midwife at her GP surgery for the rest of her pregnancy.

Case 2 Prolonged pregnancy

Presentation

Charlotte Davidson, who is 34 years old, attends a routine antenatal clinic appointment with her midwife. She is 41 weeks pregnant.

Initial interpretation

The duration of Charlotte's pregnancy is approaching 42 weeks, at which it would be defined as a prolonged (post-term) pregnancy. Such pregnancies carry an increased risk of fetal and maternal complications, although the absolute risk remains low.

Placental function decreases in a prolonged pregnancy, which compromises the supply of oxygen and nutrients to the fetus. This puts it at risk of growth restriction and stillbirth. Conversely, there is an increased chance of macrosomia (birth weight > 4.5 kg), with the attendant risks of injury during birth to both baby and mother, as well as neonatal hypoglycaemia. Meconium aspiration is also more likely; the mature fetus passes meconium (its first faeces) in utero, and this may be swallowed if it is stressed.

For the mother, a prolonged pregnancy is associated with an increased risk of difficult labour, perineal trauma and emergency caesarean section.

Further history

Charlotte has had one previous vaginal delivery. It was 3 years ago and proceeded uneventfully. No problems have been identified during her current pregnancy to date.

Examination

Abdominal palpation is carried out. The symphysis-fundal height is 40 cm.

The three stages of labour

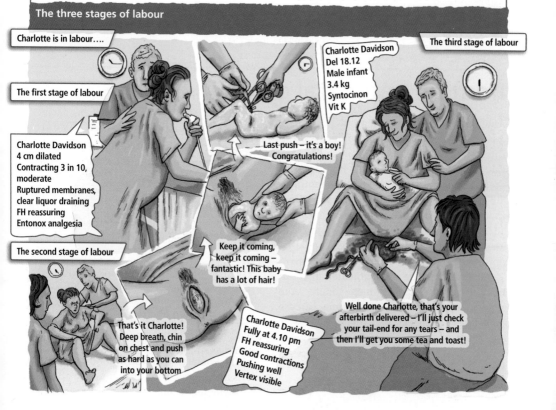

Charlotte is in labour….

The first stage of labour

Charlotte Davidson
4 cm dilated
Contracting 3 in 10, moderate
Ruptured membranes, clear liquor draining
FH reassuring
Entonox analgesia

The second stage of labour

That's it Charlotte! Deep breath, chin on chest and push as hard as you can into your bottom

Charlotte Davidson
Fully at 4.10 pm
FH reassuring
Good contractions
Pushing well
Vertex visible

Keep it coming, keep it coming – fantastic! This baby has a lot of hair!

Last push – it's a boy! Congratulations!

Charlotte Davidson
Del 18.12
Male infant
3.4 kg
Syntocinon
Vit K

The third stage of labour

Well done Charlotte, that's your afterbirth delivered – I'll just check your tail-end for any tears – and then I'll get you some tea and toast!

Case 2 *continued*

Charlotte has a singleton fetus of cephalic presentation, in the right occipitolateral position. Two fifths of the fetal head are palpable. A fetal heart rate of 120 beats/min is measured by auscultation.

The cervix is assessed. It is soft, central, 1 cm long and 1 cm dilated, with 50% effacement (thinning) and the fetal head at the −2 station. The midwife carries out a membrane sweep (see page 160).

Interpretation of findings

The examination has shown a fetus with normal growth and an engaged head. The cervix is favourable, meaning that induction of labour is likely to succeed. A Bishop score is used to assess the readiness of the cervix for induction. It is calculated by adding up individual scores for the position, consistency, effacement and dilation of the cervix and the fetal station. A score of 6 (as with Charlotte) or more indicates the cervix is favourable, 9 or more that labour is likely to start spontaneously.

Before the use of any formal induction technique, however, a membrane sweep is recommended. The procedure is offered at 40- and 41-week antenatal visits. Its purpose is to try to initiate labour by encouraging the body to release prostaglandins, which soften the cervix and stimulate contractions.

Investigations

Charlotte's blood pressure is 128/65 mmHg. Dipstick urinalysis shows no abnormalities.

Diagnosis

To reduce the risks associated with prolonged pregnancy, Charlotte is offered induction of labour between 41 and 42 weeks of gestation. The option of expectant management is also discussed with her.

She attends her local maternity unit at 42 weeks. A prostaglandin pessary is inserted to ripen (soften and dilate) the cervix. Labour and a normal vaginal delivery follow.

Routine antenatal care

Antenatal care is the care pregnant women receive before delivery. It encompasses routine care for all pregnant women, as well as the identification of those with high-risk pregnancies and their referral to appropriate specialist services. In the UK, a nulliparous woman with a low-risk pregnancy has 10 antenatal visits, and a parous woman with an uncomplicated pregnancy has 7. **Table 4.1** outlines the specific purpose of each visit.

All antenatal care is documented in hand-held notes. Pregnant women should keep these notes with them at all times in case emergency care is required.

> **'Booking visit'** is the term used in many countries for the first antenatal visit (e.g. Australia, UK).

Screening in pregnancy

Screening tests are carried out in pregnancy to identify asymptomatic women and their babies who would benefit from additional support or medical intervention. Screening also provides information on which to base difficult decisions about whether or not to continue a pregnancy.

> **Not all expectant parents will accept the offer of antenatal screening.** The advice provided by health care professionals should be non-directive.

A range of tests, including blood tests, urine tests and imaging, may be offered to all pregnant women or only those at increased risk

Routine antenatal care			
Visit	Information to provide or topic to discuss	Maternal assessment	Fetal assessment
First contact with health care professional	Folic acid supplementation, foods to avoid, smoking cessation, alcohol and drug avoidance, screening tests		
First antenatal visit, i.e. 'Booking' visit (ideally by 10 weeks)	Fetal development, diet and exercise, pathway of care, antenatal classes, entitlement to financial support and maternity leave	Take medical, surgical, drug, obstetric, family and social history to identify additional care needs Discuss mental health Measure BP Blood tests: blood group; rhesus status; haemoglobinopathy and infection screening Urine tests: proteinuria, asymptomatic bacteriuria	US to assess gestational age Down's syndrome screening US screening for structural anomalies
16 weeks	Discuss screening test results; plan pathway of care	BP, test urine for proteinuria Investigate Hb < 11 g/100 mL and consider iron supplementation	
18–20 weeks	Fetal movements: when felt, frequency, what to do if reduced/absent		Anomaly US scan
25 weeks (nulliparous women only)	Any issues that have arisen	BP, test urine for proteinuria	Measure symphysis–fundal height
28 weeks	Any issues that have arisen	Check Hb and blood group for atypical antibodies; provide anti-D if Rh-negative Investigate Hb < 10.5 g/100 mL and consider iron supplementation BP, test urine for proteinuria	Measure symphysis–fundal height
31 weeks (nulliparous women only)	Any issues that have arisen, and results of 28-week tests	BP, test urine for proteinuria	Measure symphysis–fundal height
34 weeks	Preparation for labour and birth	Offer second dose of anti-D if Rh-negative BP, test urine for proteinuria	Measure symphysis–fundal height
36 weeks	Breastfeeding, care newborn, discuss administration of vitamin K to baby at birth to reduce the risk of HDN, postnatal care and awareness of 'baby blues'	BP, test urine for proteinuria	Measure symphysis–fundal height Check baby's position; for breech presentation, offer external cephalic version
38 weeks	Recognising labour, packing a hospital bag, what to get for new baby, breastfeeding, Braxton Hicks contractions, options in prolonged pregnancy	BP, test urine for proteinuria	Measure symphysis fundal height
40 weeks (nulliparous women only)	Prolonged pregnancy	BP, test urine for proteuria	Measure symphysis fundal height
41 weeks	Offer membrane sweep and induction of labour	BP, test urine for proteinuria	Measure symphysis fundal height

BP, blood pressure; Hb, haemoglobin; HDN, haemolytic disease of the newborn; Rh, rhesus; US, ultrasound.

Table 4.1 Routine antenatal care

of a condition such as gestational diabetes. None of these tests are compulsory, so women can choose to decline them.

> It can be difficult to explain to patients the results of screening tests because these indicate only the likelihood of having a condition. For example, if a woman's Down's syndrome screening gives a risk of 1:100, she needs to be made aware this means that among 100 pregnant women with the same result 99 will have babies with a normal karyotype and one will have a baby with Down's syndrome. If the result is 1 in < 150, chorionic villus sampling or amniocentesis is offered to confirm whether or not the baby has Down's syndrome.

Screening for haematological conditions

Screening is done to identify anaemia, pregnancies at risk of haemolytic disease of the newborn, and asymptomatic haemoglobinopathies.

Anaemia

Haemoglobin concentration is checked at booking and 28 weeks to identify anaemia; a concentration of < 10.5 g/100 mL is diagnostic. If anaemia is present, investigations such as measurement of iron, vitamin B12 and folate levels, are carried out to determine the cause of the anaemia. The most common cause is iron deficiency, which is treated with oral or, if not tolerated, intravenous supplementation.

Anaemia causes tiredness and compromises the body's ability to cope with blood loss at delivery. Repeat testing is done to allow adequate time for treatment.

Blood group and alloantibodies

At the booking visit, a blood group, rhesus status and atypical alloantibody screen is carried out to identify rhesus-negative women. Detection of specific, significant atypical antibodies prompts referral to a specialist fetal medicine clinic for further investigation and monitoring. Specific atypical antibodies are associated with haemolytic disease of the newborn (see Chapter 6).

These screening tests are repeated at 28 weeks to ensure that atypical antibodies have not developed during the pregnancy.

Haemoglobinopathies

Whether haemoglobinopathy screening is offered varies from country to country, depending on the prevalence of the haemoglobinopathies. In countries like the UK the approach to screening also varies regionally, relative to local prevalence of sickle cell disease and thalassaemia. Where the prevalence is high, for example in cities where people of black and minority ethnic groups are likely to live, all women are screened at booking. If the prevalence is lower, screening is offered only to women whose pregnancies are identified through the family origin questionnaire as being at high risk. This includes the situation where the woman or the baby's father is of African, Afro-Caribbean, South and South-East Asian, Middle-Eastern or Southern European origin.

Screening for infections

Blood samples, urine samples, and in some countries vaginal samples are used to screen for infections. Infection screening enables treatment to be provided antenatally to reduce the risk of transmission to the fetus, and the results also guide postnatal management (**Table 4.2**).

Screening for fetal anomalies

This includes screening for structural abnormalities as well as Down's and other syndromes.

> For most expectant parents, the results of antenatal screening tests are reassuring; for others (about 5%), they may cause significant anxiety. These parents may face difficult decisions about whether or not to have invasive diagnostic tests, and in the case of a definitive result, whether or not to continue the pregnancy. In the UK, the charity Antenatal Results and Choices offer non-directive counselling to parents in this situation.

Screening for infections			
Infection	Type of test	When carried out	Reason for testing
Asymptomatic bacteriuria	Urine	First antenatal visit (at about 10 weeks)	Treating infection reduces risk of pyelonephritis and possibly premature labour
HIV	Blood	First antenatal visit; offered again at 28 weeks if initially declined	Enables antenatal and intrapartum intervention to reduce transmission of infection
Hepatitis B	Blood	First antenatal visit	If positive, neonatal vaccination and immunoglobulin are given to reduce risk of chronic hepatitis in the baby
Syphilis	Blood	First antenatal visit	Enables antibiotic treatment to be given to the mother to reduce transmission and its associated adverse outcomes (e.g. rash, saddle nose without a bridge, failure to thrive, abnormal teeth, skin scarring)
Rubella	Blood	First antenatal visit	Enables postnatal vaccination of non-immune women to reduce risk of infection during future pregnancies
Group B Streptococcus	Vaginal swab or urine	35–37 weeks' gestation in France, Spain, Belgium, Canada and Australia (not routine in UK, the Netherlands and New Zealand because screening is not cost or clinically effective in these countries. Intrapartum antibiotics are given if Group B Streptococcus infection is detected during screening for other infections)	Prophylactic benzylpenicillin is given to women in labour who have had a positive result any time in their pregnancy; this reduces the risk of neonatal group B streptococcal disease

Table 4.2 Screening for infections in pregnancy

Down's and other syndromes' screening

Down's syndrome (trisomy 21) is caused by the presence of an extra chromosome 21 in each cell. Screening for the condition is offered antenatally to all pregnant women as a 'combined test': a blood test to measure pregnancy-associated plasma protein-A and β-human chorionic gonadotrophin, and an ultrasound scan to measure the thickness of the fetal nuchal translucency. The test is done between the 11th and the end of the 13th week of weeks' gestation.

The nuchal translucency is the appearance on ultrasound of a collection of fluid beneath the skin at the back of the fetal neck (**Figure 4.1**). This fluid-filled sac is formed by a collection of immature lymphatic channels that dilate in response to high placental resistance. The nuchal translucency tends to be thicker in pregnancies affected by chromosomal abnormality, possibly as a result of the presence of congenital malformations.

> The thickness of the nuchal translucency can also be increased by changes in the composition of the extracellular matrix. Many extracellular matrix proteins are encoded on chromosome 21, which is why Down's syndrome is associated with increased nuchal translucency thickness.

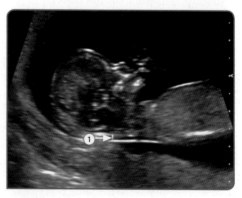

Figure 4.1 An ultrasound scan at 12 weeks' gestation showing normal nuchal thickness. ① Calipers measuring nuchal translucency (fluid filled sac).

After 14 weeks' gestation, the nuchal translucency is no longer visible, because the lymphatic system is more developed and placental resistance is reduced. Therefore the combined test is no longer useful from this time.

In Down's syndrome, the nuchal translucency is thicker, the concentration of pregnancy-associated plasma protein-A is low, and the concentration of β-human chorionic gonadotrophin is high. The combined test has a sensitivity of 82–87% and a false positive rate of 5%. The sensitivity of a test is its ability to correctly identify those with the disease, i.e. the combined test will be positive for 82–87 out of every 100 babies with Down's syndrome tested. The false positive rate is the number of times the test is positive when the disease is not present, i.e. the combined test will be positive in 5 out of 100 cases when the baby has a normal karyotype.

Other causes of increased nuchal translucency thickness include:

- Turner's syndrome (45 XO genotype)
- trisomy 18 (Edwards' syndrome)
- trisomy 13 (Patau's syndrome)
- triploidy
- blockage in the developing lymphatic system (congenital lymphoedema)
- cardiac failure
- other congenital abnormalities, including diaphragmatic hernia and skeletal dysplasia
- congenital infections
- fetal anaemia

A nuchal translucency thickness ≥ 6.0 mm on its own warrants further investigation, particularly for congenital cardiac defects.

If nuchal translucency thickness cannot be measured because of the fetal position or if screening is performed after 14 weeks gestation, women are offered serum screening for Down's syndrome at 15–20 weeks' gestation. Either the triple or quadruple test is used. The triple test comprises measurements of α-fetoprotein, unconjugated oestriol and β-human chorionic gonadotrophin; in the quadruple test, inhibin-A is also measured. Serum screening has 70–75%% sensitivity (lower than the combined test) and a 5% false positive rate. Table 4.3 shows the results of serum screening in cases of Down's syndrome and other conditions.

The combined test can be used for twin pregnancies. For triplet pregnancies, nuchal translucency thickness is measured for each baby and the results combined with the mother's age to calculate the risk of specific conditions. The risk of chromosomal abnormalities is increased in multiple pregnancies because of the greater number of fetuses present. The false positive rate is also higher as the serum markers are affected by the increased number of fetuses, leading to more women being offered invasive testing.

If the risk for Down's syndrome is 1 in < 150, diagnostic testing is offered. This is done by chorionic villus sampling before 14 weeks' gestation or amniocentesis after 15 weeks (Figure 4.2).

- In chorionic villus sampling, a small portion of placental tissue is collected through either the abdomen or the cervix
- In amniocentesis, a sample of the amniotic fluid surrounding the baby is collected transabdominally

Both procedures carry the risk of complications. These include transmission of infection, failure to obtain a sample, and injury to

Interpretation of serum screening results				
α-Fetoprotein	Unconjugated oestriol	β-Human chorionic gonadotrophin	Inhibin	Associated conditions
Low	Low	High	High	Down's syndrome
Low	Low	Low	Low	Edwards' syndrome (trisomy 18)
High	Normal	Normal	Normal	Neural tube defects, including spina bifida and anencephaly, omphalocele, gastroschisis, multiple pregnancy, and underestimation of fetal gestation

Table 4.3 Interpretation of quadruple test results

Diagnostic tests for Down's and other syndromes

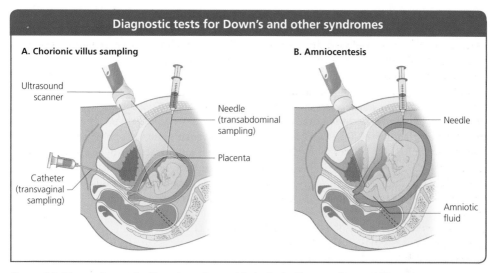

A. Chorionic villus sampling

Ultrasound scanner

Needle (transabdominal sampling)

Placenta

Catheter (transvaginal sampling)

B. Amniocentesis

Needle

Amniotic fluid

Figure 4.2 Diagnostic tests for Down's syndrome: (a) chorionic villus sampling and (b) amniocentesis.

the fetus or mother. The risk of miscarriage is operator-dependent, but is approximately 1% for amniocentesis and slightly higher for chorionic villus sampling.

> **Cell-free fetal DNA is detectable in maternal plasma and can be measured from 10 weeks' gestation.** Therefore maternal blood samples can be obtained for non-invasive fetal karyotyping. Limiting factors are cost and the availability of services to carry out these tests, but cell-free fetal DNA testing is likely to be incorporated into routine antenatal screening in the near future.

The sample (placental tissue or amniotic fluid) is sent for analysis. The results of the rapid polymerase chain reaction test are usually available within 48 h. The rapid test looks for abnormalities on specific chromosomes and provides a definitive result for the commonest genetic disorders, including Down's syndrome. To identify cases of less common chromosomal abnormalities, a full karyotype is required. This is done by polymerase chain reaction or fluorescence in situ hybridisation and takes 10–14 days.

Structural anomaly screening

An ultrasound scan to screen for fetal structural anomalies, such as cardiac abnormalities and spina bifida, is offered from the 18th to the end of the 20th week of gestation (**Figure 4.3**). Its purpose is to inform women thereby enabling them to make a choice about continuing the pregnancy and helping them prepare for the future. Based on the results of the scan, advice can be provided on place of delivery and whether or not intrauterine treatment

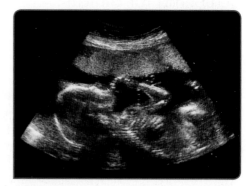

Figure 4.3 A routine ultrasound scan at 20 weeks' gestation showing no structural abnormalities. At this stage it is also possible to identify the sex of the fetus. Courtesy of Thomas Crosbie.

is warranted. Postnatal support and medical interventions can also be planned, such as feeding advice and surgery for babies born with cleft lip and palate.

> **The detection of an anomaly at the structural anomaly scan is naturally distressing for the expectant mother.** Ideally, she should be accompanied by her partner, a family member or a friend to support her in case of worrying news. Some anomalies are serious, others benign, and sometimes the significance of the anomaly is uncertain. Information and support is available from charities and organisations, such as the UK's Cleft Lip and Palate Association and ARC (Antenatal Results and Choices).

The scan is a systematic examination of the fetus. However, not all abnormalities are detected, particularly if the fetus is lying awkwardly or the mother has a high body mass index.

> **Only 50% of major cardiac abnormalities are diagnosed antenatally.** In contrast, 98% of cases of anencephaly (absence of a major portion of the brain, skull and scalp) and gastroschisis (a defect in the abdominal wall through which the abdominal contents can protrude) are detected on ultrasound before birth.

Screening for clinical conditions

Screening is also used to identify asymptomatic maternal disease and the site of the placenta (**Table 4.4**). Detection and treatment of a clinical condition, and planning of the delivery, reduce maternal and fetal morbidity.

Screening for fetal growth and well-being

Fetal growth and well-being are determined at each antenatal visit by asking about fetal movements and by measuring the symphysis-fundal height. Deviations from normal require further assessment.

Fetal growth

The symphysis-fundal height is measured at every antenatal visit after 24 weeks. The measurements are plotted on a customised growth chart in the mother's handheld notes. Maternal height, weight and ethnicity are used to estimate fetal weight using a specially designed computer programme. At 20 weeks, the uterus reaches the umbilicus, and at 36 weeks it reaches the xiphisternum.

If the symphysis-fundal height is less than expected, or if growth velocity slows, an ultrasound assessment of fetal weight and amniotic fluid volume is carried out.

Fetal presentation

This is determined by abdominal palpation from 36 weeks' gestation. Ultrasound is used if breech presentation is suspected. Assessment of presentation before 36 weeks is unreliable, because the fetus may still assume cephalic presentation with advancing gestation.

Antenatal screening for clinical conditions			
Condition	Screening test	Who is screened	When testing is carried out
Gestational diabetes	Oral glucose tolerance test	Women at increased risk of the disease (see Chapter 6)	24–28 weeks
Pre-eclampsia	Blood pressure and dipstick urinalysis for proteinuria	All women	Each antenatal visit
Placenta praevia	Ultrasound for placental site	All women	Anomaly scan (from 18th to end of 20th weeks); repeated at 32 weeks if placenta is covering internal cervical os at earlier gestation

Table 4.4 Antenatal screening for clinical conditions

Fetal well-being

Auscultation of the fetal heart is not routine. However, it may reassure the woman.

Fetal movements are usually felt from 20 weeks' gestation, although they may be noticed earlier by multiparous women. Formal counting of fetal movement is not advocated as there is a wide range of 'normal' movements, but women are advised to monitor their baby's movements and report deviations from normal. If a change in fetal movements is reported, fetal well-being is promptly assessed by cardiotocography, possibly combined with ultrasound.

Lifestyle advice

Lifestyle advice is provided to all pregnant women to allow them to improve their general health, reduce the risk of pregnancy complications and to prevent harm to the fetus. Verbal advice and leaflets are given at the first visit and reinforced throughout the pregnancy.

Nutritional supplements

All women should take folic acid before conception and for the first 12 weeks of pregnancy to reduce the risk of neural tube defects. The daily dose is 400 μg. However, a higher dose (5 mg/day) is recommended for women with:

- a previous pregnancy affected by neural tube defect
- a neural tube defect, or a partner with a neural tube defect
- epilepsy
- pre-existing diabetes
- obesity (body mass index > 30 kg/m^2)
- malabsorption (e.g. inflammatory bowel disease)
- sickle cell anaemia

A 10-μg daily vitamin D supplement is recommended, especially for women who are obese, spend much of the day indoors, have dark skin or cover their skin for religious reasons. In the UK, vitamin D is available in the Healthy Start multivitamin supplement for women on low incomes. Alternatively, it can be purchased over the counter at pharmacies.

Exercise

Exercise is encouraged during pregnancy because it helps:

- the body adapt to the physiological changes that occur during pregnancy
- the ability to cope with labour
- avoid excessive weight gain in pregnancy

Aerobic exercise such as running, walking or swimming can be continued for as long as the woman is comfortable. The woman should be able to hold a conversation while exercising; if not, she is exercising too strenuously. This can cause a reduction in blood flow to the fetus and negatively impact on growth. If the woman is taking up exercise for the first time during pregnancy it should build up gradually to a maximum of four 30 minute sessions a week. Pelvic floor exercises during pregnancy reduce the risk of stress incontinence.

Certain types of exercise should be avoided during pregnancy:

- Those that involve lying flat because this reduces venous return
- Contact sports, due to the risk of abdominal injury
- Scuba diving, because the baby is not protected from decompression sickness and gas embolism
- Exercising at heights >2500 m due to the possibility of altitude sickness

Diet

Maintaining a healthy diet has maternal and fetal benefits: it prevents excessive weight gain, provides vital vitamins and minerals, and ensures optimal fetal development and growth. Women do not need to 'eat for two'; an extra 200 calories per day are required for fetal development in the last three months of pregnancy. A healthy diet for a pregnant woman includes:

- At least 5 portions of fruit and vegetables per day (washed to avoid toxoplasmosis)
- At least one source of protein per day
- Two portions of fish a week

- Predominantly carbohydrate-based meals, particularly wholemeal foods
- Low-fat dairy products

Obese women are encouraged to lose weight before becoming pregnant to reduce the risk of obstetric complications (see Chapter 6). Weight loss should be avoided during pregnancy, along with fatty and sugary foods.

> **Public health bodies offer support to ensure that poverty does not prevent a woman having sufficient** milk and vegetables to help maintain a healthy diet during pregnancy.

Foods to avoid

Dietary modifications are recommended to reduce the risk of food-borne infections and fetal abnormalities. Pregnant women are advised not to eat:

- unpasteurised milk, ripened and blue-veined cheese, paté and undercooked food, which can cause listeriosis
- raw or partially cooked eggs or meat (particularly poultry), which can cause salmonellosis
- raw fish, because this can cause food poisoning (including hepatitis A)
- fish, such as swordfish and shark, that contain high levels of mercury, which affects the development of the fetal nervous system
- liver products, which contain teratogenic (malformation-causing) levels of vitamin A

> **If drugs need to be prescribed during pregnancy, their number and dose are minimised.** Very few drug trials have included pregnant women, and the use of most drugs prescribed during pregnancy is off-licence. Drug formularies contain sections on the use of medicines in pregnancy, and these are consulted before prescribing.

Smoking

Children born to mothers who smoke are at higher risk of preterm delivery, low birthweight and neurodevelopmental problems. Therefore women who smoke in pregnancy are routinely referred for smoking cessation advice. Nicotine replacement therapy is safe, but patches should be removed before going to bed, to reduce the dose of nicotine received. E-cigarettes are advised against until more safety data become available.

Alcohol

Excessive alcohol consumption in pregnancy is associated with miscarriage, stillbirth, preterm delivery and low birthweight, as well as fetal alcohol syndrome. Children with this condition have a small head, small and narrow eyes, and an absent philtrum; they also have learning difficulties and behavioural problems.

A safe limit for alcohol consumption during pregnancy is not known. Therefore women should avoid any alcohol in the first trimester and consume at most one to two units, once or twice a week, during the remainder of the pregnancy. Getting drunk and binge drinking are particularly harmful.

Travel

Pregnant women travelling by car should wear a seatbelt, which should be placed above and below the bump rather than over it. Long-haul air travel is associated with an increased risk of deep vein thrombosis and pulmonary embolism, so women should drink plenty of water, move around the plane at least hourly, and wear compression stockings on flights longer than 4 h. Heparin is prescribed for pregnant women at high risk, who are seen in a combined obstetric-haematology clinic. Pregnant women are advised to avoid travelling to areas where vaccinations are required, because the majority are live vaccinations which can potentially affect the fetus. If travel is vital, the risks of being vaccinated need to be weighed up against the risk of developing the disease.

Anti-D

The rhesus antigen is a protein on the surface of the red blood cells of most people; they are rhesus-positive. However, up to 15% of the population are rhesus-negative; they lack this protein. A rhesus-negative woman carrying a rhesus-positive baby can become sensitised to its blood. Her body then produces antibodies against future rhesus-positive babies, leading to haemolytic disease of the newborn (see Chapter 6). However, this is prevented by treatment with anti-D, a blood product that helps remove rhesus-positive fetal blood cells from the maternal circulation before sensitisation.

Anti-D is given at the time of sensitising events, when maternal and fetal blood may come into contact, i.e. during:

- surgical management of miscarriage at < 12 weeks, termination of pregnancy or ectopic pregnancy
- vaginal bleeding from 12 weeks
- amniocentesis
- intrauterine transfusion or surgery
- external cephalic version (attempted or successful)
- abdominal trauma (including that sustained during a car accident)
- fetal death
- delivery

Anti-D is given as a standard dose of 250 IU intramuscularly up to 19 weeks of gestation and 500 IU from 20 weeks. Anti-D is administered ideally within 72 h of the sensitising event, but it can be given up to 10 days afterwards. A Kleihauer test is carried out after 20 weeks to ensure that the dose is adequate.

One dose of anti-D provide cover for 6 weeks. Therefore in the event of recurrent sensitising events, only one dose every 6 weeks is required, as long as the Kleihauer test result is negative (see Chapter 3 for test description).

Prophylactic anti-D is also given at 28 weeks' gestation to cover 'silent sensitising events', i.e. times when maternal and fetal blood has come into contact but there have been no triggering events. It is given as either a single dose of 1500 IU or two doses of 500 IU at 28 and 34 weeks; the two options are equally efficacious. Prophylactic anti-D is given regardless of whether it has already been given after a sensitising event.

Normal delivery

Labour is the period between the onset of contractions and the delivery of the placenta. The biology of labour is discussed in detail in Chapter 1 (pages 65–67) and the complications that can arise, along with their management, are covered in Chapter 7. The following section concentrates on normal delivery and what it requires of healthcare professionals. In normal labour:

- The first stage lasts about 12–14 h for nulliparous women and 6–8 h for subsequent pregnancies
- The second stage is about 1–2 h for nulliparous women and 5–60 min in subsequent pregnancies
- The third stage is the delivery of the placenta and lasts 30–60 min

In high-income countries, birth is generally very safe for both mother and baby. Women should be offered a choice of where to give birth. In the UK the choice is: at home, in a midwife-led unit or in an obstetric unit. Support during labour, in particular one-to-one care from a midwife, increases the likelihood of a normal vaginal delivery.

Latent first stage of labour

This is the first part of the first stage of labour. It is the time between the onset of painful uterine contractions and the point at which cervical effacement and 4-cm dilation is reached. This stage of labour is not continuous; contractions occur irregularly.

Women do not need to be with a midwife or other healthcare professional during this part of labour, but they do need to be given the knowledge of how to cope with the pain associated with contractions. Antenatal education helps women cope with the pain associated with contractions. It includes advice on the use of:

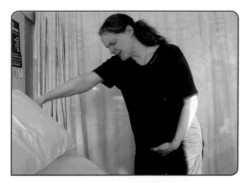

Figure 4.4 Breathing exercises performed in the latent first stage of labour provide analgesia and are a form of coping strategy.

- breathing exercises (**Figure 4.4**)
- immersion in water (a warm bath)
- massage

Staying mobile and hydrated reduces the length of the latent phase.

Established first stage of labour

In the second part of the first stage of labour, painful contractions are now regular, and the cervix dilates from 4 cm to 10 cm, which marks the start of the second stage (see Figure 1.45). At this stage a woman needs one-to-one care from a midwife. She is not left alone, except for short periods of time.

During established labour, women should eat snacks or a light meal and have something to drink (preferably isotonic drinks). However, food and drink are avoided if opioids are required for pain relief. Opioids cause nausea and vomiting and increase the risk of aspiration.

The partogram

The progress of labour is documented on a partogram. This is a graphical representation of labour, comprising records of:

- maternal observations,
- cervical dilation and
- fetal well-being.

The frequency of contractions (described as the number every 10 min, e.g. 3 in 10) is documented every 30 min. Maternal pulse rate is recorded hourly, and blood pressure and temperature every 4 h. The volume of urine passed

is also documented. These measurements help the midwife ensure that the woman is receiving adequate hydration while avoiding a full bladder, which can slow labour.

Vaginal examination

Women are offered a vaginal examination every 4 h to establish progress. Cervical dilation progresses at a rate of 2 cm every 4 h. Inadequate progress suggests delay in the first stage of labour.

Second stage of labour

This is the interval between full dilation of the cervix (10 cm) and delivery of the baby. It has two parts.

- In the passive stage, there are no involuntary expulsive contractions
- In the active phase, the baby is visible and the woman has an involuntary urge to push or is encouraged to push in the absence of such urges

A safe length for the passive stage is up to 2 h in nulliparous women and 1 h in multiparous women. This allows time for the fetal head to descend, thereby shortening the active phase. A passive stage longer than this suggests malposition of the fetus or ineffective contractions and increases the risk of postpartum haemorrhage and maternal infection. It is managed by encouraging the woman to actively push and judicious use of oxytocin in nulliparous women. Delivery is expected within 3 h of the start of the active second stage in nulliparous women, and within 2 h in multiparous women.

In the second stage of labour, maternal blood pressure measurements and vaginal examinations are carried out hourly.

When pushing, the woman are advised to avoid being supine or semisupine; these positions restrict placental blood flow and increase pain. Instead, she can adopt any other comfortable position. She is guided by her own urges to push and given encouraging words from the midwife.

Cardinal (fetal) movements

During delivery, the fetus goes through a series of cardinal movements to pass through the pelvis (see Figure 1.48):

1. Engagement: the widest part of the fetal head passes through the pelvic inlet; this can occur several weeks before the start of labour, especially in nulliparous women. It is, therefore, a sign of preparation for labour, but is not used to predict when contractions will commence
2. Descent of the head through the pelvis: this is determined relative to the ischial spines of the maternal pelvis; when the head reaches the ischial spines it is said to be at 0 station, and if it is 1 cm above or 2 cm below the ischial spines it is at −1 or +2 station, respectively. The time at which these stations are reached is recorded on the partogram
3. Flexion of the head on to the chest
4. Internal rotation: the head reaches the pelvic floor muscles and rotates to the occipitoanterior position. Failure of the head to rotate delays the second stage of labour
5. Extension: the head emerges from under the symphysis pubis and crowns, meaning that it will no longer slip back between contractions. Once this point is reached vaginal delivery is inevitable
6. Restitution and external rotation: the head rotates 45° to come to lie looking to the maternal left or right . Absence of restitution is a warning sign of shoulder dystocia
7. Expulsion: the anterior shoulder descends to the symphysis pubis, rotates under it

and is delivered, followed by the posterior shoulder and the rest of the baby. This occurs during one contraction. Shoulder dystocia is diagnosed if the baby is not delivered with normal routine traction

Episiotomy

Episiotomy (surgical incision of the perineum) to increase the size of the vaginal opening for delivery is not routine. The use of this procedure is restricted to cases of presumed fetal compromise or instrumental delivery, because it does not protect against the development of 3rd or 4th degree perineal tears (**Table 4.5**). It is performed when the head has crowned and the perineum is maximally stretched.

If episiotomy is required, usually a posterior episiotomy is done. Scissors are used to make a mediolateral cut from the fourchette (the thin fold of skin at the back of the vulva), usually towards the right. This is purely for ease in performing the incision for right-handed individuals. Adequate analgesia is required (either local or regional, i.e. epidural or spinal anaesthesia). An anterior episiotomy may be needed for women who have been subjected to female genital mutilation, which significantly narrows the vaginal opening. Suturing of an episiotomy is performed immediately after delivery of the placenta. Most heal without any problems; if a woman develops pain over her episiotomy or an offensive discharge she is advised to contact her midwife.

Classification of perineal trauma		
Degree of trauma	Vaginal deliveries affected	Description of tear
1st	16%	Involves perineal skin alone
2nd	35%	Involves perineal muscle
3rd	1% (up to 7% with forceps delivery)	Involves anal sphincter
		3a: < 50% of external anal sphincter damaged
		3b: > 50% of external anal sphincter damaged
		3c: internal anal sphincter damaged
4th	< 1%	Involves external anal sphincter, internal anal sphincter and anal epithelium

Table 4.5 Classification of perineal trauma

Third stage of labour

This stage is the interval between delivery of the baby and expulsion of the placenta and membranes. The process can be physiological, when delivery occurs by maternal effort alone, or active, when uterotonic drugs (agents that increase uterine muscle tone), cord clamping and controlled cord traction are used after signs of placental separation. These include a sudden gush of blood and lengthening of the visible umbilical cord.

During active management, oxytocin is given intramuscularly, either alone at a dose of 10 IU, or at 5 IU combined with ergometrine 500 μg as Syntometrine. The two options are equally effective for preventing haemorrhage > 1000 mL. Syntometrine is better at reducing smaller haemorrhages but can cause nausea and vomiting. The risk of postpartum haemorrhage is 5–10%. Active management of the third stage of labour reduces the risk of postpartum haemorrhage by 60% (see Chapter 7).

The third stage lasts up to 30 min after active management and 1 h with physiological management.

Perineal trauma

Over 85% of women having a vaginal delivery sustain perineal trauma, and 60–70% require stitches. Perineal trauma is classified into four groups depending on its extent (**Table 4.5**), which is assessed by carrying out a systematic examination of the perineal area, including the rectum. This needs to be done by a trained midwife or doctor in an adequately-lit room, and the mother requires appropriate analgesia, e.g. Entonox, local or regional anaesthesia. Absorbable sutures are used to reduce pain and improve healing.

Monitoring in labour

Fetal heart rate is monitored during labour to assess the well-being of the baby. Intermittent auscultation is used in low-risk pregnancies, and cardiotocography in high-risk cases (**Figure 4.5**). If abnormalities are identified by intermittent auscultation, the woman is referred to an obstetrician for review; she may need to be transferred to hospital.

Intermittent auscultation

A Pinard stethoscope or Doppler ultrasound is used to carry out intermittent auscultation once the active first stage of labour is diagnosed. It is done:

- for 1 min immediately after a contraction, and at least every 15 min, in the first stage of labour
- for 1 min after a contraction, every 5 min, in the second stage of labour

The results of intermittent auscultation are recorded as a single, average, rate on the partogram.

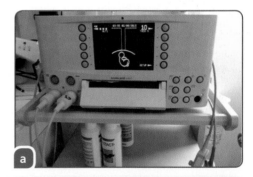

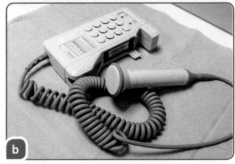

Figure 4.5 Monitoring in labour: (a) cardiotocograph and (b) handheld Doppler fetal monitor.

It is essential to distinguish between the maternal and fetal heart rates to avoid confusing the two. This is done by palpating the maternal pulse.

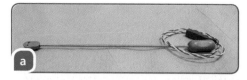

Cardiotocography

A cardiotocograph is used to monitor high-risk labours (**Figure 4.6**). These include cases of delayed first or second stage of labour, meconium–stained amniotic fluid, maternal hypertension and prolonged rupture of membranes.

An ultrasound transducer measures fetal heart rate. A pressure-sensitive contraction transducer measures the frequency of uterine contractions (although the strength and duration of a contraction can be determined only by abdominal palpation). If the fetal heart rate cannot be detected with an abdominal transducer, a fetal scalp electrode clip is used. During a vaginal examination, this small clip is inserted through the cervix, applied to the fetal scalp and attached to a monitor (**Figure 4.7**).

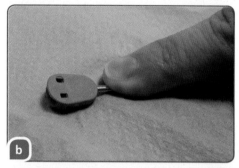

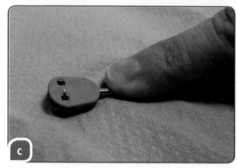

Fetal scalp electrode clips are used selectively and applied carefully, because they can cause fetal trauma. They are not used in cases of breech presentation; when the mother has a blood-borne infection, because of the risk of transmission; and when the fetus may have a bleeding disorder, such as haemophilia.

Figure 4.7 A fetal scalp electrode clip can be used to monitor fetal heart rate during labour. (a) Fetal scalp electrode. (b) When inserting the clip into the vagina the furthest end (into which the wire inserts) is rotated anticlockwise to retract the clip. This prevents causing damage to the vagina. (c) Upon application with the fetal scalp the rotation is removed. The clip is then exposed and is applied to the fetal scalp.

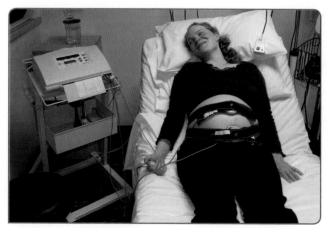

Figure 4.6 A cardiotocogram (CTG) measures fetal heart rate and uterine contractions. Before labour, women are asked to record fetal movements during the CTG using a hand-held device. Fetal movements and heart rate accelerations are signs of fetal wellbeing.

A cardiotocograph is interpreted by making an overall assessment of the trace based on the results for four variables (**Tables 4.6** and **4.7**). Management in cases of a suspicious or pathological cardiotocograph depends on the stage and progress of labour (see Chapter 7).

The use of cardiotocography does not reduce the risk of intrapartum death and disability, due to lack of a standard interpretation and poor correlation between fetal heart rate changes and adverse outcomes. However, it does increase the number of caesarean sections as a result of misinterpretation of traces and misdiagnosis of fetal distress. This is why cardiotocography is not advocated for low-risk pregnancies.

Cardiotocographic features				
Interpretation	Baseline heart rate (beats/min)	Heart rate variability (beats/min)	Decelerations (decrease in heart rate of > 15 beats/min for > 15 s)	Accelerations (increase in fetal heart rate of > 15 beats/min for > 15 s)
Reassuring	110–160	≥ 5	Absent	Present
Non-reassuring	100–109 160–180	< 5 for 40–90 min	Typical variable decelerations with > 50% of contractions for > 90 min Single prolonged deceleration for ≤ 3 min	The absence of accelerations with no other non-reassuring or abnormal features is of unknown significance
Abnormal	< 100 > 180 Sinusoidal pattern ≥ 10 min	< 5 for > 90 min	Atypical variable decelerations with > 50% of contractions for > 30 min Late decelerations with > 50% of contractions for > 30 min Single prolonged deceleration for > 3 min	

Table 4.6 Description of cardiotocographic features (National Institute for Health and Care Excellence classification)

Classification of cardiotocographic results	
Category	Definition
Normal	All four features are reassuring
Suspicious	One non-reassuring feature, all other features reassuring
Pathological	Two or more non-reassuring features, or one or more abnormal features

Table 4.7 Classification of cardiotocographic results

Analgesia and anaesthesia

Labour is painful, so analgesia is offered to all women. Several types are available (**Table 4.8** and **Figure 4.8**), but the location of the delivery may restrict choice. Local or regional analgesia is used for operative vaginal deliveries and suturing.

Analgesia during labour						
Type	Route	Mechanism	Availability	Advantages	Disadvantages	Complications
Breathing exercises, massage, acupuncture or TENS		Relaxation TENS stimulates endorphin production, reducing pain signals sent to from spinal cord to brain	All sites	No additional equipment required, low cost No adverse effects	Not effective in active labour; useful in passive phase only	None
Entonox (50:50 nitrogen: oxygen, 'gas and air'); see **Figure 4.8**	Inhalation	Possibly activation of opioid receptors in brain and spinal cord, but exact mechanism unknown	All sites	No adverse effects Minimal equipment needed, low cost Rapid relief	Short lasting Does not relieve pain completely	Light-headedness, nausea, (these wear off quickly after discontinuing)
Opioids (e.g. pethidine and diamorphine)	Intramuscular injection	Activation of opioid receptors and inhibition of transmission of nociceptive impulses	All sites (except pools: risk of impaired consciousness and drowning)	More effective pain relief Effect lasts 2–4 h	Nausea and vomiting (prophylactic antiemetic given simultaneously) Takes 20 min to become effective	Maternal drowsiness Neonatal drowsiness and respiratory depression Affects breastfeeding (feeding impaired in drowsy baby)
Regional analgesia (epidural or combined spinal–epidural)	*Epidural:* catheter inserted into epidural space between L3 and L4; opioids and local anaesthetic injected (continuously or as boluses); can be patient controlled *Combined spinal–epidural:* opioids and local anaesthetic inserted into subarachnoid and epidural space	Local anaesthetic acts on sympathetic, sensory and possibly motor fibres to block nerve transmission Opioids act as above Combined spinal–epidural: denser block, more rapid analgesia	Obstetric units only	Most effective form of pain relief Can top up for surgery Inserted at any time as long as woman can sit still	Limited availability Takes 20 min to become effective Requires fetal monitoring by cardiotocograph and more frequent maternal BP measurement Have to re-site if not wholly effective (1 in 20 cases) Increases risk of operative vaginal delivery	Maternal hypotension Loss of mobility and bladder sensation requiring catheterisation Dural puncture (1 in 1000) Pins & needles in leg (1 in 2000) Nerve injury (< 1 in 10,000) Infection at insertion site (rare)

BP, blood pressure; TENS, transcutaneous electrical nerve stimulation.

Table 4.8 Analgesic options during labour

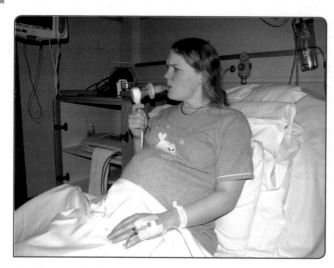

Figure 4.8 Entonox is effective pain relief during labour for many women. Deep breaths are taken from the mouthpiece as soon as a contraction starts, to allow the peak concentration of the drug to coincide with peak of the contraction. It is important to stop breathing the gas between contractions to avoid dizziness and nausea.

Induction of labour

Induction is the process of starting labour artificially. This intervention is required in many situations, most commonly to avoid prolonged pregnancy. It is necessary when the risks of continuing with the pregnancy outweigh the harms associated with delivery, e.g. in cases of pre-eclampsia after 34 weeks gestation or gestational diabetes after 38 weeks gestation. In high-income countries up to 1 in 4 labours are induced after 37 weeks' gestation. In lower-income countries induction rates are lower (as low as 1% in Niger) because fewer women have access to healthcare facilities.

The process of inducing labour takes time, particularly at the beginning, when the aim is to soften the cervix and to encourage it to dilate. Induced labour is more painful than spontaneous labour, because of the use of oxytocin. Contractions induced by synthetic oxytocin become stronger and more frequent than in spontaneous labour.

More than one third of women whose labours are induced require further intervention to give birth: 15% have an instrumental delivery and 22% need an emergency caesarean section (for a proportion because induction has failed).

Prelabour rupture of membranes at term occurs in 8% of pregnancies over 37 weeks. In 60% of such cases, labour starts within 24 h. For those women who are not labouring by 24 h after prelabour rupture of membranes at term, induction is offered because it halves the risk of serious neonatal infection (from 1% to 0.5%) without increasing the likelihood of operative delivery.

Membrane sweep

In this procedure, a finger is passed through the cervix and rotated against the wall of the uterus. This action separates the chorionic membrane from the decidua. In response, prostaglandins are released, which ripen the cervix and stimulate contractions.

Membrane sweeping is offered to women at antenatal visits from 40 weeks' gestation. It is a low-risk means of trying to start labour.

Pharmacological methods

Synthetic prostaglandins are the first-line option for inducing labour. They act in the same way as the prostaglandins released by the body in response to a membrane sweep.

These drugs are available as a tablet, gel or controlled-release pessary, which is inserted into the posterior fornix (recess of the upper vagina) of the vagina. Two doses of prostaglandin tablets or gels, 6 h apart, can be used if needed, or one controlled-release pessary inserted for 24 h. Women may be allowed home to await the effects, depending on the indication for induction and hospital policy.

A complication of the use of synthetic prostaglandins is uterine hyperstimulation; the frequent contractions cause fetal distress by reducing placental oxygenation. The treatment is removal of the source of prostaglandins and administration of tocolytic agents (drugs that inhibit uterine contractions), for example terbutaline.

If the woman is not labouring by the end of pharmacological induction, the cervix is assessed to determine whether artificial rupture of membranes is possible.

Mechanical methods

Artificial rupture of membranes (**Figure 4.9**) is the main mechanical method of inducing labour. It is used as the primary method of induction when vaginal prostaglandins are contraindicated. This may be the case when a woman has had a previous caesarean section, because prostaglandin use is associated with a higher risk of uterine rupture. Artificial rupture of membranes with or without oxytocin reduces this risk, but it remains higher than in cases in which women with a previous caesarean section labour spontaneously.

Artificial rupture of membranes releases prostaglandins which stimulate contractions. It is combined with titrated doses of oxytocin to increase their strength and frequency.

Other mechanical methods include the use of balloon catheters and laminaria tents. The latter is a thin rod containing laminaria, a member of the kelp family, which is inserted into the cervix. It slowly absorbs water and expands to dilate the cervix. Neither these nor balloon catheters are used routinely, however.

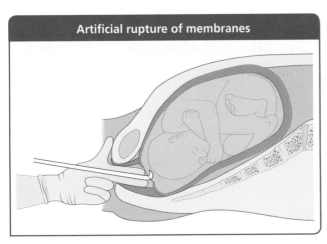

Artificial rupture of membranes

Figure 4.9 Artificial rupture of membranes. The amnihook is inserted through the cervix and 'hooked' onto the amniotic membrane, creating a hole to allow the amniotic fluid to pass through.

Postnatal care

The postnatal period lasts from delivery until 6 weeks later, by which time the woman's body has returned to normal after the physiological changes of pregnancy. The frequency of midwife visits depends on individual circumstances and varies from country to country. In the UK there is usually a visit the day after delivery, on day 5 to take the blood spot test for neonatal screening, and on day 10; care is then transferred to the health visitor. A check is carried out by the GP 6–8 weeks after delivery. A number of aspects are covered at these visits.

Maternal health

Women are advised of the signs and symptoms of postpartum haemorrhage, infection and thromboembolism, and they are encouraged to report any abnormalities. Maternal blood pressure is checked to screen for pre-eclampsia, and assessment of the perineum is offered if the woman feels any discomfort.

Assessment of the mothers wellbeing is essential in the postnatal period, because a mother who is in good mental health is better able to understand and respond to her baby's feelings. Therefore women are asked about their mood and coping strategies to enable early detection of mental health problems (see page 239).

Contraception

Contraception is discussed shortly after delivery, because ovulation can resume within 21 days of delivery for non-breastfeeding women. Breastfeeding women can use all contraceptives except the combined oral contraceptive pill, because it inhibits milk production. Full breastfeeding is a reliable contraceptive in the first 6 months after delivery if the mother's periods have not returned. Increased prolactin levels during breastfeeding inhibit production and secretion of gonadotrophin-releasing hormone, lowering oestrogen levels and preventing ovulation.

Intrauterine devices can be inserted for contraception within the first 48h or 4–6 weeks after delivery, when the uterus has reverted to its normal size. The softness of the postnatal uterus means that insertion outside these times is more likely to cause uterine perforation and expulsion of the coil.

Breastfeeding

Unrestricted breastfeeding is encouraged for all women. Midwives provide advice and support to ensure correct positioning of the baby. Breastfeeding has various benefits for both mother and baby (**Table 4.9**).

Benefits of breastfeeding	
Mother	**Baby**
Reduces risk of ovarian and breast cancer by inhibiting ovulation and reducing oestrogen exposure	Reduced risk of infective diarrhoea, chest and ear infections, eczema and sudden infant death syndrome, because of the transfer of protective immunoglobulins and cytokines
Provides contraception by inhibiting ovulation	Less constipation, because breast milk is easier to digest than formula milk
Increases calorie expenditure by 500 calories/day	Reduced incidence of type 2 diabetes in later life, possibly related to changes in glucose and insulin metabolism
Improves bonding with baby	Improves bonding with mother

Table 4.9 Benefits of breastfeeding for mother and baby

Answers to starter questions

1. This depends upon whether the woman and her baby are at low or high risk of developing complications during labour and whether she has given birth before. In the UK, all high-risk pregnancies are delivered in an obstetric led unit where appropriately skilled obstetricians and neonatologists are available. For low risk women, the risk associated with place of birth depends upon whether they are nulliparous or multiparous. For multiparous women, there is no difference in perinatal outcome whether the woman plans to deliver at home, in a midwifery led or obstetric unit: rates of stillbirth, neonatal injury or death are the same; however, in obstetric units there is a highter rate of intervention (instrumental delivery, episiotomy or caesarean section). For nulliparous women, midwifery led and obstetric units are equally safe, though again the number of normal vaginal deliveries is higher outside obstetric units. Planning to deliver at home is associated with an increase in the risk of adverse perinatal outcomes for nulliparous women, though the overall risk remains low. Almost half of all nulliparous women planning to deliver at home will be transferred into an obstetric unit, compared with 10% of women having their second baby.

2. It is unclear what stimulates labour and whether the trigger comes from the mother or the fetus. One theory is that the maternal pituitary gland produces oxytocin when the baby is ready to be born in order to stimulate contractions. Another is that the fetal adrenal gland sends a hormonal signal upon reaching maturity to the mother to stimulate labour. Researchers have also identified the β-inhibitory protein, which is thought to cause the uterus to contract. Obese women have lower levels of this, potentially explaining why they are more likely to progress slowly through labour and require a caesarean section.

3. Epidurals do not lengthen the first stage of labour or increase the risk of needing a caesarean section. However, they do increase the duration of the second stage of labour, leading to a higher chance of needing an instrumental delivery due to the loss of sensation to push.

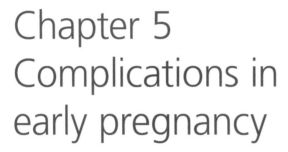

Chapter 5
Complications in
early pregnancy

Starter questions

Answers to the following questions are on page 183.

1. What causes bleeding in early pregnancy?
2. Why do some pregnancies miscarry?

Introduction

The first trimester, also known as early pregnancy, is a time of profound physiological changes as the maternal body adapts to the demands of pregnancy. These underlie the symptoms of complications of early pregnancy, which can be alarming as in cases of bleeding and pain, and also unusual, as in cases of extreme nausea and vomiting.

Bleeding in early pregnancy is most commonly caused by miscarriage. However, it is essential to exclude:

■ other disorders of pregnancy, such as ectopic pregnancy and gestational trophoblastic disease
■ local causes of bleeding, for example infection, trauma, cervical polyp and cancer

Normal, physiological bleeding at the time of blastocyst implantation, i.e. implantation bleeding, is a diagnosis of exclusion.

Abdominal pain in early pregnancy must be investigated, because it can be caused by serious pathological conditions that may or may not be related to pregnancy. These must be ruled out before attributing the pain to a corpus luteal cyst. These are physiological cysts that sometimes become large and haemorrhagic or can rupture or tort (see page 319).

■ Pregnancy-related causes of abdominal pain include miscarriage and ectopic pregnancy
■ Causes unrelated to pregnancy include appendicitis, urinary tract infection and kidney stones

In early pregnancy, increasing levels of β-human chorionic gonadotrophin (hCG) can cause mild, self-limiting nausea and vomiting. In extreme or protracted cases of nausea and vomiting, a number of potentially serious conditions must be excluded.

Case 3 Pain and bleeding in early pregnancy

Presentation

Kelly Brown, aged 24 years, has presented to the early pregnancy unit with a history of vaginal bleeding and abdominal pain at 6 weeks of pregnancy.

Initial interpretation

It is essential to establish the amount of bleeding as well as the site, nature and severity of any associated abdominal pain. Heavy bleeding and cramping suprapubic pain suggest miscarriage, whereas ectopic pregnancy typically presents with vaginal spotting and unilateral iliac fossa pain. The clinical features of faintness, shoulder tip pain and collapse are particularly useful for diagnosis; they suggest blood in the peritoneal cavity (haemoperitoneum) and large volume blood loss causing hypotension (haemodynamic compromise) after rupture of an ectopic pregnancy.

Further history

Kelly's pregnancy was unplanned. She used the morning after pill following unprotected sex 4 weeks ago. Her previous two pregnancies were terminated for social reasons. She has a history of chlamydia and smokes 20 cigarettes daily. The pain in her abdomen started a few days ago and is worsening. The vaginal bleeding started this morning.

Examination

Kelly is pale, but all clinical observations are normal. A urine test confirms that she is pregnant. She has tenderness and guarding in her left iliac fossa. On speculum examination, dark blood is found in the vagina, but no clots or products of conception (pregnancy tissue) are visible. The cervix appears healthy, and the external cervical os (orifice), is closed. Cervical excitation, i.e. marked pain on movement of the cervix, is found on digital examination, and there is left adnexal tenderness.

Interpretation of findings

This clinical picture is consistent with a diagnosis of ectopic pregnancy. Thorough history taking has identified several risk factors for the disease: failed emergency contraception, previous chlamydia infection and smoking. The examination findings of adnexal tenderness and cervical excitation are signs commonly associated with ectopic pregnancy. In a slim patient, it may be possible to palpate an adnexal mass, but undue pressure should be avoided because it can precipitate tubal rupture.

Investigations

Quantitative testing shows a serum hCG concentration of 2045 IU/L. Haemoglobin concentration is 10 g/L. Transvaginal ultrasound shows an empty uterus with a thickened endometrium, free fluid in the deepest part of the peritoneal cavity, the rectouterine pouch, and a complex left adnexal mass.

Diagnosis

This combination of scan findings and a serum hCG concentration > 1500 IU/L is

Case 3 *continued*

diagnostic for ectopic pregnancy. Kelly is haemodynamically stable at present, but she is at risk of tubal rupture. Ruptured ectopic pregnancy is a life-threatening emergency that requires urgent surgical intervention. Intravenous access is achieved, a nil-by-mouth order is imposed and the decision is made by the emergency gynaecology team to place Kelly on the emergency theatre list for laparoscopy with or without removal of the left fallopian tube (left salpingectomy).

Case 4 Spotting in early pregnancy

Presentation

Rebecca James, who is 29 years old, presents with vaginal spotting 8 weeks into her first pregnancy.

Initial interpretation

Vaginal spotting is common in early pregnancy. Pregnancy-related causes include miscarriage and ectopic pregnancy; in the latter, the bleeding is generally preceded by unilateral abdominal pain. Common causes of vaginal spotting in pregnancy that are not related to the pregnancy itself include infection, such as chlamydia, and cervical ectopy (formally known as cervical ectropion or erosion). This is a physiological change commonly

Miscarriage

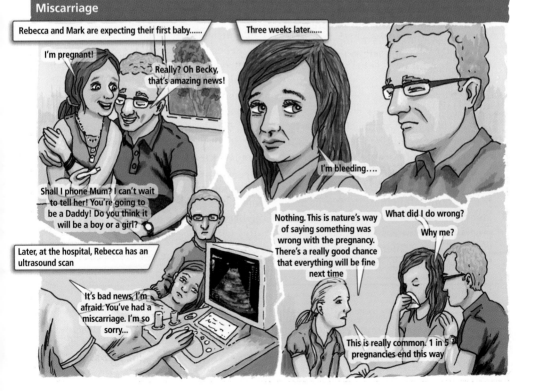

Case 4 *continued*

seen in pregnancy, where the delicate columnar epithelium of the endocervical canal extends onto the ectocervix (the portion of cervix that protrudes into the vagina) where it is prone to trauma and bleeding during intercourse. Cervical cancer is a rare cause.

It is helpful to determine if the spotting was precipitated by sexual intercourse. This would suggest bleeding originating from the lower genital tract.

Further history

The pregnancy was planned. Rebecca and her husband, Mark, had been trying to conceive for nearly a year. She had a positive result on a home pregnancy test 3 weeks ago.

The pregnancy had been uneventful until today, when she noticed dark red blood on the toilet tissue when she wiped herself. There were no precipitating factors, and there has been no pain. Rebecca had breast tenderness and urinary frequency when she first found out she was pregnant, but these symptoms have stopped. She is very worried that something is wrong with the pregnancy.

Examination

Rebecca is haemodynamically stable. Her abdomen is soft and non-tender, with no masses. Speculum examination shows a healthy cervix. There is some white discharge but no active bleeding. Bimanual pelvic examination finds the uterus to be anteverted and of a size consistent with pregnancy of 8 weeks' gestation. The cervical os is closed. There is no cervical excitation, adnexal tenderness or masses.

Interpretation of findings

The pelvic examination findings are normal for this stage of pregnancy. There are no obvious lower-genital-tract causes for the bleeding. The lack of tenderness on abdominal or pelvic examination makes an ectopic pregnancy less likely.

Investigations

A urinary pregnancy test gives a positive result. Transvaginal ultrasound finds a 30-mm irregularly shaped intrauterine gestational sac containing a yolk sac but no fetal pole. These findings are confirmed by a second sonographer.

Diagnosis

The dimensions of the gestational sac are compatible with Rebecca's dates, but a fetal pole and fetal heartbeat should be visible at this stage in the pregnancy. Therefore, the diagnosis is missed miscarriage.

Rebecca and Mark are devastated by the news. They are given time together to absorb the news privately and afterwards offered the opportunity to talk things through with a nurse. They are given contact details of the hospital bereavement service as well as the Miscarriage Association, which offers support to couples in the UK. Rebecca and Mark are provided with information on the options for management. After being given time to consider, Rebecca chooses medical management. This takes place on the gynaecology ward 2 days later.

Miscarriage

Miscarriage is the spontaneous end of a pregnancy before the fetus has reached the age of viability, i.e. the age at which it may survive outside the uterus, which is 24 weeks' gestation in the UK. The different types of miscarriage are shown in **Table 5.1**.

Epidemiology

Sporadic miscarriage occurs in 20% of all pregnancies. Miscarriage becomes less likely as pregnancy progresses. The risk is 10% after 8 weeks' gestation, and decreases to 3% once a viable intrauterine pregnancy has been confirmed by ultrasound, which is usually done by the booking scan at about 12 weeks.

Aetiology

Miscarriage has many causes, including the following:

- Genetic abnormality in the embryo: this underlies > 60% of early miscarriages
- Structural causes: uterine malformations such as large fibroids (see page 316) and uterine septum (see page 106) can prevent implantation
- Maternal infections: these include listeriosis, toxoplasmosis and parvovirus
- Maternal immunological causes: conditions such as antiphospholipid syndrome and systemic lupus erythematosus are a rare cause

Advanced maternal age is an independent risk factor for miscarriage, because oocyte quality decreases with age. Smoking, alcohol consumption, drug misuse and excessive caffeine intake also increase the risk of miscarriage.

Recurrent miscarriage, the spontaneous loss of three consecutive pregnancies, affects 1% of women. Appropriate investigations for recurrent miscarriage are shown in **Table 5.2**.

Prevention

In the absence of an established treatable cause, there is little evidence that any intervention reduces the incidence of miscarriage.

Investigations for recurrent miscarriage	
Investigation	Condition detected
Anticardiolipin antibody tests	Antiphospholipid syndrome
Parental karyotype	Balanced translocations, which can cause ≥ 75% of gametes to be unbalanced
Thrombophilia screen (protein C, protein S and factor V Leiden)	Thrombophilic defects
Ultrasound of the pelvis and/or hysteroscopy	Fibroids or congenital uterine abnormality

Table 5.2 Investigations for recurrent miscarriage

Types of miscarriage		
Type	Ultrasound findings	Typical clinical presentation
Threatened	Viable intrauterine pregnancy	Vaginal bleeding and/or abdominal pain with closed cervical os
Inevitable	Viable intrauterine pregnancy	Vaginal bleeding and abdominal pain with open cervical os
Incomplete	No intrauterine pregnancy, but thickened endometrium; or non-viable pregnancy (no fetal heartbeat)	Vaginal bleeding and abdominal pain with open cervical os and/or products of conception in cervical os
Complete	Empty uterus with non-thickened endometrium	Settling vaginal bleeding and abdominal pain with closed cervical os
Missed	No fetal heartbeat, or empty gestational sac	Can be completely asymptomatic

Table 5.1 Types of miscarriage

However, in women with antiphospholipid syndrome the use of low-dose aspirin (75 mg/day) and low-molecular-weight heparin improves the live birth rate for future pregnancies to 70%.

In women at risk of miscarriage in the second trimester as a result of cervical incompetence, ultrasound surveillance of cervical length, and insertion of a cervical suture in cases of excessive shortening of the cervix, may increase the likelihood of a live birth.

Pathogenesis

For a viable pregnancy to be established, several events must take place, including fertilisation of the oocyte, formation of the zygote, implantation of the embryo, and development of placental support for the pregnancy (see page 44). Failure at any step in this process results in miscarriage. Genetically abnormal conceptuses rarely reach full term, but the reasons for this are unclear.

Clinical features

Miscarriage generally presents with bleeding and cramping pain in the lower abdomen. It can also be diagnosed during a routine ultrasound scan in asymptomatic women. An empty gestational sac or absent fetal heartbeat at gestations where these are usually present is diagnostic (**Table 5.3**).

Early pregnancy: transvaginal ultrasound findings	
Gestation (weeks)	Findings
0–4.5	Nil
4.5–5	Small gestational sac and double decidual sign
5–5.5	Yolk sac
5.5–6.0	Fetal pole and cardiac activity
6–7	Crown–rump length: 4–10 mm Fetal cardiac activity
7–8	Crown–rump length: 11–16 mm Caudal and cephalad poles
8–9	Crown–rump length: 17–23 mm Limb buds
9–10	Crown–rump length: 23–32 mm Fetal movements

Table 5.3 Transvaginal ultrasound findings in early pregnancy

Diagnostic approach

The diagnosis of miscarriage is suspected on clinical grounds and established by examination and investigation.

Examination helps distinguish a miscarriage from the other most likely differential diagnosis, ectopic pregnancy. Speculum and pelvic examination help determine the type of miscarriage (see **Table 5.1**).

Any products of conception visible in the cervix should be removed during speculum examination to reduce blood loss and pain.

Investigations

Appropriate investigations include a urinary pregnancy test, an ultrasound scan and quantitative hCG testing.

Urinary pregnancy test

Home pregnancy tests give misleading results if carried out or interpreted incorrectly. Therefore a urinary pregnancy test is essential for all women of reproductive age presenting with symptoms that suggest miscarriage.

> **Caring for a woman with bleeding in early pregnancy is challenging, because it may be a difficult time for her.** Every woman is different, so avoid making assumptions about how she is feeling. Empathic listening will help establish how she feels.
>
> Find out whether the pregnancy was planned or unplanned. If the pregnancy was unplanned, does she want the pregnancy to continue?
>
> A woman with a history of infertility or pregnancy loss, particularly recurrent miscarriage, is likely to be extremely anxious and distressed.

Measurement of β-human chorionic gonadotrophin

Serial measurements of serum hCG concentration are useful in the absence of ultrasound confirmation of a viable intrauterine pregnancy. Absolute hCG values, especially in isolation, are less informative than the trend in values over time. Decreasing hCG concentration generally indicates miscarriage.

Ultrasound

The fetal heartbeat is auscultated by hand-held Doppler from about 12 weeks' gestation, when the uterus is just palpable above the pelvic brim. If the fetal heart is not heard, or if the pregnancy is of < 12 weeks' gestation, an ultrasound scan is the investigation of choice to determine viability, gestational age and the location of the pregnancy. Transvaginal ultrasound is more sensitive, because the probe is closer to the uterus, so it is valuable at 8 weeks' gestation or earlier (**Table 5.3**).

Management

> **Miscarriage can be an emotionally difficult time for a woman and her partner.** The way in which she is treated will determine her feelings about any future pregnancy, so a sensitive and empathic approach is essential.

Once a miscarriage is confirmed, the definitive treatment options are medical management and surgical management. A third option is expectant management, which entails waiting for the miscarriage to complete spontaneously. In general, a woman's personal preference takes precedence, although excessive, life-threatening blood loss prompts immediate surgical management.

Expectant management is an option for women who are not experiencing excessive bleeding and who would prefer to 'allow nature to take its course'. However, without intervention it may take several weeks for the miscarriage to complete, and medical or surgical management may be necessary if this fails to occur or if complications arise. If excessive ongoing bleeding does take place and it leads to haemodynamic compromise, urgent surgical evaluation is warranted (see below).

Medication

In medical management, miscarriage is induced by prostaglandins such as misoprostol administered either orally or vaginally. The use of the progesterone antagonist mifepristone administered orally 12–48 h beforehand improves the success rate for this management option. Women receive repeated doses of misprostol until their miscarriage completes; this takes 6–12 hours, during which time they remain in hospital for analgesia and emergency care in the rare event of massive bleeding.

Surgery

Miscarriage is managed surgically by dilatation of the cervix and suction evacuation of the uterus to remove the products of conception. The key risks are:

- bleeding (0.1% of cases require a blood transfusion)
- incomplete evacuation, i.e. retained products of conception, necessitating further treatment (4%)
- intrauterine infection (3%)
- uterine perforation (< 1%)

Injury to the cervix and scar tissue in the uterus (intrauterine adhesions) are rare complications. There is no evidence for an adverse effect on future fertility.

> **Emergency surgery** is required for women who are:
> - bleeding profusely
> - tachycardic, hypotensive or both
> - anaemic, with low or decreasing levels of haemoglobin
> - in need of immediate fluid resuscitation

Prognosis

After a miscarriage, most women go on to have a normal intrauterine pregnancy. However, the risk of subsequent miscarriage increases with every pregnancy loss, increasing to 40% after three consecutive miscarriages.

Ectopic pregnancy

An ectopic pregnancy is an extrauterine pregnancy. Most cases (95%) occur in the fallopian tube (**Figure 5.1**). A ruptured ectopic pregnancy is a life-threatening emergency that requires urgent surgery.

Epidemiology

1.1% of spontaneous pregnancies, and 1–3% of in vitro fertilisation (IVF) pregnancies, are ectopic.

In heterotopic pregnancy, an ectopic pregnancy and an intrauterine pregnancy coexist. Heterotopic pregnancies are extremely rare in cases of spontaneous pregnancy (1 in 30,000) but more common after IVF (1%).

Aetiology

The key risk factor for ectopic pregnancy is damage to the fallopian tube. Common risk factors are:

- pelvic inflammatory disease
- previous ectopic pregnancy
- previous tubal surgery
- an intrauterine contraceptive device (coil) in situ
- smoking
- assisted reproduction
- failed emergency contraception

Ectopic pregnancy also occurs in women with no risk factors, so a high index of suspicion is necessary.

Clinical features

Unilateral lower abdominal pain is the most common presenting complaint. There is often vaginal bleeding or spotting. Irritation of the diaphragm innervated by the phrenic nerve by subdiaphragmatic blood causes referred pain in the shoulder tips. Fainting or collapse suggests significant intra-abdominal bleeding.

Examination findings are unilateral abdominal tenderness, cervical excitation and/or an adnexal mass. Clinical signs of haemodynamic compromise or peritoneal irritation, including tachycardia, hypotension, abdominal guarding, rebound or rigidity, warrant immediate resuscitation and surgical intervention. These are indicators of tubal rupture and intra-abdominal haemorrhage.

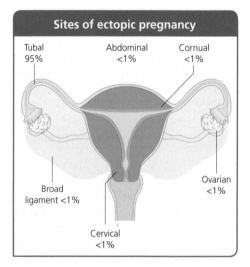

Sites of ectopic pregnancy

Tubal 95%
Abdominal <1%
Cornual <1%
Broad ligament <1%
Ovarian <1%
Cervical <1%

Figure 5.1 Proportion of ectopic pregnancies occurring at different sites. Most occur in the fallopian tubes.

> **Untreated ectopic pregnancy can result in tubal rupture, intra-abdominal haemorrhage and death.** Any woman with a positive pregnancy test result who presents with unilateral lower abdominal pain with or without vaginal bleeding is treated as though she has an ectopic pregnancy until this possibility has been excluded.

Diagnostic approach

The combination of a positive pregnancy test result and an empty uterus on ultrasound is treated as an ectopic pregnancy until proven otherwise.

Investigations

For haemodynamically stable patients, investigations include transvaginal ultrasound and serial measurements of serum hCG concentration.

> Any woman of reproductive age presenting with abdominal pain must have a urinary pregnancy test. Testing is required even if she has used contraception or does not think she could be pregnant.

Measurement of β-human chorionic gonadotrophin

In a viable intrauterine pregnancy, maternal serum hCG concentration doubles every 48 h. hCG levels that increase slowly, i.e. by < 66% over 48 h, or remain static suggest ectopic pregnancy.

Ultrasound

The most common ultrasound features of ectopic pregnancy are an empty uterus, an adnexal mass and free fluid in the rectouterine pouch. A live ectopic pregnancy is sometimes visualised on scan as an adnexal mass with a fetal heartbeat. A transvaginal ultrasound scan is more sensitive than a transabdominal scan for diagnosis of an ectopic pregnancy.

Management

Expectant management may be appropriate in some cases, provided that the woman has minimal pain, her serum hCG concentration is decreasing, and the ectopic pregnancy is not visible on ultrasound. In this option, the ectopic pregnancy fails spontaneously and resolves without any active intervention. Women are monitored carefully to ensure that their hCG levels normalise.

Medication

Medical management is an option in cases of ectopic pregnancies in which the woman has minimal pain, a small unruptured adnexal mass (< 4 cm) is visible on ultrasound, and hCG concentration is < 1500 IU/L. The fallopian tube is spared, which is an advantage for patients who wish to preserve their fertility, although there is a risk of further ectopic pregnancies in that tube.

Methotrexate, a folic acid antagonist, targets rapidly dividing cells, arrests mitosis and precipitates tubal abortion, i.e. the expulsion of the products of conception before rupture of the fallopian tube. The drug is given as a single intramuscular injection at a dose based on body surface area. hCG levels increase immediately after treatment but then decrease. About 15% of women require a second dose to complete treatment.

Women are followed up until their hCG levels decrease sufficiently (< 25 IU/L) to confirm that the ectopic pregnancy is resolving. Women must avoid a further pregnancy for 3 months after treatment, because of the teratogenic effect of methotrexate.

Surgery

Women with clinical signs of haemodynamic compromise require immediate resuscitation followed by surgery. Laparoscopic salpingectomy is carried out if the contralateral tube appears normal (**Figure 5.2**). However, if the other tube is diseased or absent, for example having been removed to treat a previous ectopic pregnancy, and the patient wishes to preserve her fertility, laparoscopic salpingostomy is preferred. In this procedure, the fallopian tube is unblocked by 'milking' the ectopic pregnancy out of the tube through a linear incision.

Open surgery is sometimes necessary, for example if the patient is haemodynamically unstable, or if a lack of facilities or staff with the necessary surgical skills precludes laparoscopic surgery.

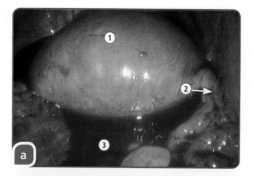

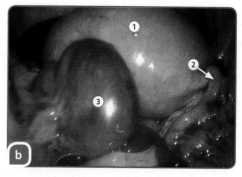

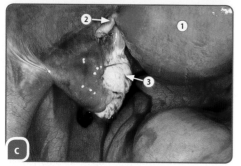

Figure 5.2 Laparoscopic appearances of left tubal pregnancy. (a) Haemoperitoneum. ①, uterus; ②, right tube; ③, blood. (b) Left tubal pregnancy and normal right fallopian tube. ① uterus; ②, right tube; ③, left tubal pregnancy. (c) Left tubal remnant after left salpingectomy. ①, uterus; ②, left tubal remnant; ③, left ovary. Courtesy of Rick Clayton.

Hyperemesis gravidarum

Nausea and vomiting are common symptoms of early pregnancy and generally harmless. However, the excessive and intractable vomiting and nausea that characterise hyperemesis gravidarum can lead to dehydration and malnutrition. In severe cases, these can result in an abnormally low level of sodium in the blood (hyponatraemia) and thiamine deficiency, and the latter can cause Wernicke's encephalopathy, a serious neurological disorder.

Between 50 and 90% of expectant mothers experience nausea and vomiting in pregnancy. The name 'morning sickness', is misleading because only 15% of women have symptoms exclusively in the morning. Symptoms start at 6–8 weeks' gestation, peak at 9–11 weeks and generally resolve by 16 weeks.

Most cases of nausea and vomiting in pregnancy are mild. However:

- 35% of pregnant women have symptoms that reduce their quality of life and limit their ability to engage in normal activities

- 1% have hyperemesis gravidarum and require hospital treatment for rehydration

Clinical features

Persistent vomiting accompanied by weight loss exceeding 5 per cent of prepregnancy body weight is diagnostic of hyperemesis gravidarum, in the absence of other causes.

Epidemiology

Hyperemesis gravidarum is more common in first rather than subsequent pregnancies. It is more likely in women who experience nausea and vomiting related to oral contraceptives, motion and migraine.

Diagnostic approach

Other causes of vomiting, such as urinary tract infection, thyrotoxicosis and liver disease, need to be excluded (**Table 5.4**).

Investigations

Investigations exclude other causes of nausea and vomiting and assess the severity of hyperemesis.

Dipstick urinalysis

Patients with significant ketonuria are usually admitted to hospital for rehydration. Protein, white blood cells or blood in the urine may indicate a urinary infection as a precipitating factor.

Blood tests

Persistent vomiting causes severe electrolyte imbalances, so levels of electrolytes in the blood are checked on admission and throughout the hospital stay (**Table 5.5**). Clinical examination for signs of thyrotoxicosis, for example goitre, eyelid lag and exophthalmia, distinguish biochemical hyperthyroidism from Graves' disease.

Ultrasound

Hydatidiform molar pregnancy and multiple pregnancies are associated with

Nausea and vomiting in pregnancy: differential diagnosis	
Category	**Diagnosis**
Disorders of the genitourinary system	Urinary tract infection
	Pyelonephritis
Disorders of the gastrointestinal system	Appendicitis
	Pancreatitis
	Cholecystitis
	Peptic ulcer
	Gastritis
Disorders of the nervous system	Migraine
	Diseases of the central nervous system
Disorders of metabolism and the endocrine system	Thyrotoxicosis
	Addison's disease
	Hypercalcaemia
	Uraemia
Disorders of the middle ear	Vestibular dysfunction
	Ménière's disease
	Labyrinthitis
Drug misuse and supplement use	Opioids
	Iron
Psychological disorder	Bulimia nervosa
Pregnancy-related complications	Molar pregnancy
	Acute fatty liver of pregnancy
	Pre-eclampsia

Table 5.4 Differential diagnosis of nausea and vomiting in pregnancy

hyperemesis. They can be excluded by ultrasound assessment.

Management

Management is predominantly supportive, with intravenous fluid therapy, antiemetics and vitamin supplementation. Prevention of deep vein thrombosis and pulmonary embolus (thromboprophylaxis) is considered for patients with extreme dehydration and limited mobility.

Hyperemesis gravidarum: blood tests	
Blood test	Rationale
Full blood count	To check for anaemia
	Increased white blood cell count indicates infection
Urea and electrolytes	Low serum sodium levels (hyponatraemia), low serum potassium levels (hypokalaemia) and low serum urea are consistent with excessive vomiting
	A metabolic alkalosis results from loss of hydrogen ions in vomitus
	A metabolic acidosis indicates severe disease
Thyroid function tests	Biochemical hyperthyroidism (high thyroxine and low thyroid-stimulating hormone) is common, because of cross-reactivity between β-human chorionic gonadotrophin and the thyroid-stimulating hormone receptor
Liver function tests	Liver function test results may be deranged (increased aspartate aminotransferase, alanine transaminase and bilirubin), but frank jaundice is rare

Table 5.5 Blood tests for hyperemesis gravidarum

Gestational trophoblastic disease

Gestational trophoblastic disease is rare in the UK (affecting 0.1% of pregnancies), and more common in South East Asia (up to 1% of pregnancies). This may relate to reduced carotene (vitamin A precursor) intake in South East Asian populations. It includes:

- benign disorders of trophoblastic proliferation, such as complete or partial hydatidiform moles
- neoplastic trophoblastic disease, for example invasive moles, choriocarcinoma and placental site trophoblastic tumours

Trophoblastic disease is more common in teenagers and women over 45 years of age.

Hydatidiform molar pregnancy

A complete hydatidiform mole is created when two spermatozoa fertilise an empty ovum, i.e. an egg containing no functional maternal DNA; it is a diploid conceptus (46XX). A partial hydatidiform mole results when two sperm fertilise a normal ovum; it is a triploid conceptus (e.g. 69XXX).

Clinical features

Vaginal bleeding in the first or second trimester is the most common presenting complaint. On ultrasound, multiple cystic areas are visible within the placental mass and contain either no recognisable fetus, in the case of a complete mole, or a grossly abnormal fetus, in the case of a partial mole. Serum hCG levels are usually extremely high. Most partial moles are diagnosed histologically after a miscarriage.

Management

Surgical evacuation of the pregnancy is recommended. In the UK, follow-up is carried out at regional trophoblastic screening centres; levels of hCG are monitored until it becomes undetectable. Persistent trophoblastic disease warrants chemotherapy (see page 116).

Prognosis

Future pregnancies are monitored for molar pregnancy, but recurrence is uncommon, with only 1% affected.

Women with a molar pregnancy are referred to the nearest regional trophoblastic screening centre. In the UK this is Charing Cross Hospital in London, Weston Park Hospital in Sheffield or Ninewells Hospital in Dundee. Monitoring of blood and urinary hCG levels is essential to exclude persistent trophoblastic disease.

Gestational trophoblastic neoplasia is considered in any woman with persistent abnormal vaginal bleeding after a miscarriage, termination of pregnancy or live birth. hCG is a reliable tumour marker for this disease, and a negative result from an hCG test excludes the diagnosis.

Gestational trophoblastic neoplasia

Invasive moles, choriocarcinomas and placental site tumours have variable presentations depending on the type and extent of the disease.

Clinical features

Irregular bleeding after a molar pregnancy, a miscarriage or, rarely, an uneventful live birth is the most common presenting complaint. Metastatic disease presents variously with bleeding, pain, coughing up blood (haemoptysis) or neurological symptoms. A high index of suspicion is key to diagnosis.

Management

Single-agent methotrexate is used to treat low-risk patients. High-risk patients require treatment with a combination of chemotherapy agents. If gestational trophoblastic neoplasia is diagnosed and treated in its early stages, the cure rate is 95–100%. Advanced stage disease is more challenging to treat and can be fatal.

Prognosis

After successful treatment, pregnancy is avoided for 12 months to reduce the risk of recurrence. A further pregnancy interferes with interpretation of hCG levels and complicates management. Barrier contraceptives (e.g. condoms) are recommended. The combined oral contraceptive pill is effective and does not alter prognosis. Intrauterine devices are associated with an increased risk of uterine perforation.

Answers to starter questions

1. Bleeding in early pregnancy is common and invariably causes distress. Most women worry that they are miscarrying and it is essential to be sensitive to this. Important pregnancy-related causes include miscarriage and ectopic pregnancy. Bleeding is only attributed to implantation or physiological changes to the cervix (cervical ectopy) in the absence of any other pathology.

2. Miscarriage affects up to 20% of pregnancies. Most occur in the first trimester as a result of genetic abnormalities. Miscarriage is more common with increasing maternal age because the proportion of genetically abnormal oocytes increases. Other causes include uterine abnormalities (e.g. submucous fibroids, bicornuate uterus), coagulation disorders (e.g. antiphospholipid syndrome), toxins (including chemotherapy drugs and alcohol) and infection.

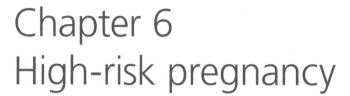

Chapter 6
High-risk pregnancy

Starter questions

Answers to the following questions are on pages 213–214.

1. Why should women who develop gestational diabetes or pre-eclampsia during their pregnancy be followed up postnatally?
2. Should macrosomic babies be induced to prevent complications during delivery?
3. Can babies with anencephaly be organ donors?
4. Are pregnancies in younger or older mothers managed differently?

Introduction

A high-risk pregnancy is one in which there is a higher than normal risk of the mother or fetus being affected by complications during or after pregnancy and birth. Reasons for this include an underlying medical problem in the mother, pregnancy-related complications and a congenital abnormality in the fetus. Pregnancies in teenagers or women older than 35 years are also high risk because of a higher risk of intrauterine growth restriction, preterm birth and maternal complications (e.g. pre-eclampsia and gestational diabetes) at the extremes of reproductive age.

The general approach to the management of high-risk pregnancies is:

■ regular review in joint clinics with obstetric and specialist input
■ stopping teratogenic medication, to minimise the risks of fetal abnormalities
■ monitoring for disease exacerbation, pregnancy-related complications, and fetal growth and well-being
■ timely delivery by the most appropriate means, to minimise maternal and fetal complications

Case 5 Diabetes in pregnancy

Presentation

Joanne Davies, aged 30 years, attends a preconception clinic with her husband, Mark. She was diagnosed with type 1 diabetes when she was 13 years old and is considering trying for a baby.

Initial interpretation

Ideally, all women with pre-existing medical disorders are seen in a preconception clinic by an obstetrician and a specialist physician. This provides the opportunity to discuss the risks of the pregnancy on the disease, the risk of the disease on the pregnancy and any potential fetal complications. It also enables disease control to be optimised before pregnancy to reduce the risk of problems arising.

Further history

Joanne manages her diabetes well in consultation with the diabetes nurse specialist and her diabetologist; she uses short-acting insulin at mealtimes and long-acting insulin before bed. She has not required hospital admission for her diabetes since diagnosis. At her most recent review 6 months ago, no complications of diabetes were found.

She takes no other medication apart from the insulin and folic acid (5 mg/day). She is generally fit and well and does not smoke.

Examination

Joanne's blood pressure is 110/70 mmHg and her body mass index (BMI), 25 kg/m^2.

Managing diabetes in pregnancy

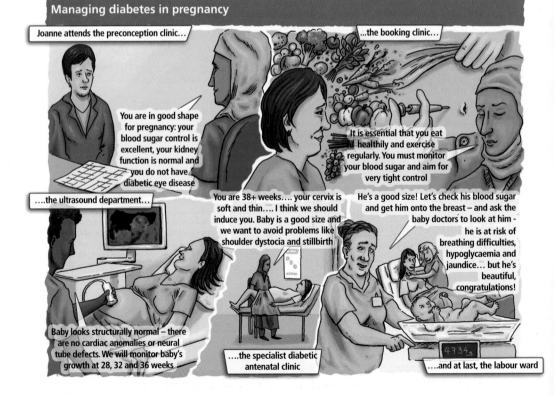

Joanne attends the preconception clinic...

...the booking clinic...

You are in good shape for pregnancy: your blood sugar control is excellent, your kidney function is normal and you do not have diabetic eye disease

It is essential that you eat healthily and exercise regularly. You must monitor your blood sugar and aim for very tight control

....the ultrasound department...

You are 38+ weeks.... your cervix is soft and thin.... I think we should induce you. Baby is a good size and we want to avoid problems like shoulder dystocia and stillbirth

He's a good size! Let's check his blood sugar and get him onto the breast – and ask the baby doctors to look at him – he is at risk of breathing difficulties, hypoglycaemia and jaundice... but he's beautiful, congratulations!

Baby looks structurally normal – there are no cardiac anomalies or neural tube defects. We will monitor baby's growth at 28, 32 and 36 weeks

....the specialist diabetic antenatal clinic

....and at last, the labour ward

Case 5 *continued*

There is no evidence of peripheral neuropathy on examination. Dipstick urinalysis shows no proteinuria.

Interpretation of findings

Joanne has well-controlled diabetes. This is supported by the absence of hospital admissions for uncontrolled blood sugars or complications from her diabetes, particularly hypertension, renal or neurological disease.

Her insulin regimen of three doses of rapid-acting insulin and an evening dose of long-acting insulin is safe to use in pregnancy, and she is not taking any teratogenic medication which would need to be reviewed to minimise the risk of fetal abnormality. Joanne is correctly taking a higher dose of folic acid than routinely advocated peri-conceptually as she is at higher risk of having a fetus affected by spina bifida due to her diabetes.

Aside from the diabetes, there are no other factors associated with increased risk of maternal or fetal complications. An HbA1C measurement is necessary to ensure Joanne's diabetic control is optimised and renal, thyroid and eye assessments are required to assess for diabetic complications, which can affect the pregnancy.

Investigations

Joanne's haemoglobin A1c value is 48 mmol/mol. Renal function is normal and her urinary albumin:creatinine ratio is within the reference range. Thyroid function is also normal. An eye screening test finds no sign of retinopathy.

Diagnosis

The haemoglobin A1c result confirms good glycaemic control; now is a good time to start trying for a baby. This is supported by the absence of kidney disease and retinopathy, which are potential complications of diabetes. The absence of any other autoimmune disease is shown by the normal results of the thyroid function tests.

Maternal diabetes can cause complications in pregnancy e.g. an increased risk of miscarriage, fetal anomalies, stillbirth and pre-eclampsia. However, the risk of developing these complications is reduced in Joanne's case, because her disease is well controlled.

Diabetes in pregnancy

Pregnancy can be complicated by either pre-existing type 1 or 2 diabetes or gestational diabetes. Gestational diabetes is the onset or recognition of glucose intolerance in pregnancy and includes undiagnosed type 2 diabetes.

Epidemiology and aetiology

Diabetes affects 0.5–5% of pregnancies. Ethnic origin influences the likelihood of developing gestational diabetes; women of South Asian and African-Caribbean origin are at greatest risk. These same individuals have a higher risk of developing type 2 diabetes, while Caucasians are more likely to be diagnosed with type 1 diabetes than African-Americans. Obesity increases the risk of both type 2 and gestational diabetes. Increasing obesity rates and higher average maternal age underlie an increase in the prevalence of the disease in recent years.

Prevention

Preconception advice and optimisation of glycaemic control prior to pregnancy reduces the risk of complications. Weight loss and lifestyle changes in women at risk of gestational diabetes reduces the likelihood of developing the disease.

Pathogenesis

Placental hormones such as human placental lactogen and growth hormone promote insulin resistance. To maintain stable glucose levels, the normal physiological response to this is increased secretion of insulin from the pancreas. However, this response is limited in women with gestational diabetes, resulting in hyperglycaemia. The rate of complications increases with increasing haemoglobin A1c levels, although why this happens is unclear.

Clinical features

Diabetes causes both maternal and fetal complications (**Table 6.1**).

Babies born to mothers with diabetes have become conditioned to high glucose levels and therefore have high basal levels of insulin. The withdrawal of the maternal source of glucose at delivery puts them at risk of hypoglycaemia. The consequent fetal hypoxia triggers erythropoiesis (red blood cell production). This leads to polycythaemia (increased haemaglobin concentration) and jaundice, resulting from the accumulation of products of the breakdown of red blood cells.

Diagnostic approach

Screening for gestational diabetes is carried out at 24–28 weeks' gestation in women with risk factors for the disease:

- BMI > 30 kg/m^2
- previous macrosomic baby (> 4.5 kg)
- first-degree relative with diabetes
- ethnic origin with high prevalence of diabetes, for example South Asian or African-Caribbean
- gestational diabetes in a previous pregnancy

Diabetes in pregnancy: complications		
Maternal complication(s)	Fetal complication(s)	Aetiology
Hyperglycaemia	Miscarriage	Insulin resistance
Ketoacidosis	Congenital anomalies, particularly sacral agenesis (abnormal development of the lower spine) and central nervous system and cardiac defects	
Increasing insulin requirements or need to start insulin for the first time		
	Macrosomia, leading to shoulder dystocia and birth injuries	
	Polyhydramnios	
	Neonatal hypoglycaemia	
Hypoglycaemia	None	Vomiting in early pregnancy
Renal nephropathy (may be irreversible)	Growth restriction	Microvascular disease
Diabetic retinopathy	Fetal hypoxia	
Pre-eclampsia	Stillbirth	
	Polycythaemia	
	Neonatal jaundice	
Increased risk of caesarean section	Prematurity	Often related to iatrogenic intervention

Table 6.1 Complications of diabetes in pregnancy

Screening is performed using a oral glucose tolerance test (OGTT).

Investigations

An OGTT is performed after a woman has fasted overnight. Firstly, her serum glucose concentration is measured. The test is then repeated 2 h after she has drunk a solution containing 75 g of glucose. Gestational diabetes is diagnosed if the fasting glucose concentration is ≥5.6 mmol/L or the glucose concentration after 2 h is ≥ 7.8 mmol/L.

Women who have had gestational diabetes before can either start monitoring their own glucose levels early in any subsequent pregnancy, or have an oral glucose tolerance test at the booking visit (first antenatal visit) and again at 24–28 weeks if the initial result is normal.

> **The threshold values for blood glucose concentration used to diagnose gestational diabetes are lower than those that define diabetes outside pregnancy.** This is because even at these glucose levels the risks to the pregnancy are increased.

Management

The aim of management of diabetes in pregnancy is to achieve or maintain tight glycaemic control.

Preconception folic acid (5 mg daily) reduces the risk of neural tube defects. The higher dose of folic acid protects against glucose induced fetal abnormalities.

Because of the risk of fetal abnormalities, angiotensin-converting enzyme inhibitors and statins, which are used to treat associated hypertension and high cholesterol levels, are discontinued and safer alternatives started, such as labetalol.

Lifestyle modification

Changes to lifestyle improve glycaemic control. Dietary improvements and moderate exercise alone are sufficient to control blood glucose levels in 80–90% of women with gestational diabetes.

Oral medication

Metformin or glibenclamide are safe to use in pregnancy for women with type 2 diabetes or gestational diabetes.

Insulin

Short-acting insulin is taken before meals and longer acting preparations at night to improve glycaemic control. Subcutaneous pumps delivering short-acting insulin are used by women with unstable disease.

> **Insulin requirements increase during pregnancy, peaking at about 36 weeks.** A sudden decrease in insulin requirements during pregnancy is a sign of placental insufficiency, so delivery is expedited to prevent stillbirth.

Screening for kidney disease and retinopathy

Screening is done early in pregnancy, or ideally before conception. Identification of kidney disease or retinopathy warrants increased monitoring during and after pregnancy.

Screening for fetal anomalies and well-being

A detailed anomaly scan is carried out at 20 weeks' gestation to screen for fetal anomalies. Growth scans are done every 4 weeks from 28 weeks' gestation to monitor fetal growth and placental function.

Delivery

Mothers with diabetes are delivered of their baby after 38 complete weeks of pregnancy to reduce the risk of late stillbirth. Macrosomic babies are delivered by caesarean section to reduce the risk of shoulder dystocia.

Postnatal management

Insulin requirements decrease rapidly once the placenta is delivered. Women with gestational diabetes stop any medication immediately after the birth, and those with pre-existing diabetes return to their prepregnancy regimen.

For women who have had gestational diabetes, fasting plasma glucose concentration is checked at their 6-week postnatal visit to the general practitioner clinic to screen for underlying type 2 diabetes. They also have annual haemoglobin A1c measurements.

Hypertension in pregnancy

Hypertension is a common medical problem in pregnancy. It is classified according to blood pressure.

- Mild hypertension: 140–149/90–99 mmHg
- Moderate hypertension: 150–159/100–109 mmHg
- Severe hypertension: > 160/110 mmHg

Severe hypertension can cause placental abruption, fetal growth restriction, cerebrovascular accident, and maternal and fetal death.

Types

Women with hypertension in pregnancy either had high blood pressure prior to pregnancy (chronic hypertension) or develop it for the first time during pregnancy. This can either be without associated proteinuria (gestational hypertension) or with proteinuria (pre-eclampsia, **Table 6.2**).

Types of hypertension in pregnancy					
Type	Incidence (%)	Significant proteinuria?	Time of onset	Aetiology	Complications
Chronic hypertension	1–2	Yes, if kidney disease present	Before pregnancy or < 20 weeks' gestation	Primary (95%): aetiology unknown Secondary (5%): ■ kidney disease (e.g. glomerulonephritis, renal artery stenosis) ■ adrenal disease (Conn's syndrome, Cushing's syndrome, phaeochromocytoma)	Fetal growth restriction, particularly if kidney disease present Superimposed pre-eclampsia End-organ disease (e.g. stroke, chronic kidney disease) Placental abruption Preterm birth
Gestational hypertension	6	No	> 20 weeks' gestation	Unknown, but may be related to abnormal placental invasion of the myometrium and reduced uteroplacental perfusion	Low risk of maternal or fetal complications
Pre-eclampsia	5–10	Yes	> 20 weeks	Genetic predisposition Failure of spiral arteries to be fully invaded by trophoblasts Maternal blood pressure increases to compensate for increased vascular resistance Endothelial damage resulting from placental hypoperfusion causes proteinuria	Fetal growth restriction Prematurity Eclampsia Haemolysis, elevated liver enzymes and low platelets (HELLP) syndrome Disseminated intravascular coagulation Maternal and fetal death

Table 6.2 Types of hypertension in pregnancy

Pre-eclampsia

This is hypertension developing after 20 weeks gestation in association with significant proteinuria.

Eclampsia

This is the onset of generalised seizures in a woman with pre-eclampsia. Only a third of women with eclampsia have hypertension and proteinuria before their first eclamptic seizure. In the other two thirds of cases, the hypertension and proteinuria may not be evident or are not identified prior to the eclamptic seizure.

Eclampsia is caused by loss of cerebral autoregulation. This leads to increased blood flow, vessel permeability and oedema.

Epidemiology

Hypertension affects 10–15% of pregnancies.

In countries like the UK, eclampsia affects 1% of women with pre-eclampsia and has an associated mortality rate of < 1% as a result of improvements in its management (see Chapter 14, page 353). In low- and middle-income countries, the incidence of eclampsia is higher (5–8%) because of limited access to health care and prophylactic treatment; the associated mortality rate is also higher in consequence (15%).

> **Failure to identify and treat hypertension in pregnancy is often identified as a shortcoming of obstetric care in inquiries into maternal deaths.** Education of health professionals about the management of severe hypertension and eclampsia, including the use of simulation, improves outcomes.

Prevention

The risk of developing pre-eclampsia is decreased by 10% when aspirin is taken from 12 weeks' gestation by women at high risk of hypertension, i.e. those with the following risk factors:

- a history of hypertension in pregnancy or a family history of pre-eclampsia
- diabetes

- chronic kidney disease
- autoimmune disease (e.g. systemic lupus erythematosus)
- first pregnancy, or an interval of > 10 years since the most recent previous pregnancy
- age ≥ 40 years
- BMI > 35 kg/m^2
- multiple pregnancy

Aspirin inhibits production of thromboxane A$_2$, (a vasoconstrictor produced by platelets) thereby reversing the vasoconstriction that underlies hypertension and improving endothelial function.

Clinical features

Hypertension is usually asymptomatic, so screening at each antenatal visit is vital. Symptoms and signs are related to increased vascular permeability and leakage of fluid into interstitial spaces. They include:

- blurred vision
- headache
- irritability
- seizures
- swollen face
- high blood pressure
- epigastric pain
- vomiting
- placental abruption
- proteinuria
- pitting oedema
- swollen feet and ankles

Diagnostic approach

The aims are first to determine the type of hypertension and then to assess its severity, including its effects on organ function and the fetus.

Investigations

Dipstick urinalysis is carried out to test for proteinuria. This is quantified using a single-spot protein:creatinine ratio test. A ratio > 30 mg/mmol indicates significant proteinuria and, in the presence of new onset hypertension in pregnancy, indicates pre-eclampsia.

Blood tests are used to identify end-organ damage and HELLP syndrome, so named because its characteristics are Haemolysis, Elevated Liver enzymes and Low Platelets. HELLP syndrome affects 15% of women with pre-eclampsia; it is a severe form of the disease and has a 25% mortality rate. Significant maternal morbidity is related to liver rupture and cerebral oedema and haemorrhage. Tests for HELLP syndrome include full blood count, urea and electrolytes, liver function tests (LFTs) and coagulation tests. In addition to the characteristics that define the syndrome, renal function is frequently impaired and the PT and APTT are prolonged in the presence of disseminated intravascular coagulation (DIC).

Management

Management depends on disease severity and gestation at diagnosis. Antihypertensive drugs are used to reduce the blood pressure and the risk of maternal intracerebral haemorrhage, buying time for the fetus to reach sufficient maturity to be delivered.

Medication

Antihypertensive drugs are used to control blood pressure and thereby reduce the risk of complications (**Table 6.3**). However, they do not treat the underlying disease.

Magnesium sulphate is given to women who are at high risk of developing eclampsia. It is given as a loading dose followed by a maintenance infusion. It is also used to treat eclamptic seizures (see Chapter 14, page 353).

Placental blood flow is not autoregulated and therefore depends on maternal blood pressure. If blood pressure control is too tight, delivery of oxygen and nutrients to the fetus is restricted. This causes growth restriction and increases the risk of stillbirth.

Monitoring

Chronic hypertension and mild and moderate gestational hypertension are managed in the community. Blood pressure is monitored as clinically indicated and proteinuria checked at each visit. Blood tests are repeated if proteinuria develops. Ultrasound is used to determine fetal growth and amniotic fluid volume at 28 and 32 weeks in cases of chronic hypertension, and at the time of diagnosis of gestational hypertension, if before 34 weeks' gestation.

Severe hypertension and pre-eclampsia are managed in hospital (see page 353). Blood pressure is checked four times daily and

Antihypertensives used in pregnancy				
Drug	Mechanism of action	Route of administration	Line of therapy	Adverse effects
Labetalol	Alpha- and beta-adrenergic receptor blockers	Oral or intravenous	First	Bronchospasm (avoid in patients with asthma) Neonatal hypoglycaemia
Nifedipine	Calcium receptor antagonist	Oral	Second	Headache Flushing Palpitations Peripheral oedema
Hydralazine	Vascular smooth muscle relaxant	Oral or intravenous	Second	Chest pain Palpitations
Methyldopa	Alpha-adrenergic agonist	Oral	Third	Nightmares Depression (avoid postnatally) Fatigue Headache

Table 6.3 Antihypertensive drugs used in pregnancy

blood tests repeated every 3–4 days to detect HELLP syndrome. Fetal growth and amniotic fluid volume are determined by ultrasound at diagnosis and assessments repeated every 2–4 weeks.

Delivery

Chronic and gestational hypertension have a good prognosis, so delivery takes place after 37 weeks. In cases of pre-eclampsia, delivery after 34 weeks reduces the risk of adverse maternal and fetal outcomes.

Prognosis

Fetal mortality is 30% after an eclamptic seizure. Hypertension resolves in women with gestational hypertension and pre-eclampsia, but this can take 6 weeks. Women with hypertension in pregnancy are at increased risk of developing it again in later life.

Obstetric cholestasis

Obstetric cholestasis is a liver disease unique to pregnancy. It develops in the third trimester and resolves after delivery.

Epidemiology

Obstetric cholestasis affects 0.5–1% of pregnant women. Its incidence is higher in women of Indian or Pakistani origin and those born in Chile and Scandinavia, for unknown reasons.

Aetiology

Genetic factors are also important, however, as not every woman develops obstetric cholestasis. One third of patients have a positive family history.

Pathogenesis

The condition arises in pregnancy when increased oestrogen levels impair sulphation of bile acids and inhibit a bile acid export pump in liver cells. This has the effect of blocking the excretion of bile salts, which are deposited in the skin and cause itching, and damages hepatocytes. Use of the combined oral contraceptive pill, which contains oestrogen, triggers a similar syndrome.

Clinical features

Women with obstetric cholestasis have severe itching, particularly of the palms and soles, in the absence of a rash. Skin excoriation occurs as a consequence of scratching. Dark urine, pale stools and jaundice result from inhibition of the intrahepatic urobilinogen cycle (process of bilirubin excretion). Steatorrhoea (fatty stools) develops because of fat malabsorption.

Diagnostic approach

Unexplained abnormalities in liver transaminases (e.g. alanine transaminase), γ-glutamyl transferase and/or bile acids are diagnostic. However, other causes should be excluded (**Table 6.4**).

> Symptoms of obstetric cholestasis can develop before LFT abnormalities. Therefore LFTs are repeated every 1–2 weeks if unexplained itching persists.

Investigations

These include blood tests and ultrasound (**Table 6.4**). LFTs are repeated weekly to monitor the disease; a return to normal is inconsistent with obstetric cholestasis, and rapid escalation prompts a search for other causes.

Acute fatty liver of pregnancy is an important differential diagnosis, because although rare, affecting only 1 in 7000–20,000 pregnancies, it has high maternal and perinatal mortality rates (2% and 11%, respectively). Severe vomiting and abdominal pain are associated with significant increases in alanine transaminase and alkaline phosphatase concentration as well as disseminated intravascular coagulation (widespread activation of the

Obstetric cholestasis: investigations		
Test(s)	Reason for test(s)	Result in obstetric cholestasis
Liver function	To assess hepatocyte damage	Increased alanine transaminase and γ-glutamyl transferase Normal bilirubin and pregnancy-adjusted alkaline phosphatase
Bile acid	Most specific test for obstetric cholestasis	Increased
Coagulation	Reduced fat absorption decreases uptake of vitamin K, preventing clotting factor production	Normal or prolonged prothrombin time
Viral hepatitis screen: hepatitis A–C, Epstein–Barr virus, cytomegalovirus	To exclude other diseases	Normal, but compared with non-infected women, those with hepatitic C are at increased risk of obstetric cholestasis and develop symptoms earlier in pregnancy.
Autoimmune hepatitis screen: anti-smooth muscle antibodies and anti-mitochondrial antibodies	To exclude chronic active hepatitis and primary biliary cirrhosis, respectively	Normal
Liver ultrasound	To exclude gallstones and acute fatty liver of pregnancy	Normal
Blood pressure measurement and dipstick urinalysis	To exclude pre-eclampsia	Normal blood pressure and no proteinuria

Table 6.4 Investigations in suspected obstetric cholestasis

coagulation system causing simultaneous clotting and bleeding due to consumption of clotting factors). Expeditious delivery of the fetus and intensive supportive care, including dialysis and ventilation, improve prognosis. In the event of fulminant (sudden and severe) liver failure and hepatic encephalopathy (confusion and loss of consciousness due to liver disease), referral to a liver unit is required for consideration of transplantation.

Delays in diagnosing acute fatty liver of pregnancy can be lethal. It can be confused with HELLP syndrome (haemolysis, elevated liver enzyme and low platelets), of which it is a variant, but hypertension and proteinuria are only mild in acute fatty liver of pregnancy. Acute fatty liver of pregnancy is distinguished by significant hypoglycaemia, a marked increase in serum uric acid concentration, and coagulopathy with a normal platelet count.

Management

Management is supportive, with medication used to relieve symptoms. Delivery of the baby is the only known cure for the disease.

Medication

Obstetric cholestasis is treated with various medications.

Topical emollients such as aqueous cream with menthol are used to soothe the skin. The cooling effect of the menthol helps reduce the perception of itch.

Antihistamines, for example chlorphenamine, may be prescribed. They block the action of histamine which is responsible for activating C-nerve fibres, which transmit the sensation of itch to the brain. However, they can be sedating.

Ursodeoxycholic acid, 500 mg taken two or three times daily, relieves itching and improves LFT results by binding bile acids. However, it is not licensed for use in pregnancy and is of no proven benefit to the fetus.

If clotting is abnormal, vitamin K may be used to correct the reduction in vitamin K dependent clotting factors (10 mg daily, orally). It is not used if clotting is normal, because large doses cause neonatal haemolytic anaemia, and there is no increase in post-partum haemorrhage rates in women with obstetric cholestasis. At delivery, babies are given vitamin K intramuscularly to prevent haemorrhagic disease of the newborn. They are at risk of this due to reduced production of vitamin K dependent clotting factors.

> Historically, obstetric cholestasis was thought to cause fetal compromise and stillbirth; however, this belief has been challenged in more recent studies. Extra fetal monitoring is not required, because it does not predict fetal death, which is sudden and occurs in the absence of placental insufficiency.

Delivery

Women with obstetric cholestasis are delivered of their baby in an obstetric-led unit, because of the increased risk of meconium and fetal distress, and premature and operative delivery. Delivery is induced after 37 weeks because of the risk of stillbirth but this causes iatrogenic prematurity, respiratory distress, neonatal unit admission and failed induction, resulting in increased operative delivery rates.

Prognosis

Obstetric cholestasis resolves with delivery, and the easing of symptoms and normalisation of biochemical abnormalities confirms the diagnosis. Resolution can take time, so repeat LFTs are performed at least 10 days after delivery. The risk of recurrence in a future pregnancy is 90%.

Polyhydramnios

Polyhydramnios, the presence of excess amniotic fluid around the fetus, affects 1% of pregnancies. It is classified according to single deepest pool depth.

- Mild polyhydramnios: 8–11 cm
- Moderate polyhydramnios: 12–15 cm
- Severe polyhydramnios: > 16 cm

Aetiology

The volume of amniotic fluid is controlled by fetal swallowing and urination. Any imbalance in this intake and output results in polyhydramnios.

Polyhydramnios has both maternal and fetal causes (**Table 6.5**). The latter include TORCH infections: Toxoplasmosis, Other (varicella-zoster virus, syphilis and parvovirus), Rubella, Cytomegalovirus and Herpes.

Clinical features

The symphysis–fundal height is greater than expected for the week of gestation, the maternal abdominal skin is stretched and shiny,

Polyhydramnios: maternal and fetal causes	
Maternal causes	Fetal causes
Gestational diabetes	Intrauterine infection (TORCH*)
Cardiac failure	
Kidney disease	Fetal anomalies:
Haemolytic disease of the newborn	■ oesophageal or duodenal atresia
Placental chorioangioma	■ tracheo-oesophageal fistula
Unexplained (> 80% of cases of mild polyhydramnios but < 10% of severe cases)	■ diaphragmatic hernia
	■ anencephaly
	Twin-to-twin transfusion syndrome
	Kidney disease (e.g. Bartter's syndrome)
	Chromosomal abnormalities (e.g. Down's syndrome, Edwards' syndrome)
	Skeletal dysplasia

*Toxoplasmosis, Other (varicella-zoster virus, syphilis and parvovirus), Rubella, Cytomegalovirus and Herpes.

Table 6.5 Maternal and fetal causes of polyhydramnios

the uterus is tense, and the different parts of the fetus are difficult to palpate. Inhibition of movement (splinting) of the diaphragm by the enlarged uterus causes shortness of breath.

Investigations

Ultrasound is used to measure the amniotic fluid pool depth and to screen for fetal anomalies. Amniocentesis is offered if a chromosomal abnormality is suspected. Maternal blood is checked for atypical alloimmune antibodies and evidence of recent infection with a TORCH organism. An oral glucose tolerance test is carried out to screen for gestational diabetes.

Management

Mild asymptomatic polyhydramnios is managed expectantly (i.e. with no intervention).

Medication

Indometacin decreases amniotic fluid volume by reducing urine production by the fetal kidneys. However, it also causes premature closure of the ductus arteriosus.

Surgery

In symptomatic women, excess fluid is drained by amniocentesis. However, the fluid reaccumulates and the procedure carries a risk of miscarriage (see Chapter 4, page 155).

Prognosis

Uterine stretch increases the risk of:

- preterm labour
- abruption
- preterm prelabour rupture of the membranes
- post-partum haemorrhage
- unstable fetal lie (where the fetus continuously changes its lie, from cephalic to breech and transverse and back again), leading to delivery complications including cord prolapse (see page 355)

Idiopathic polyhydramnios is not associated with adverse fetal outcomes. If fetal and placental abnormalities are present, the perinatal mortality rate is up to 60%.

Medical disorders in pregnancy

Women with underlying medical problems are managed in specialist clinics during pregnancy. The aim of care is to monitor for disease exacerbation, prevent long term deterioration in maternal health and minimise risks to the fetus. Optimising disease control prior to pregnancy, in conjunction with pre-conception counselling, is necessary to ensure the best possible outcome for mother and baby. Common medical disorders seen in pregnancy are:

- infections
- obesity
- epilepsy
- cardiac disease

Infections

Babies born to mothers with hepatitis B, hepatitis C and HIV are at risk of viral transmission. This can occur antenatally, intrapartum or postnatally. Perinatal infections cause 2–3% of congenital anomalies. The TORCH organisms are the commonest causes of these infections (**Table 6.6**). Maternal symptoms of infection are mild, but the potential consequences for the fetus are severe.

Epidemiology

The prevalence of HIV varies between and within countries. For example, in the UK about 1 in 700 women giving birth are HIV-positive, and the highest rates are in central London (1 in 250 women). UK rates of HIV positivity are highest in women of Sub-Saharan origin: 2–3.5%, compared with < 0.02% in women born in the UK. In parts of Southern Africa, 30% of pregnant women are infected with HIV.

TORCH infections: incidence, sources and risk of complications

Infection	Incidence	Sources	Gestation and risk
Toxoplasmosis	Varies throughout the world, 1 in 5000 pregnancies in the UK	Soil Undercooked or raw meat Lambing Cat faeces	Risk of transmission increases as pregnancy progresses, from 10–15% in first trimester to 70–80% by third trimester. Consequences become less severe with advancing gestation
Varicella-zoster virus	3 in 1000 pregnancies	Respiratory droplets Direct contact with vesicle fluid Indirect contact with objects that carry infection (e.g. skin, hair, bedding)	Fetal varicella syndrome: 1–2% risk if infection before 28 weeks, no risk after Varicella infection of the newborn: 25% risk in cases of maternal infection 1–4 weeks before birth
Parvovirus	1–3 in 100 pregnancies	Respiratory droplets	Risk of complications if < 20 weeks' gestation
Rubella	Rare (only 9 cases in England and Wales in 2014)	Respiratory droplets	Risk of complications if < 16 weeks' gestation 90% risk of fetal anomalies before 12 weeks 10–20% risk of fetal anomalies at 12–16 weeks
Cytomegalovirus	1 in 100 pregnancies	Bodily fluids (e.g. saliva, urine, sexual fluids)	Transmission risk increases as pregnancy progresses, from 40% in first trimester of pregnancy to 75–80% by third trimester, but consequences less severe with advancing gestation
Herpes	1 in 7500–15,000	Skin-to-skin contact Sexual intercourse	Third trimester, particularly within 6 weeks of delivery

Table 6.6 TORCH infections: their incidence and sources of infection. TORCH infections carry differing levels of risk depending on the gestation.

Similarly, hepatitis prevalence varies. The UK has a low prevalence of hepatitis B; 0.1–0.5% of the population are infected. In contrast, carrier rates are 10–15% in parts of Africa and Asia. Hepatitis C is transmitted by infected needles. In the UK, half of intravenous drug users are affected.

Clinical features

Toxoplasmosis

Toxoplasmosis (infection with *Toxoplasma gondii*) is asymptomatic in the mother in most cases, but presents with flu-like illness and lymphadenopathy in some patients. Infections can cause miscarriage, particularly if they occur within the first 10 weeks of pregnancy. Complications for the fetus are:

- Hydrocephalus and intellectual disabilities
- Cerebral calcifications
- Chorioretinitis causing blindness, which develops in childhood or adulthood despite vision appearing normal at birth

Varicella-zoster virus

Varicella-zoster virus infection presents in the mother with:

- fever
- malaise
- maculopapular rash (chicken pox)

Pneumonia, hepatitis and encephalitis are more common with adult infections and are associated with increased morbidity and mortality.

There is no increased risk of miscarriage, however the fetus can develop fetal varicella syndrome which presents with:

- scarring in dermatomal distribution
- eye defects (e.g. chorioretinitis)
- microcephaly
- cortical atrophy
- intellectual disability
- bladder and bowel sphincter dysfunction

Babies born with varicella infection present with the same symptoms as the mother. It has a mortality rate of 30%.

Parvovirus

Parvovirus infection is asymptomatic in the mother in 20–30% of cases. The remainder present with:

- Non-vesicular facial rash ('slapped cheek')
- Malaise
- Sore throat
- Mild fever
- Arthropathy (painful joints)
- Anaemia and anaplastic crisis (temporary cessation of red blood cell production)

Parvovirus infection carries a 15% risk of infection before 20 weeks' gestation, decreasing to 2% after 20 weeks. There is no increased risk of the fetus developing congenital anomalies. Hydrops fetalis (abnormal accumulation of fluid in two or more fetal compartments, e.g. ascites, pleural effusion, skin oedema) is a fetal complication resulting from fetal anaemia and cardiac failure.

Rubella

Rubella presents in the mother with:

- Malaise
- Fever
- Conjunctivitis
- Coryzal symptoms (e.g. runny nose, sore throat)
- Macular rash
- Arthropathy
- Post-auricular lymphadenopathy

Fetal complications are:

- Miscarriage
- Stillbirth
- Intrauterine growth restriction
- Sensorineural deafness
- Microcephaly and intellectual disability
- Cataracts
- Cardiac defects

Cytomegalovirus

Cytomegalovirus infections are asymptomatic in the mother in most cases, but present with flu-like illness, lymphadenopathy, fever and sore throat in some patients. Fetal complications are:

- Hepatosplenomegaly
- Thrombocytopenia
- Intracranial calcification
- Hearing loss
- Chorioretinitis
- Microcephaly and intellectual disability
- Intrauterine growth restriction
- Stillbirth

Of the 5–15% of infected babies acutely symptomatic at birth, 30% will die (>70% within the first year of life) and 80% have serious sequelae. Between 10% and 15% of asymptomatically-infected babies subsequently develop auditory, visual or neurological defects.

Herpes

In the mother primary genital herpes presents with painful ulcers. Disseminated herpes presents with encephalitis, hepatitis and widespread skin lesions. Patient with recurrent disease are usually asymptomatic.

Herpes infection has no increased risk of miscarriage. In the fetus, in 30% of cases it is localised to skin, eyes and mouth, and with antiviral treatment morbidity is < 2%. In 70% of cases there is disseminated disease with or without central nervous system involvement; neurological morbidity is 70% and mortality 6–30%, even with treatment.

Diagnostic approach

Pregnant women are screened for HIV and hepatitis B at the booking visit. HIV screening is reoffered at 28 weeks to those who decline initially. Screening for hepatitis C is offered to women at high risk of infection. Serological testing is carried out after exposure to TORCH organisms, as well as after ultrasound detection of congenital anomalies and severe growth restriction.

Investigations

Women known to be HIV-positive have regular (at least once every trimester) assessments of their viral load (HIV RNA) and CD4 count. The results are used to determine the timing of initiating antiretroviral therapy, as well as the mode of delivery i.e. vaginal delivery or caesarean section.

In women with hepatitis B or C, viral load is assessed because the result is used to assess the risk of fetal and neonatal transmission. This is performed early in the pregnancy and may be repeated in the third trimester.

Positive immunoglobulin M antibodies to a TORCH organism are diagnostic of recent infection. The presence of immunoglobulin G antibodies indicates previous or current infection; an increasing immunoglobulin G titre for samples taken 2 weeks apart confirms acute disease. Amniocentesis and viral detection by PCR or culture confirm fetal infection but do not identify associated fetal anomalies. Serial ultrasound scans are required to screen for complications of infection.

Management

The aim of management is to reduce the risk of transmission. Termination of pregnancy is selectively offered to women with TORCH infections, depending on the causative organism, the gestation at which infection occurred and the presence or absence of fetal anomalies.

Medication

HIV

Women with HIV who conceived while receiving antiretroviral therapy continue to use it throughout pregnancy. Women who do not require antiretroviral therapy for their own health start using it by 24 weeks. This allows time for reduction of viral load and therefore risk of transmission. Cabergoline is used postnatally to suppress lactation in women with HIV.

> **Antiretroviral medication has no significant effect on the rate of fetal anomalies, but a few types cause gestational diabetes.** Therefore women taking these drugs require an oral glucose tolerance test.

Hepatitis

Antiviral drugs are used in the third trimester for women with hepatitis B and a high viral load. There is no safe drug treatment for hepatitis C in pregnancy.

Toxoplasmosis

Spiramycin is given prophylactically to reduce the risk of parasitic transmission; it does not reduce the risk of fetal anomalies. If the fetus is infected, pyrimethamine and spiramycin are given to reduce disease severity:

- Pyrimethamine is teratogenic so is not used in the first trimester
- Pyrimethamine is a folate antagonist; folinic acid supplements are needed to reduce the adverse effects of folate deficiency

Parvovirus

There is no drug treatment available. Intrauterine transfusions are given to treat fetal anaemia.

Rubella

There is no drug treatment available. Cochlear implants and cardiac surgery may be needed for the child after birth.

Cytomegalovirus

Antiviral mediation (e.g. ganciclovir and cidofovir) is given to babies with congenital infection to reduce the risk of hearing loss.

Herpes

Primary disease is treated with aciclovir, which reduces maternal symptoms and decreases viral shedding. For women who have had primary infection in pregnancy, aciclovir is given prophylactically from 36 weeks' gestation to reduce the need for caesarean section; it is not indicated in recurrent disease.

Delivery

HIV

Women with an HIV viral load of < 50 RNA copies/mL at 36 weeks' gestation have vaginal delivery, provided there are no obstetric contraindications for this. If the viral load is > 50 RNA copies/mL at 36 weeks, caesarean section is carried out to reduce the risk of intrapartum transmission of infection. Delivery is expedited in cases of prelabour rupture of membranes at term. Intravenous zidovudine (azidothymidine, AZT) is given to women with an HIV viral load > 1000 RNA copies/mL at the time of delivery.

Traditionally, the use of artificial rupture of membranes, fetal blood sampling and fetal scalp electrodes has been avoided for HIV-positive women in labour. These practices were thought to increase the risk of mother-to-child viral transmission. However, since the introduction of antiretroviral therapy, viral loads have decreased significantly and labour is now managed along the same lines as in women without HIV.

Hepatitis

Mode of delivery has no effect on transmission rates for hepatitis B and C. Therefore, there are no recommendations regarding vaginal delivery or caesarean section.

Herpes

For women who have primary infection in the third trimester, delivery by caesarean section is indicated to decrease the neonatal viral transmission. For women with recurrent herpes, vaginal delivery is recommended even if lesions are present because the risk of transmission is only 0–3%.

TORCH infection

Mode of delivery has no effect on transmission of TORCH organisms, therefore there are no recommendations regarding vaginal delivery or caesarean section.

Breastfeeding

This increases the risk of postnatal HIV transmission, so it is avoided in high-income countries. In middle and low-income countries, the risk of sickness and death from infected water used to make up formula milk outweighs the risk of HIV infection from breast milk.

Women with hepatitis B and C are encouraged to breastfeed, because transmission through breast milk is very rare. Transmission of TORCH organisms in breast milk is rare, with the exception of CMV. Even in this case, infection is highly unlikely and women are encouraged to breast feed even if they have been infected antenatally.

Neonatal vaccination

No HIV or hepatitis C vaccine is available. Babies born to mothers with hepatitis B receive the first dose of the hepatitis B vaccine and a dose of hepatitis B immunoglobulin within 12 h of birth. Further doses of vaccine are given at 1 and 6 months of age. Mothers identified antenatally as rubella non-immune are offered rubella vaccination following delivery. There are no vaccines currently available as prophylaxis against infection with the other TORCH organisms.

Prognosis

Antiretroviral therapy, appropriate management of delivery and avoidance of breastfeeding reduce the risk of mother-tochild transmission of HIV from 25% to 1%.

Immunisation of neonates born to mothers with hepatitis B is 85–95% effective at preventing infection, which would otherwise lead to chronic hepatitis B in > 90% of cases.

The risk of hepatitis C transmission is 10%. This is increased in the presence of coinfection with HIV. TORCH infections are not associated with long-term maternal complications; the fetal sequelae are discussed above.

Obesity

Obesity, defined as BMI >30 kg/m², is increasingly prevalent worldwide. For example 20% of pregnant women in the UK had a BMI ≥ 30 kg/m² in 2015. It is associated with adverse outcomes for both mother and baby (Table 6.7).

Prevention

A woman with a BMI > 30 kg/m² is advised to achieve or maintain a weight-neutral

Risks of maternal obesity	
Risks to mother	**Risks to fetus**
Gestational diabetes	Miscarriage
Gestational hypertension and pre-eclampsia	Fetal anomalies, particularly neural tube defects, cardiac defects and omphalocele (an abdominal wall defect)
Operative vaginal delivery and caesarean section	
Difficulty siting epidurals and carrying out intubation	Stillbirth
Wound infection and breakdown	Prematurity
Post-partum haemorrhage	Undiagnosed small-for-gestational-age fetus
Venous thromboembolism	Shoulder dystocia
	Childhood and adolescent obesity

Table 6.7 Maternal and fetal risks associated with obesity

pregnancy, i.e. one without significant weight gain or loss. This reduces the risk of further problems during the pregnancy. Light exercise and dietary modification is recommended. The following prophylactic drugs are advised:

- folic acid 5 mg/day to reduce the risk of neural tube defects
- vitamin D to prevent deficiency
- aspirin to reduce the risk of pre-eclampsia

Diagnostic approach

Body mass index is calculated at the booking visit. Women whose BMI is more than 35 kg/m^2 are referred to a specialist antenatal service.

Investigations

Investigations are done to screen for complications of obesity in pregnancy.

- Ultrasound is used for:
  - early detection of miscarriage
  - screening for fetal abnormalities, although this is technically challenging in women with obesity
  - assessment of growth, because symphysis-fundal height measurement is inaccurate in this group of patients
- Blood pressure is measured and dipstick urinalysis carried out to detect pre-eclampsia
- An oral glucose tolerance test is done for the diagnosis of gestational diabetes

- A manual handling and tissue viability assessment are carried out in the third trimester to ensure that appropriate equipment and personnel will be available at delivery. This is carried out by completing the relevant questionnaire.

> **A cuff of appropriate size is needed for blood pressure measurements in women with obesity.** This avoids over- or underestimation as a result of a cuff that is too tight or too loose, respectively.

Management

The babies of women with BMI ≥ 35 kg/m^2 are delivered in obstetric-led units, because of the higher risk of intrapartum complications.

Medication

Low-molecular-weight heparin reduces the risk of venous thromboembolism in obese women with additional risk factors. Women with BMI > 40 kg/m^2 receive heparin injections for at least 1 week after delivery, regardless of mode. The dose is weight-adjusted.

Delivery

Women with BMI > 40 kg/m^2 are referred to an anaesthetist antenatally for planning of analgesia and anaesthesia in labour.

A fetal scalp electrode is used if abdominal auscultation of the fetal heart rate is not possible. Intravenous access is secured early in labour in case of emergency. This allows intravenous anaesthetic drugs to be given if a caesarean section is required and oxytocic drugs to treat postpartum haemorrhage.

The third stage of labour is managed actively (see Chapter 4, page 162) to reduce the risk of post-partum haemorrhage.

Breastfeeding

Women with obesity are given extra encouragement and support to breastfeed. They benefit from the increased calorie expenditure and reduction in childhood diabetes but are less likely to breastfeed because of perceptions of difficulty in positioning and impaired prolactin response to suckling.

Epilepsy

Epilepsy is the commonest neurological disorder in pregnant women.

Epilepsy affects 0.5% of women of childbearing age.

Aetiology

There are several types of epilepsy, which differ in age of onset and type of seizure. Most cases are of unknown aetiology, but a family history is reported in a third of cases. Epilepsy can also be secondary to brain tumour, surgery or head trauma.

> **Epilepsy is usually diagnosed before pregnancy.** A first seizure in pregnancy is due to eclampsia until proven otherwise.

Investigations

A first seizure in pregnancy prompts screening for pre-eclampsia by measuring blood pressure and using dipstick urinalysis to test for proteinuria. Blood samples are taken for a platelet count, renal and liver function tests, coagulation tests, measurement of glucose and calcium concentration, and a drug screen, to investigate other causes of seizure. CT or MRI of the head is carried out to exclude mass lesions or haemorrhage as a cause of the seizure or complication of pre-eclampsia. Electroencephalography is required if epilepsy is suspected.

Management

Epilepsy in pregnancy is managed by balancing the teratogenic risk from antiepileptic medication against worsening seizure control.

Medication

Many antiepileptic drugs cause fetal abnormalities, including neural tube defects, cleft lip and palate and congenital heart abnormalities. The risk of abnormalities increases with the number of drugs prescribed.

- Sodium valproate has the highest rate of congenital anomalies: 6–11%, twice that of other antiepileptic drugs
- Carbamazepine and lamotrigine have a 2–2.5% incidence of malformations, just above the background rate

Generally, antiepileptic drugs should continue to be used in pregnancy, because the risk of seizures generally outweighs the risk of teratogenicity.

> **Women with epilepsy are encouraged to switch from sodium valproate to another antiepileptic drug before pregnancy,** unless it is the only drug able to control their seizures. If it is used, the daily dose is split into multiple doses to reduce peak concentration and, therefore, teratogenic potential.

All antiepileptic drugs have the potential to cause fetal anticonvulsant syndrome. Symptoms and signs include a reduction in IQ and dysmorphic features:

- small palpebral fissures
- short nose
- flat mid-face
- indistinct philtrum
- thin upper lip
- epicanthal folds
- low nasal bridge
- minor ear abnormalities
- maxillary hypoplasia
- micrognathia

Folic acid 5 mg/day reduces the risk of neural tube defects. It is started before conception and continued throughout pregnancy, because antiepileptic drugs cause folate deficiency.

Women prescribed liver enzyme-inducing antiepileptic drugs, for example carbamazepine, also take vitamin K (10–20 mg orally) from 36 weeks' gestation, to prevent vitamin K-dependent clotting factor deficiency. Vitamin K is also given intramuscularly to the baby at birth to reduce the risk of haemorrhagic disease of the newborn.

Delivery

Epilepsy is not an indication for induction of labour or caesarean section. The risk of seizures during labour is 1–2%; they are stimulated by pain, anxiety and sleep deprivation. An early epidural is beneficial in reducing these triggers.

Prognosis

Seizure frequency is not affected by pregnancy. Deterioration in seizure control results from poor adherence to drug regimens because of fears about teratogenicity.

The fetus is resistant to the short periods of hypoxia associated with single seizures. There is a 4–5% risk of the child also developing epilepsy.

Cardiac disease

Cardiac disease is classified as:

- congenital, for example transposition of the great arteries, atrial and ventricular septal defects
- acquired, for example coronary artery disease, rheumatic fever

Epidemiology

The incidence of cardiac disease in pregnancy is increasing as more women with congenital cardiac disease are surviving into adulthood. In high-income countries, 80% of cardiac disease in pregnancy is congenital, this proportion is smaller in other countries. Outside Europe and North America, rheumatic heart disease is the commonest cause of cardiovascular disease.

Aetiology

Congenital cardiac disease is caused by malformation of the heart during development.

Acquired cardiac disease caused by coronary artery disease is increasing due to the rising incidence of obesity and diabetes in an ageing population.

Peripartum cardiomyopathy is a dilated cardiomyopathy of unknown aetiology that causes loss of cardiac function. It is unique to pregnancy and presents between the last month of pregnancy and 6 months after birth with breathlessness, peripheral oedema and palpitations as a result of heart failure. It is a diagnosis of exclusion.

Clinical features

The symptoms experienced by women with cardiac disease during pregnancy depend upon the underlying disease, the impact this has on cardiac function and whether they have pulmonary hypertension (a poor prognostic sign). They range from being assyptomatic to symptoms of heart failure, i.e. breathlessness on exertion, orthopnoea (breathless when lying flat) and peripheral oedema. In general, symptoms increase in pregnancy as the circulating blood volume increases and greater demands are placed on the heart.

Investigations

The aim of investigations is to assess maternal and fetal well-being (**Table 6.9**).

> Exercise testing is carried out informally in clinic by monitoring the distance that can be walked before breathlessness develops. Worsening exercise tolerance can warrant a change in medication or even delivery of the fetus.

Management

The management of cardiac disease in pregnancy is based on the same ethos as used in other medical conditions. The extent of intervention and frequency of review is dependent on cardiac function.

Cardiac disease in pregnancy is managed in joint obstetric–cardiology clinics.

Medication

Aspirin is used prophylactically in women with coronary artery disease. It is safe at doses

Cardiac disease in pregnancy: maternal and fetal assessment

Investigation	Reason for investigation
Maternal	
Electrocardiography	To detect palpitations or arrhythmias
Echocardiography	to assess ventricular and valve function
Exercise testing	To assess functional capacity and detect heart failure
Fetal	
Cardiac ultrasound	To detect congenital heart disease (2–5% risk)
Genetic testing	To identify specific chromosomal abnormalities or mutations associated with congenital heart disease, e.g. Down's syndrome
Serial assessment of fetal growth and well-being by ultrasound from 28 weeks	To detect placental dysfunction and fetal compromise, for which there is an increased risk

Table 6.9 Cardiac disease in pregnancy: assessment of maternal and fetal well-being

of 150–300 mg in the rare event of an acute myocardial infarction during pregnancy.

Antibiotic prophylaxis during labour to prevent endocarditis in women with cardiac defects is no longer recommended.

Women with metallic heart valves require thromboprophylaxis to reduce the risk of valve thrombosis. Warfarin is used outside pregnancy but is teratogenic and, therefore, avoided if possible; it causes miscarriage, cerebral haemorrhage, central nervous system defects, hypoplasia of the nasal bridge, shortened fingers resulting from epiphyseal stippling (abnormality of bone ends) and growth restriction. High-dose heparin is safe, but the risk of valve thrombosis is higher.

Treatment of peripartum cardiomyopathy is the same as that for heart failure in general, with diuretics, beta-blockers, digoxin and angiotensin-converting enzyme inhibitors (the last of these after delivery). Anticoagulation reduces the risk of left ventricular thrombosis. Cardiac transplantation is the only option if severe ventricular dysfunction does not improve with delivery and medical support.

Delivery

This takes place in an obstetric-led unit with cardiology and anaesthetic expertise. Vaginal delivery is preferred, as this has the best outcome for mother and baby, and induction used to time delivery, particularly for women receiving anticoagulant drugs. Arterial lines are used for invasive maternal monitoring of blood pressure and heart rate.

Early epidural reduces pain associated increased sympathetic nerve activity. A prolonged second stage of labour is avoided by resorting to operative vaginal delivery, if necessary. Use of the Valsava manoeuvre during pushing reduces venous return.

Prevention of maternal haemorrhage after delivery is necessary to prevent decompensation. Low-dose oxytocin infusions are used to avoid peripheral vasodilation, tachycardia and fluid retention, which occur with boluses. Ergometrine is contraindicated, because it causes hypertension and increases the risk of myocardial infarction and pulmonary oedema.

Prognosis

The outcome is good if a left-to-right shunt is present and the woman has minimal symptoms, but women with stenotic valvular lesions and reduced ventricular function do less well. Pulmonary hypertension is a contraindication to pregnancy, because the maternal mortality rate is 30–50%. Therefore termination of pregnancy is offered to women with this disorder.

Peripartum cardiomyopathy has a maternal mortality rate of 6–10%. Half of patients make a full recovery, with prognosis depending on residual left ventricular dysfunction at 6 months. The risk of recurrence and death is significant in future pregnancies if ventricular function does not return to normal.

Haemolytic disease of the newborn

Haemolytic disease of the newborn is a severe form of anaemia caused by incompatibility between maternal and fetal blood types. It is caused by the passage of red blood cell antibodies across the placenta from mother to fetus, which have been generated in response to previous exposure to incompatible blood. The rhesus group of red blood cell antigens is the commonest target for the antibodies, but others, including ABO and Kell and Duffy antigens, are also causative.

Epidemiology

Atypical antibodies are detected in 1.2% of pregnancies, though only 0.4% are clinically relevant. Severe haemolytic disease of the newborn affects 7–8 per 100,000 pregnancies.

Aetiology

IgM antibodies are produced when cells of the maternal immune system are exposed to a 'foreign' antigen on fetal red blood cells. This sensitisation occurs in fetomaternal haemorrhage (see Chapter 4, page 159), blood transfusion or exposure to environmental antigens found in food, bacteria and viruses.

The current pregnancy is not affected, because the mother's immune system is exposed to a low dose of antigen. However, the response of the now sensitised immune system is amplified with repeated antigen exposure in a subsequent pregnancy. The resulting immune-mediated hemolysis, i.e. the destruction of fetal red blood cells, and the fetal response to it, underlies hemolytic disease of the newborn.

Prevention

Prophylactic anti-D reduces the risk of severe haemolytic disease of the newborn in rhesus-negative women (see Chapter 4, page 159).

Pathogenesis

Haemolytic disease of the newborn is most commonly caused by rhesus antibodies. These are produced when a rhesus negative woman becomes pregnant by a rhesus positive father and the fetus is rhesus positive. The rhesus incompatibility between the mother and the fetus results in sensitisation of the maternal immune system in the first pregnancy and destruction of fetal red blood cells in any subsequent rhesus-positive pregnancy (**Figure 6.1**). IgG antibodies cross the placenta and mediate this effect.

Clinical features

Damage to fetal red blood cells causes:

- anaemia
- increased erythropoiesis and hepatosplenomegaly
- jaundice arising from hyperbilirubinaemia
- oedema and polyhydramnios as a consequence of high-output heart failure

In severe cases, fetal death in utero or neonatal death can occur.

Diagnostic approach

Blood group screening to detect atypical antibodies is offered at the booking visit and 28 weeks' gestation. Women with clinically significant antibodies are referred to a fetal medicine department for further investigation.

Investigations

Antibody titres are used to guide further management. If antibody levels are significantly increased, the fetal genotype is determined using cell-free fetal DNA testing (see Chapter 4, page 155). If the gene is absent, no further monitoring is required because there is no risk of haemolytic disease of the newborn.

To detect anaemia in at-risk pregnancies, Doppler ultrasound is used weekly to measure the velocity of blood flow in the middle cerebral artery of the fetus. An anaemic fetus tries to maintain adequate tissue oxygen delivery by increasing its cardiac output. Also, its blood viscosity is reduced as a consequence of loss of red blood cells. These effects increase blood

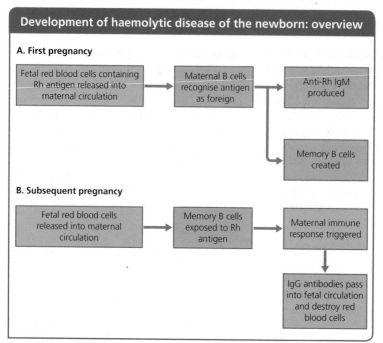

Development of haemolytic disease of the newborn: overview

A. First pregnancy

Fetal red blood cells containing Rh antigen released into maternal circulation → Maternal B cells recognise antigen as foreign → Anti-Rh IgM produced

→ Memory B cells created

B. Subsequent pregnancy

Fetal red blood cells released into maternal circulation → Memory B cells exposed to Rh antigen → Maternal immune response triggered

→ IgG antibodies pass into fetal circulation and destroy red blood cells

Figure 6.1 Overview of development of haemolytic disease of the newborn: production of maternal antibodies in response to exposure to 'foreign' rhesus (Rh) antigen on fetal red blood cells in a first Rh-positive pregnancy in a Rh-negative mother. Anti-Rh, anti-rhesus Ig, immunoglobulin.

flow velocity in the middle cerebral artery.

If the velocity is > 1.5 multiples of the median for the gestation, a sample of fetal blood is taken from the placental cord insertion site or intrahepatic vein to determine haemoglobin concentration, and blood transfusion is carried out simultaneously.

Management

Management depends on the gestation of the fetus and the degree of fetal compromise.

Delivery

Delivery is expedited when the risk of the fetus remaining in utero is deemed higher than the risk of prematurity; this is usually at 37–38 weeks' gestation. Senior paediatric support is needed at delivery, along with facilities for fetal blood transfusion.

Intrauterine transfusion

This can be carried out weekly if required to treat significant anaemia and fetal compromise. However, it is not used after 35 weeks, because delivery is more appropriate from that time.

Prognosis

The severity of haemolytic disease of the newborn is variable: 50% of affected babies have normal haemoglobin, 25% have moderate disease requiring blood transfusion and 25% have severe disease. Overall survival is 84–90%, but is <40% for those fetuses whose cardiac failure is not reversed by in utero transfusion.

Multiple pregnancy

In multiple pregnancies, two or more fetuses develop in the womb simultaneously. These pregnancies have an increased risk of most pregnancy-related complications, including pre-eclampsia, growth restriction and pre-term birth. If twins share a single placenta, abnormal blood flow can result in twin-to-twin transfusion syndrome. This is where connections between blood vessels in the placenta result in one fetus receiving too little blood and becoming growth restricted and the other receiving too much and developing heart failure.

Epidemiology

Multiple pregnancies currently account for 1–2% of all births, but this proportion is increasing with the use of fertility treatments. About 1 in 80 naturally conceived pregnancies produce twins, and 1 in 6400 (1:80) produce triplets.

Aetiology

One third of twins are monozygotic; they are formed from one fertilised oocyte and are therefore identical. The remaining two thirds are dizygotic: they develop from two separate fertilised oocytes (if two oocytes have ovulated simultaneously) and are non-identical. When the embryo divides after fertilisation determines whether monozygotic twins have one or two amnions and chorions or are conjoined (**Figure 6.2**).

The cause of monozygotic twin pregnancies is unknown. Dizygotic twin pregnancies are more common in older women (for unknown reasons), after fertility treatment (due to transfer of multiple embryos in IVF), Africans and when there is a maternal family history of twins (genetic predisposition).

Diagnostic approach

Chorionicity is determined by ultrasound most accurately before 14 weeks' gestation. The presence of the lambda or twin peak sign (triangular appearance of the chorion in the inter-twin space) indicates dichorionic pregnancy, whereas the T sign (right-angle junction between the inter-twin membrane and external rim) indicates monochorionic twins. Monochorionic pregnancies are at

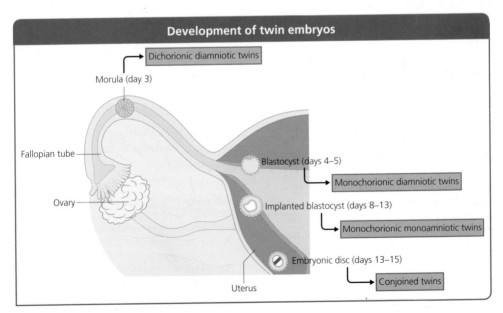

Development of twin embryos

Dichorionic diamniotic twins

Morula (day 3)

Fallopian tube

Ovary

Blastocyst (days 4–5)

Monochorionic diamniotic twins

Implanted blastocyst (days 8–13)

Monochorionic monoamniotic twins

Embryonic disc (days 13–15)

Conjoined twins

Uterus

Figure 6.2 Embryological development of twin pregnancies.

higher risk of complications than dichorionic pregnancies.

Investigations

The combined test (combined ultrasound and serum testing for β-human chorionic gonadotrophin and pregnancy associated plasma protein A) is used to screen for Down's syndrome in twin pregnancies, and nuchal thickness and maternal age are used in triplet pregnancies. Both are performed before 14 weeks' gestation. Second trimester serum screening is used if the nuchal thickness cannot be measured; it has a higher false positive rate and lower sensitivity in twin pregnancies than in singleton pregnancies and is not used in triplet pregnancies. As in singleton pregnancies, ultrasound is used between 18 and 20 weeks' gestation to screen for fetal anomalies.

Fetal growth is difficult to assess clinically in multiple pregnancy. Serial ultrasound is used instead from 24 weeks. A size discordance of ≥ 25% between twins or triplets is clinically significant, and warrants referral to a fetal medicine unit for further investigation and monitoring.

Monitoring is more frequent in the early stages of monochorionic pregnancies, because of the risk of twin-to-twin transfusion syndrome. Fortnightly ultrasound scans are carried out from 16–24 weeks.

Management

Twin pregnancies are managed in an obstetric-led unit. Monoamniotic twin and triplet pregnancies require referral to a tertiary fetal medicine unit, as the risk of complications is even higher in these pregnancies.

Delivery

Preterm delivery is common in multiple pregnancies; 60% of twins and 75% of triplets are delivered spontaneously before 37 and 35 weeks, respectively. To reduce the risk of late stillbirth in uncomplicated monochorionic diamniotic and dichorionic pregnancies, delivery is by induction of labour or caesarean section at 36 and 37 weeks, respectively.

Labour is induced for twin pregnancies when the first twin presents cephalically, regardless of the presentation of the second twin. Caesarean section is recommended to reduce perinatal morbidity and mortality when the first twin is in a breech or transverse presentation. Monochorionic monoamniotic twins are the exception. They should be delivered at 32 weeks by caesarean section to avoid the risk of cord entanglement.

Antepartum haemorrhage

Antepartum haemorrhage is any vaginal bleeding from 24 weeks' gestation until delivery. The most serious diagnoses are:

- placental abruption, i.e. separation of the placenta from the uterine wall before birth
- placenta praevia, a placenta partially or wholly covering the cervix
- placenta accreta, a placenta that is abnormally adherent to the myometrium, usually at the site of the scar from a previous caesarean section
- vasa praevia, i.e. bleeding from fetal vessels

Epidemiology

Antepartum haemorrhage complicates 3–5% of pregnancies. It is associated with up to 25% of preterm births.

> **For pregnancies affected by placenta accreta, up to 33% of caesarean sections result in hysterectomy.** Partial detachment of the placenta causes massive haemorrhage. Planned hysterectomy with the placenta left in place reduces bleeding but prevents further pregnancies.

Antepartum haemorrhage: causes		
Bleeding from external genitalia and vagina	Bleeding from cervix	Bleeding from uterus
Trauma	'Show'	Placental abruption
Infection	Cervicitis	Placenta praevia and accreta
Vulval or vaginal cancer (rare in women of childbearing age)	Cervical polyp	Vasa praevia
	Cervical cancer	Uterine rupture

Table 6.10 Causes of antepartum haemorrhage

Aetiology

Bleeding can arise from the external genitalia, cervix or uterus (**Table 6.10**). The cause is unknown in 40% of cases.

Risk factors for abruption include:

- abdominal trauma
- multiple pregnancy
- polyhydramnios
- premature rupture of membranes
- smoking
- cocaine use
- previous abruption (4% if one abruption, 25% if two previous abruptions)

Clinical features

Abruption presents with pain and bleeding. Fetal compromise and maternal collapse, disproportionate to the visible amount of blood lost, can occur.

Placenta praevia and vasa praevia are painless bleeds. Bleeding secondary to vasa praevia occurs after rupture of membranes, either artificial or spontaneous.

Diagnostic approach

Maternal well-being is assessed and resuscitation started, if appropriate (see page 350). Observations including blood pressure, pulse and respiratory rate are carried out and the results used to guide management. Abdominal and speculum examinations are done to help diagnose the cause of bleeding and quantify the blood loss.

The placental location on previous ultrasound scans is reviewed.

A digital vaginal examination is not carried out until the placental location has been determined by ultrasound. In the case of placenta praevia, the examination triggers significant bleeding.

Investigations

Ultrasound is used to exclude placenta praevia. It is not helpful for the diagnosis of abruption or screening for vasa praevia.

Intravenous access is gained when blood loss is estimated to be > 50 mL. Blood samples are sent for:

- full blood count to diagnose anaemia
- crossmatch in case transfusion is necessary
- coagulation tests, because disseminated intravascular coagulopathy follows massive haemorrhage

Fetal heart rate is monitored by cardiotocography once the mother's condition has stabilised.

An acid elution (Kleihauer) test is carried out for rhesus negative women; the results are used to guide the amount of anti-D required. It is not useful for the diagnosis of abruption.

Management

Management is supportive, with hospital admission for significant bleeds until they have settled. In the case of massive bleeding or fetal or maternal compromise, delivery is expedited.

Antepartum haemorrhage increases the risk of post-partum haemorrhage, so active management of the third stage of labour and increased vigilance are required. This is because of retained tissue in cases of placenta accreta; uterine atony after abruption, and depletion of clotting factors with massive haemorrhages (see Chapter 7, page 231).

Unexplained antepartum haemorrhage is associated with adverse perinatal outcomes. Therefore serial growth scans are required to screen for growth restriction and oligohydramnios.

Medication

Corticosteroids are given if significant antepartum haemorrhage occurs before 35 weeks, in case delivery is needed.

Anti-D is required for non-sensitised rhesus-negative women.

Small-for-gestational-age fetus

Small-for-gestational-age (SGA) is an estimated fetal weight or abdominal circumference < 10th centile for gestation when adjusted for maternal height, weight and ethnicity. If these measurements decrease to < 3rd centile, the condition is classified as severe.

The term SGA is not synonymous with fetal growth restriction, in which the fetus fails to reach its genetic growth potential. Not all fetuses whose growth is restricted meet the definition of SGA; the growth restriction may just cause them to be smaller than they would have been but still within the normal range. However, fetal growth restriction is more common in fetuses who are extremely small for gestational age.

SGA fetuses are at higher risk of stillbirth, intrapartum hypoxia, neonatal complications, e.g. hypoglycaemia, necrotising enterocolitis, impairment of neurodevelopment and, in later life, obesity, diabetes and cardiovascular disease (Barker's hypothesis). The majority of SGA fetuses are healthy, however, the risk of complications is higher in very small fetuses and those that are growth restricted. Identification of SGA fetuses allows increased monitoring and intervention to be introduced to improve outcomes.

Epidemiology

By definition, 10% of fetuses are diagnosed as SGA. Between 50 and 70% of these are constitutionally small, with no underlying pathology.

Aetiology

Growth restriction can be placental-mediated or non-placental mediated (**Table 6.11**).

Diagnostic approach

Growth restriction is suspected on palpation of a symphysis–fundal height that is smaller than expected for the gestation. It is diagnosed by ultrasound screening of women whose pregnancies are at high risk of growth restriction.

Fetal growth restriction: causes	
Placental mediated	Non-placental mediated
Low maternal weight	Structural anomaly
Substance abuse	Chromosomal anomaly
Pre-eclampsia and hypertension	Inborn error of metabolism
Diabetes	Congenital infection (e.g. TORCH organisms*)
Kidney disease	
Autoimmune disease (e.g. systemic lupus erythematosus)	
Thrombophilia	

*Toxoplasmosis, other (varicella-zoster virus, syphilis and parvovirus), rubella, cytomegalovirus and herpes.

Table 6.11 Causes of fetal growth restriction

Investigations

Fetal weight is estimated based on ultrasound measurements of abdominal circumference and femur length. This is plotted on a customised chart (**Figure 6.3**). Placental-mediated growth restriction is associated with oligohydramnios, i.e. single deepest pool of amniotic fluid < 2 cm. This is because in cases of reduced nutrient transfer across the placenta from mother to fetus, the fetus maintains blood flow to the brain in order to preserve neurodevelopment in preference to non-essential organs, such as the kidney. This results in poor renal perfusion and reduced urine output. Umbilical artery Doppler may show reduced, absent or reversed end-diastolic flow.

If a severe case of SGA is diagnosed at < 23 weeks' gestation, further investigation is required to try to identify the cause:

- karyotyping
- detailed anomaly scan
- uterine artery Doppler

- serological screening for cytomegalovirus and toxoplasmosis
- screening for syphilis and malaria in high-risk women (i.e. women at risk of sexually transmitted disease and those who have traveled to endemic countries, respectively).

Management

If the results of umbilical artery Doppler are normal, serial growth assessment is carried out every 2–4 weeks, with planned delivery at 37 weeks' gestation.

If the results of umbilical artery Doppler are abnormal, more regular monitoring with up to daily scans are carried out or the baby is delivered, depending on the gestation.

Fetuses with abnormal umbilical artery Doppler results are delivered by caesarean section, because they do not tolerate labour. If end-diastolic flow is still present, labour is induced, with continuous fetal monitoring to detect signs of distress.

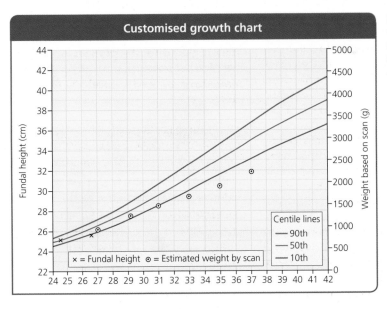

Figure 6.3
Customised growth chart showing a small-for-gestational-age fetus.

Stillbirth

Stillbirth is the death in utero of a fetus from 24 weeks' gestation onwards. It affects 1 in 200 pregnancies.

The diagnosis is preceded by reduced fetal movements. Maternal disease, such as severe sepsis, pre-eclampsia, cholestasis or the presence of fetomaternal haemorrhage, is associated with fetal death. Stillbirth is confirmed, by the absence of fetal heart activity on ultrasound. This must be verified by two sonographers.

Investigations

Investigations take place after stillbirth has been confirmed, and include blood tests, microbiological tests on swab samples, post-mortem examination and genetic testing (**Table 6.12**). The results provide useful information for future pregnancies to try to prevent recurrence. However, no cause can be determined in half of cases.

> **Parental consent is required for investigations to try to determine the cause of a stillbirth.** Post-mortem examinations provide the greatest amount of information, but many parents do not wish their baby to undergo this procedure. Discussions with grieving parents need to be handled sensitively and with compassion, and are difficult for all concerned.

Investigations offered after stillbirth	
Investigation	**Reason for test or condition detected**
Full blood count, urea and electrolytes, urates, C-reactive protein, bile salts	Screening for: ■ Pre-eclampsia ■ sepsis ■ obstetric cholestasis
Coagulation profile, including fibrinogen	Disseminated intravascular coagulation
Kleihauer test	Fetomaternal haemorrhage Determination of dose of anti-D required
Maternal microbiology: blood cultures, midstream specimen of urine, vaginal swabs	Sepsis secondary to bacterial infection, including listeriosis
Maternal serology: ■ viral screen (parvovirus B19, rubella, cytomegalovirus, herpes simplex and *Toxoplasma gondii*) ■ syphilis serology	Occult fetal infection
Random blood glucose	Occult maternal diabetes mellitus
Haemoglobin A1c	Gestational diabetes
Maternal thrombophilia screen*	Thrombophilia
Fetal and placental microbiology: swabs from placenta, fetus and fetal blood for culture	Fetal infection
Fetal karyotype (tissue or cord sample)	Aneuploidy or single-gene disorders
Post-mortem examination†	Congential abnormalities, metabolic disease, placental disease

*Most tests are affected by pregnancy, so abnormal results are confirmed by repeating tests 6 weeks after the birth.

†Requires parental consent (written), and includes external examination, autopsy, microscopy, radiography and examination of the placenta and cord.

Table 6.12 Investigations offered after a stillbirth

Management

Management consists of preventing the mother's condition from deteriorating, trying to determine the cause of death, delivery of the baby, psychological support and follow-up.

Medication

Labour is induced by the administration of mifepristone and misoprostol. Vaginal delivery avoids a scar on the uterus and its potential effect on subsequent pregnancies or births i.e. uterine rupture and increased risk of further stillbirths.

Surgery

Caesarean section is used to deliver the baby if the maternal condition necessitates this. e.g. she is septic or bleeding heavily. The procedure is also warranted if there is an obstetric reason such as more than two previous caesareans.

Psychological support

Families are given the opportunity to hold their baby; not doing so is often regretted afterwards. Parents are warned about potential changes in appearance if their baby died some time ago.

They are also given time to take photographs, locks of hair, impressions of the baby's hands and feet, and other mementoes. Memory boxes are offered in which to keep these items, which can be helpful to them in their bereavement.

Parents may wish to understand why the stillbirth happened, and if it has any implications for future pregnancies. These issues may be discussed, along with the results of any tests and the post-mortem examination, at a follow-up appointment several weeks after the birth.

Parents may also be referred to a bereavement support worker and made aware of patient organisations (e.g. Sands, the UK stillbirth and neonatal death charity).

Prognosis

The risk of stillbirth affecting a future pregnancy in women with a previous unexplained stillbirth is 12 times higher than that of women who have had a previous live birth.

> **Parents, siblings and other family members struggle to cope with the loss of a baby to stillbirth.** Its profound effects may last from the time of diagnosis to many years afterwards, and be exacerbated during any subsequent pregnancy. Interventions based on supportive counselling, understanding and explanation have been designed to help health care professionals provide the best care for those affected.

Answers to starter questions

1. Pregnancy is biologically stressful for the mother and can temporarily expose subclinical diseases which may return in later life. Women diagnosed with gestational diabetes have a 35–60% chance of developing type 2 diabetes within 10–20 years of pregnancy. Likewise, women with pre-eclampsia have a higher risk of developing cardiovascular disease in the future. More understanding of these risks has led to closer postnatal follow up to identify modifiable risk factors that can be addressed.

2. A macrosomic baby has a birth weight >4.5 kg. They are considered in two groups: those born to mothers with diabetes and those who are macrosomic due to genetic factors, ethnicity and their sex (male babies weigh more than females). Babies born to diabetic mothers have a higher risk of experiencing shoulder dystocia. They are delivered at 38 weeks by caesarean section to reduce this risk. However, estimating fetal weight by ultrasound in macrosomic babies is inaccurate and most are born without any problems. Inducing labour at term of non-diabetic women for suspected macrosomia does not improve maternal or fetal outcomes, and is not performed.

Answers *continued*

3. Anencephaly is absence of most of the brain, skull and scalp and occurs during embryological development. Affected babies usually die in utero or, if born alive, do not survive more than a few days. Parents who do not wish to terminate the pregnancy often ask whether their baby's organs can be used for transplantation. The problem is that defining death in these babies is difficult because they have a functioning brainstem. Waiting for the loss of all brain function results in the deterioration of tissues to the extent that they cannot be used. Recent changes in the legal definition of death have allowed anencephalic babies to successfully donate organs.

4. Teenage pregnancies are often unplanned and complications are more common. They are looked after in dedicated teenage pregnancy clinics that provide increased support and access to social services, including housing. An older mother is > 35 years old when pregnant. Older mothers also have an increased risk of complications and are screened regularly in obstetric-led antenatal clinics. Induction of labour is offered at 39–40 weeks to women >40 years to reduce the risk of stillbirth.

Chapter 7
Complications in delivery and the postnatal period

Starter questions

Answers to the following questions are on page 240.

1. Should women be able to request a caesarean section with no clinical justification?
2. What is the chance of a baby surviving if born at 24 weeks' gestation?
3. What is the safest instrument to use for an operative vaginal delivery?
4. How can wound infection following caesarean section be reduced?
5. Why has litigation for intrapartum fetal compromise not decreased with the introduction of CTGs?

Introduction

Most deliveries are uneventful, but complications can arise in a small minority. An obstetrician is required in cases of any deviation from normal delivery, for example if there is a delay in labour or suspicion of maternal or fetal compromise. As in other specialities, the aims are to identify the problem, diagnose the underlying cause and provide safe and effective treatment. The only difference in obstetrics is that there are two patients to consider, the mother and the fetus, with potentially conflicting interests. This makes management decisions more complex.

Case 6 Slow progress in labour

Presentation

Katie Atkinson presented to her local maternity unit 4 h ago with regular, painful contractions. At that time, she was found to be 5 cm dilated. A repeat vaginal examination has just been carried out by the midwife, and there has been no change in cervical dilation.

Initial interpretation

Katie is in the established first stage of labour; her contractions are regular and painful and her cervix is between 4 and 10 cm dilated. During this time, an increase in cervical dilation of ≥ 2 cm in 4 h is expected (see Chapter 4, page 160). The lack of change suggests delay in the first stage of labour.

Further history

This is Katie's first pregnancy, and she is now at 38 weeks. The antenatal period was uneventful. There is no history of membrane rupture. She is using Entonox ('gas and air') for pain relief but is starting to struggle with the strength of the contractions.

Examination

Symphysis-fundal height is 36 cm. The fetus is in a longitudinal lie, cephalic presentation and left occiput posterior position.

The contractions have decreased in strength and frequency to two in every 10-min period. A repeat vaginal examination confirms that Katie is 5 cm dilated,

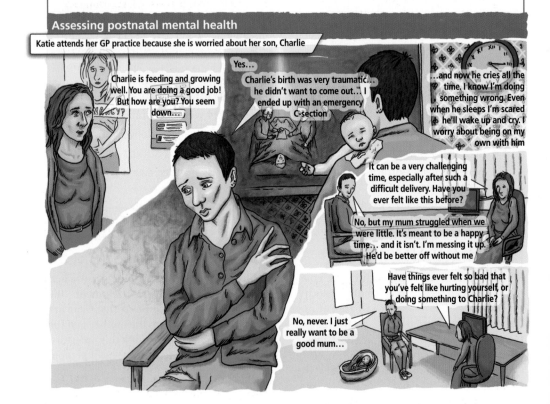

Assessing postnatal mental health

Katie attends her GP practice because she is worried about her son, Charlie and bulging membranes are felt. Artificial rupture of membranes is carried out with an amnihook.

Interpretation of findings

The fetus is appropriately grown and there is no evidence of malpresentation. The decrease in strength and frequency of contractions and the malposition of the fetus are the causes of the suspected delay in the first stage of labour. The occipito-posterior position is more difficult to deliver vaginally as the head is deflexed, meaning that a wider diameter has to pass through the pelvis. In contrast, in an occipito-anterior position, the head is flexed and narrower, making delivery easier.

Investigations

Fetal wellbeing is assessed by auscultation of the fetal heart beat after a contraction every 15 minutes with a sonicaid (see Chapter 4, page 162). The heart rate is normal indicating that there is no sign of fetal distress. Artifical rupture of the membranes causes release of prostaglandins and an increase in the strength and frequency of contractions. An assessment of Katie's contractions reveals that they have increased in frequency to three in every 10 minute period but that they remain short lasting and incoordinate (irregular). This means that labour is unlikely to progress without further intervention, e.g. synthetic oxytocin administration.

Diagnosis

A repeat vaginal examination is carried out 2 h after the artificial rupture of membranes to determine whether progress has been made; the cervix is still 5 cm dilated. An epidural catheter is sited to provide analgesia and an infusion of synthetic oxytocin (Syntocinon) started. This will increase the strength and frequency of contractions and, hopefully, result in increased cervical dilatation. The dose is up-titrated until there are four strong contractions every 10 min.

Four hours later, Katie is having regular contractions but there is still no change in cervical dilation. Failure to progress in the first stage of labour is diagnosed because there has been no change in cervical dilatation, despite the use of synthetic oxytocin. Given that the frequency and strength of contractions have been optimised, fetal malposition is the most likely cause of the failure to progress. A caesarean section, therefore, is carried out.

Case 7 Breech presentation

Presentation

Ishaani Singh is visiting her midwife at 36 weeks' gestation for a routine antenatal appointment.

Initial interpretation

A routine antenatal appointment is made for this gestation to discuss ongoing issues, preparation for labour, breastfeeding and care of the newborn. It also allows an assessment of fetal presentation.

Further history

This is Ishaani's second pregnancy, and it has been uneventful. She has had one previous vaginal delivery and wishes to discuss with the midwife the possibility of a home birth.

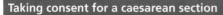

Case 7 *continued*

Taking consent for a caesarean section

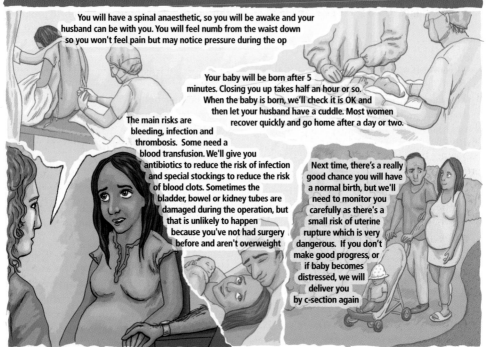

You will have a spinal anaesthetic, so you will be awake and your husband can be with you. You will feel numb from the waist down so you won't feel pain but may notice pressure during the op

Your baby will be born after 5 minutes. Closing you up takes half an hour or so. When the baby is born, we'll check it is OK and then let your husband have a cuddle. Most women recover quickly and go home after a day or two.

The main risks are bleeding, infection and thrombosis. Some need a blood transfusion. We'll give you antibiotics to reduce the risk of infection and special stockings to reduce the risk of blood clots. Sometimes the bladder, bowel or kidney tubes are damaged during the operation, but that is unlikely to happen because you've not had surgery before and aren't overweight

Next time, there's a really good chance you will have a normal birth, but we'll need to monitor you carefully as there's a small risk of uterine rupture which is very dangerous. If you don't make good progress, or if baby becomes distressed, we will deliver you by c-section again

Examination

The symphysis-fundal height is 37 cm, and the fetus is in a longitudinal lie. The midwife palpates the fetal head at the fundus and locates the heartbeat above the umbilicus.

Interpretation of findings

The findings of the fetal head at the fundus and the heartbeat above the umbilicus are consistent with a breech presentation. Ishaani is referred to her local maternity assessment unit to confirm the diagnosis by ultrasound scan and discuss management options. This is because there are increased risks for the fetus of undergoing a vaginal breech delivery.

Investigations

Ultrasound confirms breech presentation with the fetal legs in an extended position. Estimated fetal weight is on the 50th centile on Ishaani's customised growth chart, and liquor volume is normal. These findings indicate that the fetus is normally grown for the gestation and that there are no contraindications to performing external cephalic version.

Diagnosis

The fetus is presenting as a frank breech as the legs are extended. An obstetrician discusses with Ishaani the pros and cons of vaginal breech delivery, external cephalic version (ECV) and elective caesarean section, and gives her the opportunity to discuss these options with

Case 7 *continued*

her partner. She opts for an ECV, but this is unsuccessful. After further discussion, Ishaani decides to have an elective caesarean section, because it carries a lower risk of fetal morbidity and mortality than a vaginal breech birth.

Premature labour

A baby is born prematurely if it is delivered before 37 weeks' gestation. In the UK, 7–8% of babies are born before term. Subcategories of preterm birth are:

- moderate to late preterm (32 to < 37 weeks)
- very preterm (28 to < 32 weeks)
- extremely preterm (< 28 weeks)

Viability is the stage of development at which there is a reasonable chance of the fetus surviving outside the uterus. This is about 24 weeks' gestation and with a birthweight of ≥ 500 g. Resuscitation is considered by a few neonatal units for babies delivered between 23 and 24 weeks, if they are born in good condition and at a good weight. However, survival at this gestation is frequently complicated by significant disabilities and multi-organ dysfunction.

Aetiology

Preterm birth occurs either spontaneously or as a consequence of medical intervention. Spontaneous premature labour is initiated by multiple interacting factors, including infection, inflammation, haemorrhage and uterine over-distension. The exact cause of spontaneous preterm labour is unknown, but risk factors for a particular pregnancy include:

- previous preterm birth (the strongest risk factor for preterm labour)
- multiple pregnancy
- short interval between pregnancies (< 6 months)
- low body mass index
- smoking

- infection, including ascending genital tract infections (e.g. bacterial vaginosis) and urinary tract infections
- previous cervical trauma or surgery, for example multiple loop excisions for treatment of cervical intraepithelial neoplasia
- antepartum haemorrhage

The likelihood of premature labour also depends on ethnic group. In the developed world , the rate of preterm birth is 16–18% in black women, compared with 5–9% in white women. This effect was initially thought to be due to socioeconomic factors, but other, unexplained, mechanisms must also be important because university-educated black women continue to have a higher rate of preterm labour compared with their white counterparts.

Premature labour is preceded by preterm prelabour rupture of membranes in 40% of cases. It can be necessary to induce labour prior to 37 weeks if the risks to the mother and/or fetus from remaining pregnant are higher than those associated with premature delivery. This is the case with severe pre-eclampsia and small for gestational age fetuses with abnormal umbilical artery Dopplers.

Prevention

Women with risk factors for premature labour are referred early in pregnancy to specialist clinics. To assess the likelihood of preterm delivery, ultrasound is used to measure cervical length. Women with a cervix < 25 mm long are at higher risk of preterm birth.

In women at high risk, a cervical suture is inserted to prevent delivery before 24 weeks (**Figure 7.1**). This procedure, known as cervical cerclage, is indicated on the basis of any of the following:

- a history of three or more previous preterm births (history-indicated cerclage)
- cervical shortening to < 25 mm on ultrasound (ultrasound-indicated cerclage)
- premature cervical dilation with exposed fetal membranes (rescue cerclage)

If premature delivery occurs despite vaginal cerclage, an abdominal suture is inserted either laparoscopically or via laparotomy, preferably between pregnancies, to protect subsequent pregnancies. Abdominal sutures are permanent, so delivery is by caesarean section.

Clinical features

Premature labour presents with painful contractions and backache with or without increased vaginal discharge. Bleeding or loss of fluid vaginally is also present, if the preterm labour is triggered by antepartum haemorrhage or preterm, prelabour rupture of the membranes, respectively.

Diagnostic approach

Cervical dilation is assessed either digitally or by direct visualisation with a speculum. Premature labour is diagnosed by examination alone once cervical dilation is > 3 cm. Investigations are used to exclude premature labour in symptomatic women with no cervical dilation on examination.

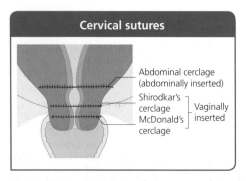

Cervical sutures

Abdominal cerclage (abdominally inserted)

Shirodkar's cerclage ⎤ Vaginally
McDonald's ⎦ inserted
cerclage

Figure 7.1 McDonald's, Shirodkar's and abdominal vaginal sutures.

Investigations

The fibronectin test or Actim Partus test is used to predict preterm birth (**Table 7.1**). The proteins detected are absent from the vagina and cervix between 22 and 34 weeks'

Tests to exclude premature labour		
Feature	Fibronectin test	Actim Partus test
Site of swab	Vaginal	Cervical
Protein detected	Fetal fibronectin	Phosphorylated insulin-like growth factor–binding protein–1
Positive predictive value (%)	20–50	58
Negative predictive value (%)	99	92–98
Contraindications	Cervical dilation > 3 cm	Cervical dilation > 3 cm
	> 35 weeks' gestation	> 35 weeks' gestation
	Ruptured membranes	Ruptured membranes
	Previous digital vaginal examination	
	Sexual intercourse within past 24 h	
	Ongoing bleeding	
Management of a positive result	Hospitalisation, corticosteroids, and tocolysis to reduce neonatal morbidity and mortality in the event of preterm birth	
Management of a negative result	Reassurance that preterm birth is highly unlikely in the next 10–14 days; no medical intervention required	

Table 7.1 Comparison of tests to exclude premature labour

gestation, but they leak from the uterus when the decidua and chorion start to detach in premature labour. These tests reduce unnecessary medical intervention and conserve resources.

In cases of suspected preterm labour, a urine sample and vaginal swabs are taken to screen for infection.

After preterm prelabour rupture of membranes, a full blood count and C-reactive protein test are carried out to monitor for infection.

> **A fibronectin swab must be taken before a digital vaginal examination,** otherwise a false positive result is likely.

Management

The aim is to prolong time to delivery to allow the administration of corticosteroids and in utero (before delivery) transfer to a hospital with appropriate neonatal intensive care facilities (**Figure 7.2**).

Medication

Corticosteroids improve neonatal outcomes by reducing the risk of:

- neonatal death
- respiratory distress syndrome (by stimulating surfactant production)
- intraventricular haemorrhage
- necrotising enterocolitis
- intensive care admission and need for respiratory support
- systemic infections

They are given intramuscularly between 24 and 34 weeks' gestation as two doses of betamethasone 12 mg 24 h apart or four doses of dexamethasone 6 mg every 6 h. They are given up to 35 weeks if the fetus is affected by growth restriction. Both regimens are equally efficacious and have no known maternal adverse effects. Administration is considered

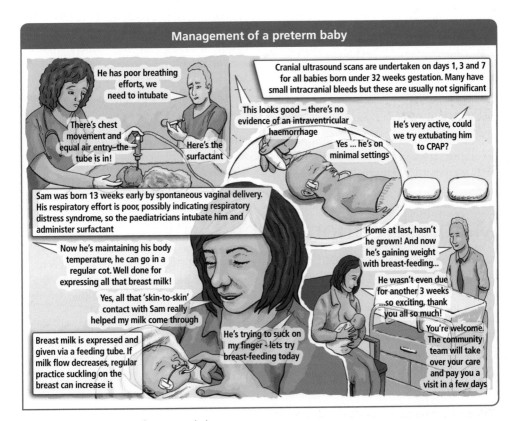

Figure 7.2 Management of a preterm baby.

Tocolytics					
Drug	Route of administration	Mechanism of action	Licensed indication?	Adverse effects	Contraindications
Atosiban	Intravenous	Oxytocin receptor antagonist	Yes	Nausea Headache Injection site reactions	None
Nifedipine	Oral	Calcium receptor antagonist	No	Flushing Palpitations Nausea and vomiting Hypotension	Cardiac disease Use with caution in multiple pregnancies and diabetes because of risk of pulmonary oedema

Table 7.2 Comparison of tocolytics

from 23 weeks' gestation if preterm birth is highly likely.

The beneficial effects of corticosteroids are apparent if the baby is born 24 h after the second dose and the effects last for 7 days.

Tocoloytics inhibit uterine contractions and delay delivery (**Table 7.2**). Tocolytics have no beneficial effect themselves on neonatal outcome, but allow time for a complete course of corticosteroids to be administered.

Erythromycin is given for 10 days after preterm prelabour rupture of membranes to prevent infection, thereby delaying birth and protecting neurodevelopment.

Prognosis

Babies born before term have difficulty breathing, feeding and maintaining their body temperature (**Figure 7.2**). In the short term, they are at risk of necrotising enterocolitis (NEC) and intracranial haemorrhage, and need careful monitoring. They are also at risk of long-term disabilities, including cerebral palsy, developmental delay and problems with vision and hearing. The earlier a baby is born, the higher the risk of serious disability and death. For example, the chance of survival at 23 weeks is 15%, compared with 80% at 25 weeks. Babies born before 26 weeks, however, have a significant risk of disability; cerebral palsy rates are 50% with only 20% having no disabilities. This contrasts with babies born between 29 and 32 weeks, where 70% will have no health problems, 20% will have mild visual impairment or cerebral palsy and only 10% will have severe cerebral palsy, blindness or deafness.

Malpresentation of the fetus

Malpresentation is any non-cephalic presentation i.e. when any part of the fetus other than the head is closest to the maternal pelvis. Breech presentation is the commonest malpresentation, affecting 3–4% of fetuses at term (**Figure 7.3**). This is where the bottom is the closest part of the fetus to the maternal pelvis. Other presenting parts include the shoulders in a transverse lie, the face or the brow.

■ Vaginal delivery is possible with breech and face presentations, but they are associated with increased perinatal morbidity and mortality
■ Vaginal delivery is not possible with transverse lie and brow presentations, because the fetus will not pass through the pelvic canal

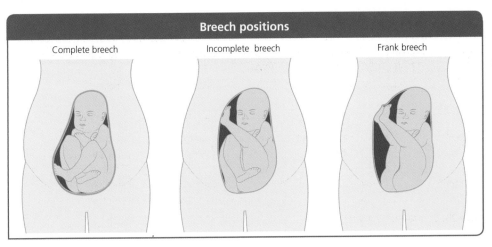

Breech positions

Complete breech   Incomplete breech   Frank breech

Figure 7.3 Complete, incomplete and frank breech positions.

Predisposing factors for malpresentation	
Maternal	Fetal
Pelvic tumours or fibroids	Prematurity
Congenital uterine anomalies (e.g. arcuate or septate uterus)	Fetal anomalies (e.g. hydrocephalus)
Oligohydramnios	Multiple pregnancy
Placenta praevia	Intrauterine death

Table 7.3 Maternal and fetal predisposing factors for malpresentation

Aetiology

Most cases are of unknown aetiology. However, there are maternal and fetal predisposing factors for malpresentation (**Table 7.3**).

Clinical features

Malpresentation is suspected antenatally on abdominal palpation when the fetal head is not lying over or in the pelvis. During digital examination in labour, landmarks other than the vertex and fontanelles are felt.

Diagnostic approach

If malpresentation is suspected, the diagnosis is confirmed by ultrasound.

Investigations

As well as determining presentation, ultrasound is used to assess fetal growth, anatomy and amniotic fluid volume as potential causes of malpresentation and to inform management.

Management

External cephalic version is manipulation of the fetus into a cephalic presentation by applying pressure to the maternal abdomen (**Figure 7.4**). It is used for breech presentation and transverse lie. The success rate is 50% overall but higher in multiparous women and if the uterine relaxant terbutaline is used. Complications are rare (0.5% of cases), but include fetomaternal haemorrhage, abruption, precipitation of labour, fetal distress and cord prolapse. Spontaneous reversion back to breech occurs in 3% of cases after successful ECV.

> For ECV to be attempted, facilities must be available to carry out an immediate caesarean section in case a complication arises. Fetal heart rate is monitored before and after the procedure, and anti-D prophylaxis given to rhesus-negative mothers to reduce the risk of complications.

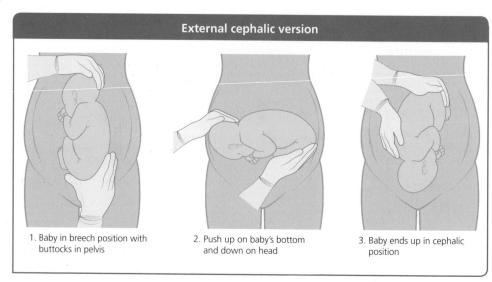

External cephalic version

1. Baby in breech position with buttocks in pelvis

2. Push up on baby's bottom and down on head

3. Baby ends up in cephalic position

Figure 7.4 External cephalic version for breech presentation and transverse lie.

> Discuss the pros and cons of ECV, vaginal breech delivery and caesarean section with mothers and allow her to choose. There is no right or wrong answer, and individuals will choose differently. It is essential to offer appropriate support whatever the decision.

If ECV is unsuccessful or declined, delivery is by vaginal breech delivery or caesarean section. Perinatal morbidity and mortality is increased with a vaginal breech delivery compared with a caesarean section, because of difficulties delivering the fetal head and the increased risk of cord prolapse. The absolute risk of poor perinatal outcome is nonetheless very low, and women with an otherwise low-risk pregnancy and in spontaneous labour can be supported to have a vaginal breech delivery if appropriately trained birthing attendants are available.

Failure to progress in labour

Failure to progress is defined differently depending on the stage of labour and whether the woman has had children previously (**Table 7.4**; see Chapter 4).

Aetiology

Failure to progress in the first two stages of labour is the result of one or more of the three P's: power, passenger or passage.

Power

This is the efficiency of contractions, and is assessed by the effect the contractions have on cervical dilatation. Contractions are stimulated by oxytocin; intravenous administration of the synthetic drug, syntoncinon, increases oxytocin levels and thus contraction strength and frequency. The supine position reduces the efficiency of contractions.

Passenger

The passenger is the fetus; its size, presentation or position may underlie failure to progress. The outlet of the maternal pelvis is 11 cm wide and the fetal skull, at its widest part, is 9.5 cm in diameter. Therefore there is just enough room for the head to pass through the pelvic canal.

Passage through the pelvic canal requires the fetal head to be flexed and with the chin

Failure to progress in labour: definitions

Stage of labour	Definition
Established first stage	Suspected if < 2 cm change in cervical dilation in a 4-h period, or slowing of progress in a multiparous woman
	Confirmed if there is no change in cervical dilation 2 h after artificial rupture of membranes
Second stage	Primiparous woman: failure to deliver within 2 h of active pushing
	Multiparous woman: failure to delivery within 1 h of active pushing
Third stage	Passive management: failure to deliver placenta within 1 h of birth
	Active management: failure to deliver placenta within 30 min of birth

Table 7.4 Definitions of failure to progress in labour

tucked on the chest, in the occipito-anterior position. Malposition increases the size of the head relative to the pelvic canal, thereby causing delay. Malpresentation delays or precludes delivery because the fetus is not in the ideal position for birth.

Passage

This is the birth canal. Mismatches in size between the pelvis and the fetus are caused by:

- abnormalities of the bony pelvis as a result of malnutrition, trauma or polio
- abnormalities of the soft tissue, caused by tumour or scarring from female genital mutilation

Cephalopelvic disproportion is failure of the fetal head to pass through the pelvis because of discrepancies in size. It is more common in areas of the world where women have inadequate nutrition, have limited access to health care or at risk of female genital mutilation. It is rare in high-income countries, where for most women the size of the pelvis is adequate for the size of the fetus.

Retained placenta is the consequence of failure of the uterus to contract, trapping of the placenta in a closed cervix or an abnormally adherent placenta that fails to detach.

Diagnostic approach

Failure to progress is a clinical diagnosis. It is confirmed by serial vaginal examinations to assess cervical dilation and fetal descent.

The frequency and strength of contractions are determined by abdominal palpation. Fetal size, presentation and position are assessed by abdominal palpation and vaginal examination.

Investigations

Ultrasound is used to determine fetal presentation and position if clinical examination is unhelpful.

Assessment of pelvic size by clinical examination or MRI is inaccurate and is not done. Hormone-induced relaxation of ligaments and sitting or squatting positions significantly increase pelvic outlet dimensions. The only way to determine whether a woman is able to give birth vaginally is for her to try.

Management

Artificial rupture of membranes is carried out for women with suspected failure to progress and intact membranes (see Chapter 4). It increases the strength and frequency of contractions.

Medication

Synthetic oxytocin (Syntocinon) is used if failure to progress in labour is confirmed. It is given intravenously, with the dose up-titrated every 30 min to increase the strength and frequency of contractions to a maximum of four or five strong contractions in 10 min. It expedites delivery but does not influence the mode of delivery. Fetal heart rate is monitored by cardiotocograph to detect fetal compromise.

> **Contractions become more painful after starting oxytocin.** Extra analgesia, including an epidural, is offered before it is administered.

> **Synthetic oxytocin is used judiciously in the second stage of labour, particularly in multiparous women.** Failure to progress in the second stage is usually because of fetal malposition rather than inefficient contractions. Although use of oxytocin can facilitate rotatation of the fetus into the occipito-anterior position, it can also cause uterine hypercontractility and even uterine rupture in rare cases.

Vaginal examination is done 4 h after starting oxytocin. If cervical dilation has not increased by at least 2 cm, then a caesarean section is carried out. Caesarean section is also necessary if there is delay in the second stage of labour and operative vaginal delivery is not appropriate, as in cases of a head above station 0.

Operative vaginal delivery

This is carried out when there is delay in the second stage of labour and if the fetal head is low enough (see page 229). In cases of malposition, a rotational delivery is necessary. This can be done manually or using an instrument such as a ventouse or Kielland's forceps.

> **Caesarean section in the second stage of labour has a higher complication rate than in the first stage.** Extra care is needed to prevent uterine angle extensions and bladder injury when disimpacting the fetal head. Surgical trauma and uterine atony cause post-partum haemorrhage.

Retained placenta is managed by manual removal. This is done by separating the placenta from the uterine wall during vaginal examination. Adequate analgesia is required, because the procedure is uncomfortable. Intravenous access is gained and a full blood count and identification of blood group and antibody profile (group and save) carried out because of the risk of post-partum haemorrhage. Antibiotic prophylaxis prevents endometritis.

Fetal compromise in labour

Fetal compromise in labour is suspected on the basis of fetal heart rate changes detected on cardiotocograph and the passage of meconium. The overall risk of needing a prompt caesarean section for fetal concern is 3%, but this figure is higher in specific subgroups.

Aetiology

Fetal compromise in labour is caused by maternal and fetal factors.

- Maternal factors include:
  - diabetes, hypertension and pre-eclampsia causing uteroplacental vascular disease
  - hypotension reducing placental blood flow
  - post-term pregnancy
  - cord prolapse
- Fetal factors include:
  - multiple pregnancy
  - growth restriction
  - prematurity
  - oligohydramnios
  - sepsis

A fetus with reduced reserves of energy is unable to tolerate the intermittent reduction in placental blood flow that occurs with contractions.

Clinical features

Fetal movements are reduced as the compromised fetus conserves its limited energy resources.

Meconium is faecal material passed by the fetus or newborn baby. Passage of meconium in utero is normal for a mature gastrointestinal system, but it is also a sign of fetal distress, because hypoxia relaxes the anal sphincter. Amniotic fluid leaking from the vagina is dark green or brown.

Diagnostic approach

Distinguishing a compromised fetus from

one that is coping well in labour is difficult and associated with interpreter error. Fetal heart rate monitoring is supplemented with invasive tests of acid balance (fetal blood sampling) to improve diagnostic accuracy.

Investigations

Cardiotocography is used to monitor fetal heart rate. Assessment is based on four variables (see page 164):

- baseline rate
- variability
- presence of accelerations
- presence of decelerations

A suspicious cardiotocograph is not associated with fetal compromise. Reduced variability in the short term (< 40 min) occurs when the fetus sleeps. Early and variable decelerations reflect head and cord compression during contractions. Prompt recovery indicates good fetal oxygen reserves.

A pathological cardiotocograph indicates fetal hypoxia in 50% of cases (**Figure 7.5**).

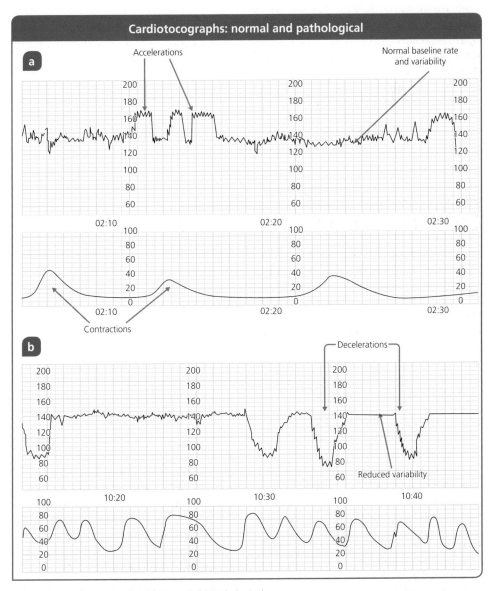

Figure 7.5 Cardiotocographs. (a) Normal. (b) Pathological.

Decelerations are deep, prolonged and slow to recover.

Fetal blood sampling is carried out when a cardiotocograph is pathological and delivery is not imminent. A small scratch is made on the fetal scalp, and a few droplets of blood are collected in a capillary tube. Cervical dilation of ≥ 3 cm is required to access the fetal scalp with the aid of a speculum. The results of measurement of pH and lactate are used to guide management.

Management

Management depends on the degree of fetal compromise and the stage and progress of labour (**Table 7.5**).

Women with meconium-stained liquor before labour require immediate induction rather than waiting for contractions to start spontaneously.

Fetal blood sampling		
Lactate concentration (mmol/L)	pH	Management
≤ 4.1	≥ 7.25	Repeat fetal blood sampling in 1 h if cardiotocograph abnormalities persist or sooner if they worsen
4.2–4.8	7.21–7.24	Repeat fetal blood sampling in 30 min if cardiotocograph abnormalities persist or sooner if they worsen
≥ 4.9	≤ 7.20	Urgent delivery

Table 7.5 Fetal blood sampling: results and management

Operative vaginal delivery

An operative vaginal delivery is required in 10–13% of all births. A ventouse or forceps are used (**Figure 7.6**). The aim is to use the instrument to facilitate the same cardinal movements of the fetus during delivery as occurs in spontaneous vaginal birth.

Indications

Indications for operative vaginal delivery are maternal or fetal and include the following.

- Maternal
  - Failure to progress in the second stage of labour
  - Contraindications to prolonged second stage (e.g. maternal cardiac disease)
  - Maternal fatigue

- Fetal
  - Suspected fetal compromise

The prerequisites for operative vaginal delivery are listed in **Table 7.6**.

Instrument choice

Use of a ventouse causes less perineal trauma. However, it is more likely to fail than forceps and is also more likely to cause neonatal cephalohaematoma and retinal haemorrhage. Contraindications to the use of a ventouse are:

- prematurity (< 34 weeks' gestation)
- face presentation
- suspected fetal bleeding disorder or predisposition to fracture (e.g. osteogenesis imperfecta)
- maternal HIV or hepatitis C

Complications

Perineal trauma, including third- and fourth-degree tears, is common with operative vaginal delivery (see pages 161–162). Episiotomy is done to widen the vaginal outlet and thereby assist with birth in up to 90% of cases of operative delivery.

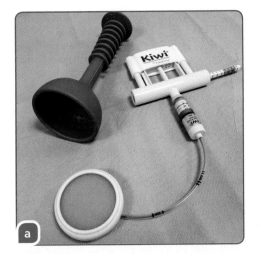

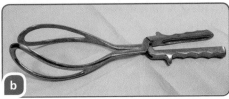

Figure 7.6 Instruments used in operative vaginal delivery. (a) Ventouse. (b) Forceps.

Operative vaginal delivery: prerequisites	
Characteristic	Prerequisite
Maternal	Informed consent
	Adequate analgesia
	Good contractions (i.e. at least 3 every 10 minutes)
	Empty bladder
	Adequate pelvis
	Fully dilated cervix and ruptured membranes
Fetal	Vertex presentation
	Head less than or equal to one fifth palpable abdominally
	Position known
	Minimal swelling (caput) on fetal head if ventouse used
Staff	Appropriately trained
	Facilities to carry out immediate caesarean section if delivery unsuccessful
	Staff able to deal with complications, including neonatal resuscitation, shoulder dystocia and post-partum haemorrhage

Table 7.6 Prerequisites for operative vaginal delivery

Post-partum haemorrhage occurs in 10–40% of operative vaginal deliveries. It is caused by perineal trauma and uterine atony.

The type and frequency of fetal injury depends on the instrument used. Forceps leave temporary marks on the face and rarely cause facial nerve palsies. A ventouse delivery results in a chignon, a swelling on the baby's head that settles in 48 h.

Shoulder dystocia is more common after an operative vaginal delivery. Traction applied during an operative vaginal delivery causes the fetal head to deflex and the shoulders to abduct, thereby widening their diameter and making entrapment in the maternal pelvis more likely (see page 358).

Caesarean section

Caesarean section is a surgical procedure to deliver the baby through an incision in the woman's abdomen and uterus. It is done electively or as an emergency.

Rates of caesarean section

Mortality and morbidity in mothers and babies can be reduced when caesarean section is carried out for the appropriate indications. However, it also carries a risk of various complications, so the World Health Organization recommends that it should be used only when medically necessary.

By international consensus, the ideal rate for caesarean sections is 10–15%, but they are becoming more common in low-, moderate- and high-income countries. The lowest caesarean section rates are in Africa, where there are barriers to obstetric care in terms of availability, affordability and acceptability in many countries. The highest rates are in Brazil, where 46% of all births are by caesarean section, increased to 80–90% if performed in a private hospital. This is because of cultural and medical pressure on women to have their babies delivered at convenient times. In the UK, the rate has doubled over the past 25 years and is now 25%. This is because of a rising rate of elective caesarean sections, the most common indication being a previous caesarean section.

> **Various explanations have been proposed for the increasing rates of caesarean section worldwide.** These include a greater proportion of complicated births as a result of increasing average maternal age and prevalence of obesity, the perception of caesarean section as an indication of high-quality care, and some obstetricians favouring the procedure because it requires less time commitment than a vaginal delivery.

Indications

Elective caesarean sections are carried out for many reasons, including:

- previous caesarean section, the commonest reason
- breech presentation
- multiple pregnancy
- placenta praevia or accreta
- previous third-degree tear, to prevent further anal sphincter dysfunction
- HIV, to reduce vertical transmission if viral load is > 50 copies/mL
- maternal request

Emergency caesarean sections are carried out if there is:

- fetal compromise
- failure to progress despite synthetic oxytocin administration
- cord prolapse

The urgency with which a caesarean section is carried out depends on the indication (**Table 7.7**). Elective caesarean sections are done after 39 weeks' gestation, to reduce the risk of respiratory distress in the baby.

> **Transient tachypnoea of the newborn is a short-term respiratory problem caused by increased fluid in the lungs.** The fluid is normally squeezed out during vaginal delivery, but this does not occur with caesarean section. Transient tachypnoea of the newborn increases the risk of admission to a neonatal intensive care unit.

Types of incision

A Joel Cohen incision is used to gain entry into the abdomen (**Figure 7.7**). It is quicker and associated with less blood loss, pain and infection than a Pfannenstiel's incision,

Caesarean section: classification of urgency			
Category	Indication	Example	Interval from decision to delivery
1	Immediate threat to the life of the woman or the fetus	Fetal blood sampling shows pH ≤ 7.20 Cord prolapse	Within 30 min
2	Maternal or fetal compromise that is not immediately life-threatening	Pathological cardiotocograph and fetal blood sampling is not possible	Within 75 min
3	No maternal or fetal compromise but early delivery required	Failure to progress in labour	Within 24 h
4	Delivery timed to suit woman or staff	Elective procedure	Variable (depends on convenient time)

Table 7.7 Classification of urgency of caesarean section

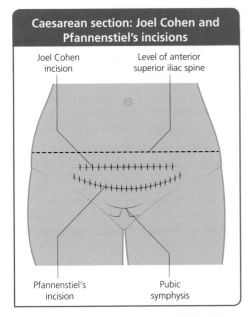

Caesarean section: Joel Cohen and Pfannenstiel's incisions

Joel Cohen incision

Level of anterior superior iliac spine

Pfannenstiel's incision

Pubic symphysis

Figure 7.7 Joel Cohen and Pfannenstiel's incisions.

has yet to form. However, this type of incision is associated with a higher risk of uterine rupture in future labours – 10% versus < 1% with a transverse, lower segment uterine incision – so future labours are contraindicated.

Complications

Maternal and fetal complications can arise during a caesarean section, and occur more frequently in emergency than in elective procedures. Measures are taken to reduce these risks (**Table 7.8**).

> **When discussing the potential complications of a procedure such as caesarean section,** it is helpful to divide them into those common to all surgical interventions, for example bleeding, infection and thrombosis, and those specific to the operation in question. This is done, for example, when obtaining a patient's consent.

because blunt rather than sharp dissection is carried out. A transverse, lower segment uterine incision then allows access to the fetus.

In a classic caesarean section, a vertical uterine incision in the upper segment of the uterus is made. This is necessary if the lower segment cannot be accessed because of fibroids or placenta praevia, or in cases of extreme prematurity, when the lower segment

A woman trying for a vaginal birth after a caesarean section has a 75% chance of success if she has had only one previous caesarean section. Success is more likely if she has had a previous vaginal delivery, and less likely if she has been induced or if her caesarean section was for failure to progress in labour.

Post-partum haemorrhage

Post-partum haemorrhage is blood loss > 500 mL after delivery. It is:

- primary, occurring in the first 24 h, or
- secondary, occurring between 24 h and 12 weeks postnatally

And the degree of blood loss is:

- minor (500–1000 mL), or
- moderate (> 1000 to 2000 mL)
- severe > 2000 mL

It complicates 6–10% of pregnancies and is a major cause of maternal morbidity and mortality worldwide. Most deaths related to

post-partum haemorrhage are preventable. They are the result of a lack of skilled birth attendants at deliveries, limited use of active management of the third stage of labour and poor access to uterotonic drugs.

Aetiology

Primary post-partum haemorrhage is caused by the four T's.

- Tone (70% of cases): lack of uterine contractility
- Trauma (20% of cases): perineal tears or surgical trauma

Caesarean section: complications and risk reduction		
Complication	Frequency	Measures taken to reduce the risk
Bleeding	Common: blood loss > 1000 mL in 4–8 of 100 women	Intravenous access secured Preoperative full blood count and group and save in case of significant bleeding Cross-matched blood available in case of placenta praevia Oxytocin 5 IU intravenously after baby is delivered, to contract the uterus
Infection	Common: 6 in 100 women	Single dose of intravenous antibiotics before starting procedure Placenta delivered by controlled cord traction rather than manual removal, to reduce risk of endometritis
Thrombosis	Rare: 4–16 in 10,000 women	TED stockings Early mobilisation and hydration Assessment of thrombosis risk: all women having emergency caesarean sections require subcutaneous heparin for 7 days
Anaesthetic-related-aspiration pneumonitis	Uncommon: 1 in 660 women	Ranitidine preoperatively to reduce gastric acidity Regional anaesthesia in preference to general anaesthesia Rapid sequence induction if general anaesthesia required
Damage to bladder, bowel, ureters	Rare: 1 in 1000 women	Indwelling catheter inserted before starting procedure reduces bladder injuries and also prevents bladder over-distension caused by loss of sensation with regional anaesthesia
Fetal laceration	Common: 2 in 100 babies	Care taken when entering uterus Blunt rather than sharp dissection
Return to theatre or readmission to hospital	Common: 5 in 100–1000 women	As for infection and bleeding
Emergency hysterectomy	Rare: 7–8 in 1000 women	Senior physician present if complicated procedure anticipated Uterine artery embolisation in case of placenta praevia
Future pregnancies: antepartum stillbirth	Uncommon: 1–4 in 1000 women	Fetal monitoring by cardiotocograph, with or without ultrasound, if fetal movement is reduced
Repeat caesarean section in labour	Very common: 25 in 100 women	Delivery in obstetric-led unit
Uterine rupture during future labour	Uncommon: 2–7 in 1000 women	Await spontaneous labour, because risk is lower Care taken if prostaglandins used for induction Judicious use of synthetic oxytocin as the enhanced strength and frequency of contractions increases the risk of uterine rupture Continuous fetal heart rate monitoring in labour, because a pathological cardiotocograph is the commonest sign of uterine rupture One-to-one midwifery care and prompt delivery if there is continuous abdominal pain over the scar between contractions
Placenta praevia or accreta in future pregnancies	Uncommon: 4–8 in 1000 women	Advise against multiple repeat caesarean sections, because risk increases with number of procedures Placental localisation on ultrasound at 18–20 weeks' gestation; MRI scan if anterior placenta praevia found at 32 weeks and woman has had a previous caesarean section, to identify placenta accreta Plan for caesarean hysterectomy in cases of placenta accreta; requires gynaecologist and, if available, interventional radiologist to deal with potential massive haemorrhage

Table 7.8 Maternal and fetal complications of a caesarean section, and risk reduction

- Tissue (10% of cases): retained placental tissue
- Thrombin (< 1% of cases): clotting factor deficiency, either primary (e.g. haemophilia) or secondary to massive blood loss and disseminated intravascular coagulation

Secondary post-partum haemorrhage is caused by infection (endometritis) or retained placental tissue.

Prevention

Active management of the third stage of labour reduces the risk of post-partum haemorrhage by 60% (see Chapter 4, page 162).

Clinical features

The features of post-partum haemorrhage relate to the volume of blood lost. Acute loss of a significant volume (> 1000 mL) of blood causes maternal collapse. Loss of lesser volumes causes hypotension, tachycardia and tachypnoea.

Severe post-partum haemorrhage results in hypoperfusion of end organs, acute kidney injury in particular.

> **Assessment of blood loss is notoriously difficult and is usually significantly underestimated.** Weighing swabs and pads improves accuracy. The presence of clotted blood needs to be taken into account; double the volume of clotted blood to determine the actual blood volume lost.

Diagnostic approach

Resuscitation is carried out using the ABC approach (see page 350). The source of bleeding is identified by clinical examination. Uterine contractility is assessed abdominally, the perineum and vagina examined for trauma and the placenta evaluated for completeness.

Management

The emergency management of postpartum haemorrhage is covered in Chapter 14 (see page 360).

Anaemia after delivery is treated with iron replacement, either orally or intravenously. Blood transfusion is required in cases of significant blood loss, to quickly replace volume, increase oxygen-carrying capacity and relieve symptoms. Fresh frozen plasma containing clotting factors is transfused at a ratio of 1:1 with red blood cells for women with severe post-partum haemorrhage, to prevent disseminated intravascular coagulation and worsening haemorrhage.

Postnatal infection

Sepsis, i.e. infection plus systemic manifestations of that infection, is a leading cause of maternal deaths worldwide. Severe sepsis is sepsis and sepsis-induced end organ dysfunction, and septic shock is refractory hypotension despite adequate intravenous fluid replacement.

The number of cases of invasive group A streptococcal infection has increased in many countries recently; it has a high mortality rate.

> **An increased body temperature is not always present in cases of sepsis.** In patients with sepsis, the temperature can also be normal, as a result of treatment with non-steroidal anti-inflammatory drugs, or low. Hypothermia is a particularly concerning sign, because it is associated with poor prognosis.

Postnatal infection: commonest causative organisms	
Organism	Infection(s)
Group A *Streptococcus*	Perineal infection, endometritis
Escherichia coli	Pyelonephritis
Staphylococcus aureus	Mastitis, wound infection
Streptococcus pneumoniae	Pneumonia
Methicillin-resistant *Staph. aureus* (MRSA)	Hospital-acquired wound infection

Table 7.9 The commonest causative organisms in postnatal infection

Aetiology

The commonest causative organisms in postnatal infections are listed in **Table 7.9**. Antibiotic-resistant bacteria are becoming more prevalent, including extended spectrum β-lactamases as a cause of co-amoxiclav- and cephalosporin-resistant urinary tract infections. They affect treatment because they limit the number of effective antibiotics that are available to treat the infection.

Prevention

Antibiotic prophylaxis is given before caesarean section to reduce the risk of endometritis and wound infections.

Women receive information on perineal hygiene after delivery. They are advised to wash their hands before and after using the toilet.

Clinical features

General features of infection include fever, lethargy, myalgia and loss of appetite. Signs include tachycardia, tachypnoea, hypotension, oliguria, hypoxia and impaired consciousness. A generalised maculopapular rash is present in staphylococcal and streptococcal infections.

Other features are specific to the infection.

- Mastitis causes breast pain and erythema, and there is a palpable lump in the breast; it is a common and often overlooked cause of sepsis

- Endometritis is a cause of secondary post-partum haemorrhage; the blood is offensive-smelling, there is abdominal pain and the uterus fails to involute as expected
- Perineal infection presents with pain, discharge and wound breakdown
- Pyelonephritis leads to dysuria, loin pain and vomiting
- Deep infection, particularly necrotising fasciitis, is suggested by severe pain disproportionate to the clinical signs. This requires urgent surgical debridement of the dead tissue as delay is associated with an increase in the mortality rate.

> **Do not assume that diarrhoea and vomiting are caused by gastroenteritis.** They are also symptoms of sepsis and warrant systematic assessment to exclude other causes of infection.

Diagnostic approach

Prompt assessment, investigation and treatment with antibiotics within 1 h of presentation improves outcome. Multidisciplinary input, including from intensivists and microbiologists, and support from senior colleagues are required to optimise care.

An ABC approach is used for resuscitation. This is followed by systematic examination and investigations to locate the source of infection.

> **The UK has a Surviving Sepsis Campaign 'bundle';** this lists the core elements of care that improve outcome in cases of sepsis (a 'bundle' is a set of elements of care that, implemented together, have an effect on outcomes beyond that of the individual elements alone). Recommended investigations and care pathways are described, including evidence-based time limits for the completion of tasks. Each hospital has their own version of the bundle.

Investigations

Table 7.10 lists the investigations carried out in cases of suspected sepsis. Blood samples are obtained for culture, but antibiotic treatment is not delayed while the results are awaited.

Suspected sepsis: investigations	
Test	Reason
Blood culture	Identity causative organism
Full blood count	High or low white cell count and thrombocytosis are present in sepsis
Urea and electrolytes	To assess end organ function; acute kidney injury occurs in severe sepsis and septic shock
Liver function tests	To assess end organ function
C-reactive protein test	C-reactive protein concentration increased in sepsis
Lactate	Prognostic marker: lactate > 4 mmol/L is treated with prompt fluid replacement A persistent increase despite adequate fluid administration is associated with poor outcome
Urine culture	To identify source of infection and guide antibiotic choice
Wound, perineal, high vaginal swabs	To identify source of infection and guide antibiotic choice
Throat swab	To identify source of infection and guide antibiotic choice Group A *Streptococcus* is a common cause of pharyngitis
Nose swab	To screen for methicillin-resistant *Staphylococcus aureus* (MRSA)
Stool sample	To identify source of infection and guide antibiotic choice
Breast milk culture	To identify source of infection if mastitis suspected
Chest radiograph	To identify source of infection and look for signs of acute respiratory distress syndrome
Pelvic ultrasound or CT	To identify source of infection and guide antibiotic choice, particularly if pelvic abscess suspected

Table 7.10 Investigations in suspected sepsis

Management

Broad spectrum intravenous antibiotics are given within 1 h of presentation to hospital with signs and symptoms of sepsis. Delays in treatment are associated with worse outcome. Co-amoxiclav and metronidazole in combination or piperacillin-tazobactam (Tazocin) is commonly used.

Every hospital has a different antibiotic guideline for the management of sepsis. This is because causative organisms and their sensitivities to antibiotics vary depending on geographical location. Before a chosen antibiotic is prescribed, it must be checked that it is safe for breastfeeding women.

Not all cases of mastitis require antibiotic treatment. It is caused by the accumulation of milk as a consequence of incorrect attachment of the baby when breastfeeding, leading to inflammation of the breast tissue. If the woman is systemically well, non-steroidal anti-inflammatory drugs and continued feeding may relieve symptoms. Midwives offer advice on breastfeeding technique to reduce the risk of recurrence. Antibiotics are required only to treat superimposed infection.

Intravenous fluid replacement is guided by maternal observations, including blood pressure, heart rate and urine output, as well as serial lactate measurements.

Breast and pelvic abscesses are drained either radiologically or surgically if there is no improvement with antibiotics.

Admission to an intensive care unit is needed for women with sepsis and organ failure.

> **The paediatrician must be informed if a woman has postnatal sepsis**. The baby will need a septic screen and may need antibiotic prophylaxis.

Prognosis

Severe sepsis has a mortality rate of 20–40%, which increases to 60% if septic shock develops. The Surviving Sepsis Campaign aims to reduce mortality by 25% through better awareness and improved management.

Venous thromboembolism

Venous thromboembolism, the development of a blood clot in a vein, is a potentially life-threatening condition. Rates of venous thromboembolism are up to 10 times higher during pregnancy and the puerperium, and it remains one of the leading direct causes of maternal deaths in countries such as the UK, Australia and in Europe. In low- and middle-income countries, venous thromboembolism causes only 2% of maternal deaths as other causes, such as postpartum haemorrhage, are more common.

Aetiology

Venous thromboembolism is the collective name for deep vein thrombosis (DVT) and pulmonary embolism (PE). In DVT, a blood clot forms in a deep vein. This can lead to a potentially fatal pulmonary embolism if part of the clot becomes detached and lodges in a pulmonary artery, thereby obstructing blood flow.

Blood clots form because of static blood, hypercoagulability and endothelial injury; this is known as Virchow's triad. Pregnancy and childbirth increase susceptibility to blood clots, because all three of these factors are present: blood flow is reduced by compression of the iliac veins by the gravid uterus, clotting factor production is increased to prevent post-partum haemorrhage and endothelial injury occurs during delivery.

Other risk factors for venous thromboembolism are:

- thrombophilia, either inherited or acquired disorders of clotting factor production or function
- previous venous thromboembolism or family history in first-degree relative
- obesity
- surgery particularly emergency caesarean sections and immobilisation
- medical comorbidities, such as cancer, systemic lupus erythematosus and cardiac failure
- sepsis
- haemorrhage (blood loss > 1 L)
- prolonged labour
- older age (> 35 years)
- multiparity (three or more babies)
- smoking
- dehydration, for example as a consequence of ovarian hyperstimulation syndrome or hyperemesis

Prevention

Low-molecular-weight heparin, an anticoagulant, is given during and after pregnancy to women considered to be at high risk of developing venous thromboembolism based on known risk factors.

Anti-embolism stockings are worn to reduce the risk of DVT during immobilisation after recent surgery or prolonged sitting while travelling by aeroplane. They improve venous blood flow when combined with the pump action of the calf muscles.

Clinical features

Deep vein thrombosis presents with an acutely swollen, painful lower limb. Pulmonary embolism presents with chest pain, dyspnoea and in severe cases collapse.

Pregnant women are more likely than non-pregnant women to develop pelvic DVT. This causes constant lower abdominal pain and can be difficult to diagnose. A high index of clinical suspicion is needed, particularly if there is not an associated red, hot, painful, swollen lower limb.

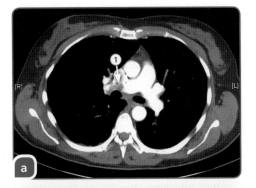

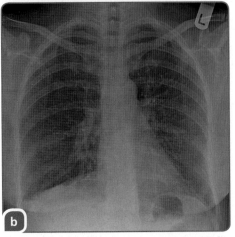

Investigations

Investigations are used to confirm a diagnosis of venous thromboembolism and to determine the dose of anticoagulation required for treatment.

Imaging

Lower limb Doppler ultrasound is carried out for women with symptoms and signs of DVT or pulmonary embolism. This investigation has no radiation risk, and if a DVT is found the treatment is the same whether or not a pulmonary embolism is also present.

If the Doppler is negative and pulmonary embolism is suspected, a chest X-ray followed by a ventilation–perfusion (V/Q) scan or CT pulmonary angiography (CTPA) is carried out (**Figure 7.8**). CT pulmonary angiography is more accurate than a VQ scan if the chest X-ray is abnormal. It also exposes the fetus to less radiation compared with a V/Q scan, but increases the risk of breast cancer in later life by up to 13%.

Figure 7.8 (a) CT pulmonary angiogram showing large pulmonary embolus. ① Filling defect in pulmonary artery. The chest X-ray (b) showed slight elevation of the right hemidiaphragm. Courtesy of Phil Crosbie.

Blood tests

Renal and liver function tests and a platelet count are necessary before treatment with low-molecular-weight heparin, because the results are used to determine the dose.

Measurement of D-dimer, a marker of blood clot formation and breakdown, is unhelpful in pregnancy. D-dimer levels are increased even in the absence of venous thromboembolism in pregnant women.

Management

Low-molecular-weight heparin is the mainstay of treatment and is started while investigations are ongoing. If the results are negative, it can be easily stopped, with minimal adverse effects.

Anti-embolism stockings reduce oedema and pain and help prevent post-thrombotic syndrome, a long-term complication of DVT associated with aching, skin discoloration and ulceration of the leg. The stockings are worn for 2 years on the affected leg and do not increase the risk of a pulmonary embolism.

Medication

Low-molecular weight heparin is given subcutaneously at weight-adjusted doses, taking into account renal and liver function.

No monitoring is required, and clotting function returns to normal within 24 h of a dose. If venous thromboembolism is diagnosed postnatally, oral anticoagulants such as warfarin can be used safely, even for breastfeeding women as these drugs are not found in significant levels in breastmilk.

Unfractionated heparin or thrombolytic therapy, for example streptokinase, are given intravenously if a massive pulmonary embolism causes maternal collapse. They are more effective and have more rapid onset of action than low-molecular weight heparin.

Surgery

In women who have venous thromboembolism despite adequate anticoagulation, a temporary inferior vena cava filter is inserted after discussion with a haematologist.

Embolectomy is carried out by cardiothoracic surgeons in seriously ill patients and those who are unsuitable candidates for thrombolysis.

Prognosis

Up to 60% of women develop post-thrombotic syndrome after venous thromboembolism, and have persistent symptoms of swelling and heaviness in the affected limb.

Maternal and perinatal death

Maternal deaths are those that occur within pregnancy or in the immediate postnatal period, i.e. within 42 days from delivery. Perinatal deaths are those that occur after 24 completed weeks of gestation and before 7 completed days after birth. They therefore include stillbirths.

Maternal death

The world's most comprehensive study in this field is the UK's annual report, *The Confidential Enquiry into Maternal Deaths*. This produced by MBRRACE-UK, Mothers and Babies: Reducing Risk through Audits and Confidential Enquiries. Under this programme, all maternal deaths in the UK are reported and analysed, and recommendations are made based on common themes that emerge from the data.

Deaths are classified by MBRRACE-UK as follows (2011–2013 data):

- Direct deaths caused by a complication of pregnancy or delivery, for example post-partum haemorrhage (3 deaths per 100,000 maternities or pregnancies that have been reported to a doctor)
- Indirect deaths resulting from exacerbation by pregnancy of a pre-existing or newly

developed health problem, for example cardiac disease (totalling 6 deaths per 100,000 maternities)
- Incidental deaths, i.e. those for which the cause is unrelated to pregnancy, for example injuries sustained in a road traffic accident (1 death per 100,000 maternities)

In the UK, the maternal mortality rate is about 9 per 100,000 maternities (direct and indirect deaths, incidental deaths not included). Even with this low rate, it is generally believed that unfortunately many of the women who die do so as a result of substandard care.

For comparison, the rate is 920 per 100,000 live births in sub-Saharan Africa, a risk of death of nearly 1%. This high rate is attributable to lack of access to health care and help from adequately trained health care professionals.

> **Since 1990, the number of maternal deaths worldwide has almost halved.** However, about 800 women die every day from preventable causes related to pregnancy and childbirth. The great majority of maternal deaths occur in low- and middle-income countries.

Perinatal death

According to the MBRRACE-UK *Perinatal Mortality Surveillance Report* for 2013, the overall perinatal mortality rate has continued to decrease, consistent with the trend from 2003 onwards. The rates of stillbirths and neonatal deaths up to 28 days were 4.2 and 1.8 per 1000 births, respectively. Perinatal mortality rates vary considerably between countries, for similar reasons to those for differences in maternal mortality rates.

Postnatal mental health

Having good mental health ensures mothers are able to understand and respond to their baby's needs. Short-term postnatal problems are common; fortunately most are short-lasting and have minimal impact on the relationship between mother and child. More significant mental health problems are rarer, but have significant sequelae.

Baby blues

'Baby blues' are characterised by tearfulness, irritability, low mood and anxiety. They occur shortly after giving birth and are thought to be related to maternal hormonal changes that trigger alterations in chemical signalling within the brain. The symptoms last only a few days and resolve spontaneously without treatment. Women should be reassured that these feelings are normal; 50% of mothers develop them.

Postnatal depression

Postnatal depression affects up to 1 in 10 women and up to 4 in 10 teenage mothers. It usually occurs 2–8 weeks after birth and can last up to 1 year. Women with postnatal depression feel increasingly depressed and despondent. They:

- lose interest in their baby
- feel hopeless and unable to cope
- can develop somatic symptoms such as loss of appetite, aches and pains, and extreme tiredness

Postnatal depression is distinguished from 'baby blues' by the duration and severity of symptoms: 'baby blues' resolve quickly and do not affect the mother's ability to lead a normal life. Mild cases of postnatal depression are treated with counselling; more severe cases require antidepressant medication. Pre-existing mental health problems and previous postnatal depression are both risk factors.

Symptoms of postnatal depression should be asked about specifically because many women do not confide their concerns to friends, family and healthcare professionals.

Suicide is one of the commonest causes of maternal death and is often associated with infanticide (infant homicide). In postpartum suicide attempts, there is a tendency for violent methods such as strangulation to be used, rather than overdose. Specialist mother-and-baby units keep the woman and her child together, thereby preventing disturbances in bonding.

Postnatal psychosis

Postnatal psychosis is the most severe postnatal mental health problem, affecting 1 in 1000 women. It develops within hours of childbirth and requires urgent attention due to the risks that a mother may pose to herself and her baby. Other people usually notice symptoms first: the mother may have symptoms of depression or mania that change rapidly, including hallucinations or delusions. Treatment is with admission to a specialist mother and baby unit and with antidepressant, mood-stabilising and antipsychotic drugs. Electroconvulsive therapy is used in rare circumstances. As with postnatal depression, pre-existing mental health problems increase the risk of postnatal psychosis.

Answers to starter questions

1. This area of obstetrics is controversial and open to individual interpretation. The safest mode of delivery for mother and baby is a vaginal delivery, but this is not always achievable. A caesarean section without labour protects the pelvic floor from damage and reduces the risk of stress incontinence and prolapse, but is not risk-free. Some women are referred to mental health services with tocophobia (fear of childbirth); refusing a caesarean section can impact on their mental wellbeing.

2. The chance of a baby born at 24 weeks surviving until discharge from hospital is 40%. However, less than 25% will have no disabilities. The outlook is much better after 27 weeks where over 90% of babies survive to discharge. Severely premature babies have difficulties with breathing and ventilation, infection, ventricular haemorrhage and necrotising enterocolitis.

3. One instrument is not inherently safer than another; it depends upon the indication for delivery, operator experience, maternal effort and fetal position, station and the degree of caput and moulding (the degree of overlapping of the fetal skull bones caused by pressure as the head passes through the pelvis in labour). A ventouse is associated with less perineal trauma than forceps, but has a higher chance of failing, particularly if a silastic cup is used. There is also an increase in maternal concerns about her baby, due to the presence of a chignon, and fetal complications such as cephalohaematoma and retinal haemorrhage are more common.

4. Wound infection rates following a caesarean section are reduced by a single dose of intravenous antibiotics given at the start of the procedure, avoiding incisions under folds of skin, use of absorbable sutures, avoidance of suturing tissues under tension and closure of subcutaneous fat >2 cm in depth.

5. A CTG is a sensitive tool to detect intrapartum fetal compromise but is not specific; only 50% of pathological CTGs are due to hypoxia. This is why it is combined with fetal blood sampling to accurately distinguish a compromised fetus from one that is coping well with labour. A caveat to this is that fetal blood sampling is relatively contraindicated in the presence of sepsis; the scalp pH is likely to be normal but the fetus is at an increased risk of harm by not being delivered even if normoxic.
A CTG is open to interpretation error and this is its main fault. Computerised CTGs are used antenatally and are better at detecting fetal compromise than human assessment, particularly before term. The fetal sympathetic and parasympathetic nervous systems are not fully developed until the third trimester meaning that the characteristic accelerations and baseline variability which are reassuring of fetal well-being are often absent earlier in pregnancy. The computerised CTG compares the fetal heart rate with CTGs of other fetuses of the same gestation, taking these differences into account and reporting on the probability of fetal compromise. Unfortunately they have not been validated for use intrapartum and fetal oximetry and computerised assessment of the ST waveform (STAN) have yet to be conclusively shown to improve neonatal outcome.

Chapter 8
Reproductive endocrinology

Starter questions

Answers to the following questions are on page 258.

1. Why do children who go through puberty early become short adults?
2. Why does anorexia delay puberty?
3. Why do some drugs cause excessive milk production?

Introduction

Hormones govern development of the reproductive system prenatally and in childhood. They also drive sexual maturation at puberty. In girls, hormonal changes during puberty lead to menarche, which marks the onset of regular menstrual cycles and the period of life when childbearing is possible. Disorders that affect development before and during puberty cannot always be cured. However, various treatments are available to alleviate their effects, and pregnancy is possible in a significant proportion of patients.

Hormonal changes can also disrupt the regular menstruation that underlies reproductive function, and fertility is impaired or lost in consequence. These changes occur naturally at menopause, the permanent cessation of ovarian activity at about the age of 50 years. However, they can also be pathological, as in premature menopause, and the infertility associated with this disorder can be devastating for women who want to start a family or to have another child.

Although the subspecialty of reproductive endocrinology focuses on the diagnosis and treatment of disorders that reduce fertility in women, it also manages other conditions with a hormonal basis that produce symptoms and require treatment, including galactorrhoea and premenstrual syndrome.

The role of the clinician is to use a systematic approach for assessment and diagnosis. Once a disorder is diagnosed, appropriate referrals are made to fertility specialists, surgeons and counselling services.

Case 8 Absent menarche

Presentation

Stephanie Mullins attends the gynaecology clinic with her mother. She is 16 years old and has not started her periods.

Initial interpretation

Absent menarche, or primary amenorrhoea, is always investigated in girls over 16 years old, as well as in girls over 14 years old if they also lack other secondary sexual characteristics. It is caused by anatomical, hormonal or karyotype abnormalities.

A detailed history must include growth and pubertal development.

- Cyclical abdominal pain suggests anatomical obstruction to menstrual flow
- A history of chronic illness, weight loss, eating disorder or heavy exercise suggests hypothalamic dysfunction

Constitutional delay is a diagnosis of exclusion. It is relatively uncommon in girls.

History

Stephanie says that all her friends have started their periods, and that she thinks she is the only girl in her class who has not. She also reports that she has not developed breasts, or pubic or axillary hair.

She was not worried at first, but now she feels 'like a freak' and feels embarrassed when getting changed for sport at school. She has always enjoyed spending time with her friends, but lately she has been making excuses to avoid sleepovers and other situations in which she would have to change clothes in front of others. She has never had a boyfriend.

Stephanie has always been shorter than her peers, but the difference has become more obvious. She likes sport but prefers other activities and does not exercise excessively. She denies any eating disorders.

Stephanie's 12-year-old sister is the same height as her and started having periods 4 months ago. This has 'made everything worse', and Stephanie has been crying herself to sleep at night. She desperately wants 'everything to be OK' but is terrified that something is wrong.

Interpretation of history

Puberty entails rapid physical and emotional changes, which most people find challenging. There is also great variation in the rate at which individuals develop during this period in their life. However, Stephanie has significant concerns and the degree of difference in development between her and her sister is unusual. Further investigation is warranted.

Further history

Stephanie is doing well at school and is otherwise fit and well. There is no medical history, medication history or family history of note. Stephanie has no headaches, visual disturbances, abdominal pain, lethargy, tiredness, breathlessness, or urinary or bowel dysfunction.

Examination

Stephanie is 150 cm tall, which places her in the 3rd centile according to a growth chart for height, standardised for girls of her age. Her body mass index is 24 kg/m². She has a low hairline and low-set ears.

General respiratory and cardiovascular examinations are normal. Stephanie has a broad chest with widely spaced nipples and small breast buds (Tanner stage 2; see **Table 8.3**). She has normal female external genitalia. She has downy hair over the labia majora but none in the axillae (Tanner stage 2; see **Table 8.3**).

Case 8 continued

A pelvic examination is not carried out. This is because Stephanie is virgo intacta; she has never been sexually active.

Interpretation of findings

Stephanie's short stature and underdeveloped secondary sexual characteristics suggest an underlying endocrine disorder. This may be caused by hypothalamic, pituitary or ovarian pathology. A hormonal profile will differentiate between hypergonadotropic and hypogonadotropic hypogonadism and direct further investigations. Stephanie's broad chest and widely spaced nipples is concerning for a chromosomal abnormality called Turner's syndrome (45XO).

Investigations

Pelvic ultrasound shows a normal uterus and adnexa.

The results of a full reproductive hormonal profile show high levels of the gonadotrophins follicle-stimulating hormone (FSH) and luteinising hormone (LH), and low levels of oestradiol. This profile is consistent with hypergonadotrophic hypogonadism, which manifests in females as primary ovarian dysfunction (see page 251).

The rest of Stephanie's hormonal profile is normal. Serum concentrations of prolactin, testosterone and thyroid-stimulating hormone are all within their normal range.

A blood sample is taken for chromosomal analysis, which shows that Stephanie's karyotype is 45XO.

Investigation of primary amenorrhoea

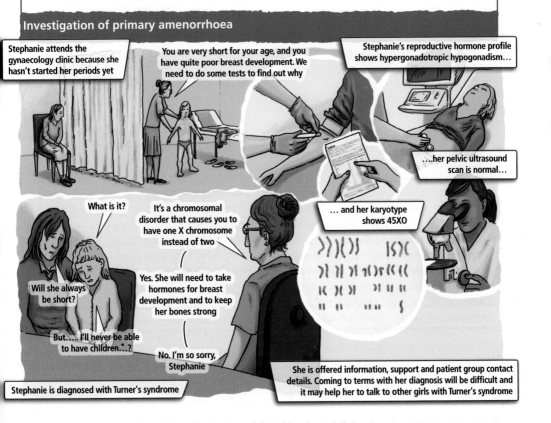

Stephanie attends the gynaecology clinic because she hasn't started her periods yet

You are very short for your age, and you have quite poor breast development. We need to do some tests to find out why

Stephanie's reproductive hormone profile shows hypergonadotropic hypogonadism...

....her pelvic ultrasound scan is normal...

What is it?

It's a chromosomal disorder that causes you to have one X chromosome instead of two

... and her karyotype shows 45XO

Will she always be short?

Yes. She will need to take hormones for breast development and to keep her bones strong

But..... I'll never be able to have children...?

No. I'm so sorry, Stephanie

Stephanie is diagnosed with Turner's syndrome

She is offered information, support and patient group contact details. Coming to terms with her diagnosis will be difficult and it may help her to talk to other girls with Turner's syndrome

Case 8 *continued*

Diagnosis

Absent menarche associated with lack of breast development and a high serum concentration of FSH is caused by chromosomal abnormalities resulting in gonadal dysgenesis (e.g. Turner's syndrome), congenital insensitivity to FSH or defects in the enzymes involved in ovarian biosynthesis of oestrogen. The most common congenital cause is Turner's syndrome. Surgery, trauma, infection, toxins, radiation or drugs are acquired causes of primary ovarian dysfunction that are usually suggested by the history and therefore unlikely in Stephanie's case. Stephanie's karyotype is 45XO, which means that she has only one X chromosome, instead of the usual two. Therefore Stephanie has Turner's syndrome.

> **Turner's syndrome has a classic phenotype (Figure 8.1) and is associated with a range of potentially serious conditions that affect some, but not all, patients.** Patients require screening for cardiovascular malformations, diabetes, renal abnormalities, hypothyroidism, hypertension, ophthalmic abnormalities and hearing dysfunction. This is done at diagnosis and annually thereafter, depending on clinical risk.

Stephanie and her mother are extremely upset by this diagnosis. They had suspected that something was wrong but now their worst fears have been realised. They know that there is no cure for

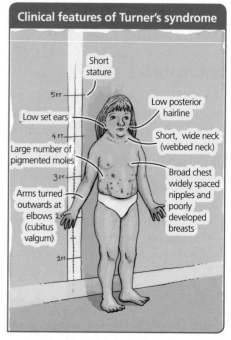

Clinical features of Turner's syndrome

Short stature

Low set ears

Low posterior hairline

Short, wide neck (webbed neck)

Large number of pigmented moles

Broad chest widely spaced nipples and poorly developed breasts

Arms turned outwards at elbows (cubitus valgum)

Figure 8.1 Clinical features of Turner's syndrome.

Turner's syndrome, and that Stephanie will never be able to have biological children. However, they are relieved to learn that the effects of the disorder on sexual development can be treated. Stephanie is started on low dose oestrogen therapy to promote breast development. When the time is right, it will be possible for her to conceive using donated oocytes and assisted reproductive techniques. The family are offered psychological support and given written information including contact details for support groups and patient forums.

Disorders of puberty

Precocious or delayed puberty can reflect normal variation or be the consequence of an underlying disease process.

Precocious puberty

In girls, precocious puberty is the development of secondary sexual characteristics before 8 years of age. It is more common in obese girls and is classified as central or peripheral.

- Central precocious puberty results from early maturation of the entire hypothalamic-pituitary-gonadal axis (see page 4)
- Peripheral precocious puberty is much less common and is gonadotrophin-independent (**Table 8.1**)

Clinical features

Table 8.2 summarises the expected ages at which pubertal milestones are reached. In cases of precocious puberty, the child may have:

- all the physical signs of puberty
- an isolated sign of puberty, for example:
  - breast development (thelarche)
  - development of axillary hair and pubic hair (pubarche)

Increased height is usually the first observable change. Children with central nervous system lesions often complain of headaches and visual disturbances.

Pubertal development is quantified using the Tanner staging system (**Table 8.3**).

> **A sensitive approach is essential when carrying out intimate examinations on young girls.** Inspection of the external genitalia is more likely to yield useful information if the child is relaxed. Speculum examinations in clinic are never appropriate for children or adolescents who are not sexually active.

Diagnostic approach

Early sexual development is evaluated to distinguish children in whom it has a serious

Precocious puberty: causes	
Central precocious puberty (gonadotrophin-dependent)	Peripheral precocious puberty (gonadotrophin-independent)
Idiopathic (90% of cases)	Oestrogen-secreting tumour (e.g. granulosa cell tumour of the ovary, ovarian follicular cyst, thecoma)
Central nervous system lesions (10% of cases)	
■ Infection (e.g. encephalitis, tuberculosis)	McCune–Albright syndrome (characterised by cystic bone lesions, café-au-lait spots and sexual precocity)
■ Tumour (e.g. hypothalamic hamartoma, craniopharyngioma, astrocytoma, neurofibromatosis)	Iatrogenic (consumption of oestrogens)
■ Trauma (e.g. head injury)	Others
■ Other (e.g. hydrocephalus, epilepsy, cranial irradiation)	■ Hypothyroidism ■ Congenital adrenal hyperplasia

Table 8.1 Causes of precocious puberty

Pubertal milestones: definitions and normal timing in girls			
Milestone	Definition	Age at which milestone occurs*	
		Median (years)	Range (years)
Thelarche	Breast development	10	8–13
Pubarche	First appearance of pubic hair	11	8.5–13.5
Growth spurt	Accelerated phase of growth in height	11	10–12.5
Menarche	First menstrual bleed	12.5	10.5–14.5
Achievement of adult height	No further growth in height	15.5	-

*UK data.

Table 8.2 Definitions and normal timing of pubertal milestones in girls

Tanner staging system		
Stage	Breast development	Pubic hair
1	Childlike breasts	No pubic hair
2	Breast buds, each an elevated areola and papilla on a small mound	Sparse, straight, downy hair over and along the labia majora
3	Great enlargement of the breasts and areolae without contour development	Hair becomes darker and coarser but is still sparse around the pubic region
4	Further enlargement of breast tissue and areolae, with development of contour above the breast	Pubic hair of adult type but no spread to inner thighs
5	Adult breasts: recession of the areolae to the mound of the breast	Adult quantity and distribution of pubic hair extending to inner thighs

Table 8.3 The Tanner staging system

underlying cause from the majority who are naturally developing more quickly than their peers.

Investigations

Appropriate investigations include blood tests and imaging.

Blood tests

Thyroid function tests, measurement of serum oestradiol and the result of the gonadotrophin-releasing hormone (GnRH) stimulation test usually establish the diagnosis (**Table 8.4**). The GnRH stimulation test measures serum LH levels before and after intravenous GnRH administration. In pre-pubertal girls, low LH levels will be observed but in girls with precocious puberty, high LH levels are diagnostic.

Imaging

The following may provide useful information.

■ A radiograph of the wrist determines bone age; this is useful to confirm the diagnosis and monitor the child during treatment; bone age reflects oestrogen levels, so when

Precocious puberty: evaluation and diagnosis					
Type of precocious puberty	Baseline LH	GnRH stimulation test result	Oestradiol, testosterone, DHEA, DHEA-S	Pelvic ultrasound	MRI of the brain
Central precocious puberty (gonadotrophin-dependent)	Pubertal (high)	LH increases	Pubertal levels	Enlarged uterus and ovaries	Normal (> 90% of cases) May identify central nervous system lesion
Peripheral precocious puberty (gonadotrophin-independent)	Prepubertal (low) or suppressed	Absent LH response	Pubertal or very high levels, depending on cause	Enlarged uterus and ovaries May find ovarian cyst	Normal

DHEA, dehydroepiandrosterone; DHEA-S, dehydroepiandrosterone sulfate; GnRH, gonadotrophin-releasing hormone; LH, luteinising hormone.

Table 8.4 Evaluation and diagnosis of precocious puberty

bone age begins to 'normalise', treatment is taking effect
- A pelvic ultrasound scan may exclude an ovarian tumour as the underlying cause
- An MRI scan of the brain is required if an intracranial lesion is suspected

Management

The aims of management are to treat any serious underlying pathology and to delay sexual maturity in young children to protect their final height as an adult.

Medication

Idiopathic central precocious puberty is treated with GnRH agonists, which reduce LH and FSH secretion through negative feedback. Treatment is usually discontinued at 10–11 years of age.

Surgery

Ovarian tumours and intracranial lesions are managed by a specialist team. One or more of surgery, chemotherapy and irradiation are usually necessary.

Prognosis

Idiopathic central precocious puberty is a benign process with an excellent prognosis. The main consequence of precocious puberty is oestrogen-driven early epiphyseal fusion of the long bones, resulting in shorter stature in adulthood. The decision to treat with GnRH agonists takes into account patient age and stage of pubertal development, as well as their current growth velocity and bone age.

Delayed puberty

In girls, delayed puberty is the absence of secondary sexual characteristics by 16 years of age, past the age at which most pubertal milestones have been reached (see **Table 8.2**).

Clinical features and diagnostic approach

Delayed puberty presents with complete lack of sexual development or the absence of menarche (see page 11).

The Tanner staging system is used to assess development (see **Table 8.3**). Examination findings and serum concentration of FSH indicate possible causes of absent menarche (**Table 8.5**).

Management

The treatment of delayed puberty depends on the underlying cause but includes oestrogen therapy (Turner's syndrome, primary ovarian dysfunction), and surgery (imperforate hymen, vaginal septum) where appropriate.

Delayed menarche: assessment			
Absence of breast development		**Breast development**	
Low serum FSH concentration	High serum FSH concentration	Uterus absent	Uterus present
Constitutional delay	Turner's syndrome (45XO)	Müllerian agenesis	Constitutional delay
Chronic illness, stress, heavy exercise, weight loss, anorexia	Premature ovarian failure (46XX)	Androgen insensitivity syndrome (46XY)	Vaginal septum
			Imperforate hymen
Prolactinoma			Polycystic ovary syndrome
Kallmann's syndrome			
Congenital adrenal hyperplasia			
FSH, follicle-stimulating hormone.			

Table 8.5 Assessment of delayed menarche

Hirsutism

Hirsutism is excess hair growth in a male distribution in women. Most cases are caused by benign disorders such as polycystic ovary syndrome (PCOS). Serious causes of hirsutism include androgen-secreting tumours, Cushing's disease, acromegaly and certain drugs.

Clinical features and diagnostic approach

Hirsutism is evaluated by using the Ferriman-Gallwey scoring system (**Figure 8.2**).

Additional signs of hyperandrogenism (androgen excess) are worrying features:

- acne
- deepening voice
- enlarged clitoris
- oligomenorrhoea
- increased aggression and libido

These warrant further investigation to exclude an androgen-secreting tumour.

Hirsutism is a sign rather than a diagnosis. Although the unwanted hair is removed using various cosmetic methods, serious underlying pathology must always be excluded.

Management

The aim of management is to treat the underlying cause. In cases of hirsutism with a benign cause, simple cosmetic measures usually suffice. The options are shaving, waxing, bleaching, electrolysis and laser hair removal.

Medication

Use of a combined oral contraceptive (e.g. Dianette) corrects the hormonal imbalance of PCOS. Antiandrogens such as cyproterone acetate, or topical treatments such as eflornithine, are necessary in severe cases.

Treatment of obesity and insulin resistance reduces androgen production and increases levels of sex hormone-binding globulin. This in turn reduces levels of circulating free, i.e. active, testosterone, leading to an improvement in hirsutism and acne.

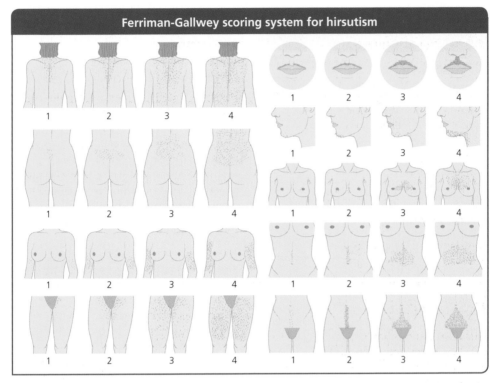

Figure 8.2 The Ferriman–Gallwey scoring system for hirsutism. The extent of excessive hair growth in nine areas of the body is scored from 1 to 4. Normal, total score < 8; mild hirsutism, score 8–15; moderate or severe hirsutism, score > 15.

Polycystic ovary syndrome

Polycystic ovary syndrome is a leading cause of subfertility. It affects up to 10% of women of childbearing age, making it the commonest endocrine disorder in this group. It is more common in women of South Asian origin.

Aetiology and pathogenesis

The trigger for PCOS is unknown. The condition is characterised by chronically increased LH and suppressed FSH levels, which replace the cyclical rise and fall that occur in the normal menstrual cycle. High LH stimulates the production of androgens, which are converted in peripheral fat to oestrogen; excess androgens and oestrogen causes chronic anovulation. Hyperinsulinaemia and insulin resistance further contribute to increased androgen levels and ovarian dysfunction.

Clinical features

The clinical features of PCOS are summarised in **Figure 8.3**. The condition is characterised by menstrual cycle disturbance and features of hyperandrogenism, i.e. hirsutism, acne and alopecia. Fertility problems are present in 75% of cases, and obesity in 50%. Women with PCOS may also experience mood swings and depression.

Diagnostic approach

Two of the Rotterdam criteria must be present for a diagnosis of PCOS:

- infrequent (oligomenorrhoea) or absent (amenorrhoea) periods
- hyperandrogenism (clinical features of androgen excess, e.g. hirsuitism) or

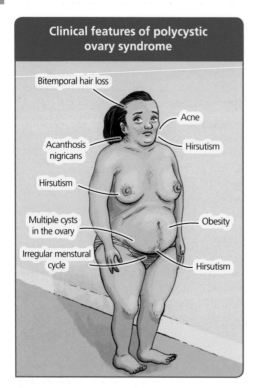

Clinical features of polycystic ovary syndrome

Bitemporal hair loss

Acne

Acanthosis nigricans

Hirsutism

Hirsutism

Multiple cysts in the ovary

Obesity

Irregular menstrual cycle

Hirsutism

Figure 8.3 Clinical features of polycystic ovary syndrome.

hyperandrogenaemia (elevated serum testosterone)
- polycystic ovaries on ultrasound

Investigations

Blood tests and pelvic ultrasound establish the diagnosis.

Blood tests

An LH:FSH ratio of 3:1 within the first 5 days of the menstrual cycle is consistent with a diagnosis of PCOS. Oestrogen, testosterone and androstenedione levels are all increased.

Ultrasound

The classic picture is of a 'necklace' of several small follicles positioned along the periphery of the ovary, which is usually enlarged.

Management

There are several approaches to management, depending on the patient's wishes for:

- fertility
- treatment of hirsutism, acne or both
- normal menstruation

Lifestyle modification

If PCOS is associated with overweight or obesity, weight loss through dietary improvements and exercise is the most effective way of normalising ovulation and menstruation. It also improves pregnancy rates, hirsutism, hyperandrogenism, insulin resistance, hyperlipidaemia and quality of life. However, many patients find it difficult lose weight.

Medication

Clomifene citrate is used to induce ovulation in women seeking fertility. This selective oestrogen receptor modulator increases production of gonadotrophins by inhibiting negative feedback on the hypothalamus. The use of the combined oral contraceptive pill provides regular withdrawal bleeds and improves symptoms of hyperandrogenism.

Cyproterone acetate, an antiandrogen, is effective in some patients with excessive hirsutism or acne. Metformin, an insulin-sensitising agent, improves glucose tolerance, decreases androgen levels and improves ovulation rates.

Surgery

Ovarian drilling (laparoscopic puncture of 10–12 small ovarian follicles using electrocautery) temporarily improves ovulation rates in women with PCOS who fail to conceive with clomifene treatment.

Prognosis

The long-term sequelae of PCOS are:

- obesity
- insulin resistance and type 2 diabetes mellitus
- hypertension
- cardiovascular disease
- dyslipidaemia
- cerebrovascular accident

Women with PCOS are also at risk of endometrial hyperplasia or cancer if they have persistent oligomenorrhoea or amenorrhoea and high levels of circulating oestrogen.

Hypogonadism

In females, hypogonadism is the term used to describe non-functioning ovaries. The consequences of hypogonadism are:

- failed oestrogen production, leading to defective primary or secondary sexual development in children and premature menopause in adults
- failed oocyte development, leading to subfertility

Aetiology and pathogenesis

Hypogonadism is caused by:

- a defect in the ovaries, i.e. primary ovarian dysfunction, also known as premature ovarian failure
- a defect in the brain, i.e. primary hypothalamic-pituitary dysfunction

Primary ovarian dysfunction is a type of hypergonadotrophic hypogonadism in females. Low oestrogen levels fail to down-regulate the secretion of gonadotrophins by the hypothalamus and pituitary gland, which leads to high levels of FSH.

Primary hypothalamic-pituitary dysfunction is a form of hypogonadotrophic hypogonadism. Decreased gonadotrophic stimulation of the ovaries leads to failed folliculogenesis and low levels of oestrogen.

The most common causes of hypogonadism are shown in **Table 8.6**. Examples are:

- gonadal dysgenesis, including Turner's syndrome
- Kallmann's syndrome
- Sheehan's syndrome
- Prolactin-secreting adenoma

Gonadal dysgenesis, including Turner's syndrome

In gonadal dysgenesis, the ovaries fail to develop. Instead of ovaries, patients have characteristic underdeveloped streak gonads, where the ovaries are replaced by non-functional fibrous tissue. Streak gonads do not contain follicles or produce oestrogen.

Turner's syndrome (45XO) affects 1 in 2500 live births. It accounts for more than half of cases of gonadal dysgenesis. Patients with Turner's syndrome typically present in their late teenage years with an absence of secondary sexual characteristics and menarche (primary amenorrhoea; see page 284). They have a recognisable phenotype (see **Figure 8.1**). Besides ovarian dysfunction, abnormalities associated with Turner's syndrome include spina bifida, deafness and coarctation of the aorta.

Hypogonadism: causes		
Primary ovarian dysfunction (hypergonadotrophic hypogonadism)	Primary hypothalamic–pituitary dysfunction (hypogonadotrophic hypogonadism)	Others
Genetic cause ■ Turner's syndrome (45XO)	Hypothalamic causes ■ Kallman's syndrome ■ Stress, weight loss, anorexia, excessive exercise ■ Brain tumour	Polycystic ovary syndrome Congenital adrenal hyperplasia Hypothyroidism
Acquired causes ■ Chemotherapy ■ Radiotherapy ■ Infection ■ Autoimmune diseases	Pituitary causes ■ Prolactinoma ■ Sheehan's syndrome	

Table 8.6 Causes of hypogonadism

Kallmann's syndrome

This is hypogonadotrophic hypogonadism caused by failure of migration of fetal GnRH neurones to the hypothalamus. These neurones secrete GnRH, which stimulates the release of LH and FSH from the pituitary gland. It is usually associated with anosmia and midline facial anomalies. Kallman's syndrome is generally inherited as an autosomal recessive condition, but some cases are X-linked.

Sheehan's syndrome

This is acquired pan-hypopituitarism caused by pituitary ischaemia and necrosis resulting from massive post-partum haemorrhage. It presents after childbirth with failed lactation with or without failure to resume menses. Prolactin, gonadotrophin and growth hormone production are affected.

Prolactin-secreting adenoma

This is a benign tumour of the pituitary gland that produces prolactin. Hyperprolactinaemia causes ovulatory dysfunction (see page 254).

Clinical features

The clinical features of hypogonadism depend on the timing of ovarian failure.

- If the ovaries have never functioned, puberty is delayed and secondary sexual characteristics do not develop
- Failure in later life leads to premature menopause

Most patients present with amenorrhoea (see page 284) or difficulty conceiving (see page 271).

Investigations

Investigations include karyotyping and imaging as well as blood tests.

Blood tests

Gonadotrophin levels distinguish hypergonadotrophic from hypogonadotrophic hypogonadism.

- High serum FSH indicates hypergonadotrophic hypogonadism
- Low serum FSH indicates hypogonadotrophic hypogonadism

Gonadotrophin levels are normal in PCOS (page 249), congenital adrenal hyperplasia, hyperprolactinaemia (page 254) and hypothyroidism.

Karyotyping

Chromosomal analysis is indicated in patients with hypergonadotrophic hypogonadism to exclude Turner's syndrome and other chromosomal disorders.

Imaging

Magnetic resonance imaging of the brain is indicated in hypogonadotrophic hypogonadism to diagnose hypothalamic or pituitary tumours (**Figure 8.4**).

Management

Management depends on the underlying cause.

Behaviour modification

If the hypothalamic dysfunction is caused by stress, excessive exercise or weight loss, behavioural modification normalises gonadotrophin production in most cases. In anorexia nervosa, ovarian function returns upon restoration of a healthy body weight.

Medication

Girls and young women are treated with hormone replacement therapy (HRT) to promote breast development and maintain bone health. The combined oral contraceptive pill is a suitable alternative to HRT. Older women may not need treatment, but HRT is always offered because premature menopause is associated with an increased risk of osteoporosis.

> **Empathy and patience are extremely important when dealing with children and adolescents with hypogonadism.** Insensitivity can be psychologically devastating to a girl who is, for example, finding out that she is genetically male or unable to have biological children. Directing families to accurate sources of information and support is an essential part of the clinical management of this condition.

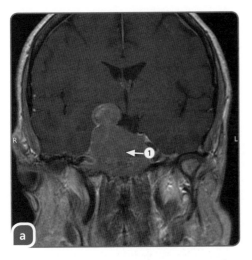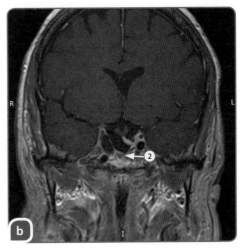

Figure 8.4 Prolactinoma. (a) ① Before and (b) ② after treatment, showing a reduction in the size of the prolactinoma and restoration of brain anatomy.

Surgery

Large brain tumours require surgical excision. Intra-abdominal gonads are removed in patients who have a Y chromosome to prevent the malignant transformation that occurs in up to 25% of cases.

Prognosis

Oestrogen deficiency is easily treated with HRT, thereby enabling the patient's sexual development to proceed appropriately. However, fertility may not always be possible. Great care is needed when informing a patient, particularly a child or adolescent, that they have a disorder that causes permanent infertility. Counselling is essential.

Assisted conception is tailored to meet the needs of the individual patient.

- Clomifene citrate improves pregnancy rates in women with normal gonadotrophin levels
- Pulsatile GnRH or gonadotrophins are used to treat women with low gonadotrophin levels
- Donor oocytes and in vitro fertilisation (see page 275) offer the best chance of pregnancy in women with high gonadotrophin levels, in whom ovulation is unlikely

Galactorrhoea

Lactation is the production of breast milk. In pregnancy, high levels of oestrogen and progesterone stimulate the development and subsequent enlargement of the breast alveoli and milk duct system (see page 71).

Breastfeeding is controlled by two key hormones.

- Prolactin, released from the anterior pituitary gland, stimulates milk production
- Oxytocin, released from the posterior pituitary gland, stimulates milk ejection

Milk ejection is triggered by suckling, which stimulates the myoepithelial cells of the areola. Women with pituitary necrosis, i.e. Sheehan's syndrome, do not lactate.

Lactation is normal when it follows childbirth, and abnormal when it does not. Abnormal lactation is called galactorrhoea.

Aetiology

Common causes of galactorrhoea are shown in **Table 8.7**. Most are associated with hyperprolactinaemia.

Hyperprolactinaemia is caused by decreased dopaminergic inhibition of prolactin secretion by the pituitary gland, or by prolactin-secreting tumours. Galactorrhoea is a complication of:

- certain hypothalamic and pituitary diseases
- dopamine antagonist drugs, such as certain antipsychotics (e.g. haloperidol)
- gastric motility drugs (e.g. metoclopramide)
- some antihypertensives (e.g. methyldopa)

Stress may mildly increase prolactin levels. In up to 40% of cases of galactorrhoea, no cause is identified.

Clinical features

Patients usually present with bilateral milky nipple discharge from several ducts. They also have menstrual irregularities and difficulty conceiving.

Clear or milky discharge from the nipple is normal in pregnancy and after giving birth. Yellow or green discharge from the nipple is a sign of infection, usually in a breastfeeding woman. Blood-stained discharge in a non-breast feeding woman is a sinister sign and prompts investigations to exclude breast cancer.

Diagnostic approach

A detailed drug history enables identification of any medications that could be responsible for the discharge. Headaches and visual disturbances suggest an intracranial lesion.

A recent pregnancy should always be excluded. Milky discharge from the nipples may continue for up to 6 months after cessation of breastfeeding.

Investigations

Blood tests

Measurement of serum prolactin concentration is helpful.

- Mildly increased prolactin levels are caused by stress
- Moderately increased prolactin levels reflect decreased dopaminergic inhibition of prolactin secretion by the pituitary gland
- Grossly increased prolactin levels are found in patients with pituitary prolactinoma

Blood tests are also done to exclude hypothyroidism and chronic renal failure, because both can cause galactorrhoea.

Imaging

If prolactin levels are grossly increased, imaging of the pituitary stalk is required to exclude a prolactinoma (pituitary microadenoma) (see **Figure 8.4**).

Management

The management of galactorrhoea depends on the underlying cause.

Galactorrhoea: causes	
Cause	Description
Prolactinoma	Benign tumours of lactotrophs in the anterior pituitary gland
Decreased dopaminergic inhibition of prolactin secretion	Tumours of the hypothalamus or pituitary gland
	Head trauma
	Infiltrative disease of the hypothalamus (e.g. sarcoid)
	Use of dopamine antagonists (e.g. risperidone, haloperidol, metoclopramide, domperidone, methyldopa, reserpine, verapamil)
Others	Hypothyroidism
	Chest wall injury
	Chronic renal failure

Table 8.7 Causes of galactorrhoea

Medication

Drugs that could be causing the galactorrhoea are discontinued.

Idiopathic hyperprolactinaemia and pituitary microadenomas are treated with a dopamine agonist, either bromocriptine or cabergoline. Adverse effects include nausea, postural hypotension and clouding of consciousness.

Surgery

Large prolactin-secreting pituitary tumours (macroprolactinomas) (e.g. **Figure 8.5**) that do not respond to treatment with dopamine agonists require trans-sphenoidal surgery and rarely post-surgical irradiation.

Prognosis

This depends on the underlying cause. Drug treatment normalises serum prolactin levels and therefore menstruation in 90% of women.

Premenstrual syndrome

Premenstrual syndrome (PMS) is a myriad of distressing physical, behavioural and psychological symptoms that occur during the luteal phase of each menstrual cycle:

- 5% of women experience no premenstrual symptoms
- 5–10% of women experience severe premenstrual symptoms at some point in their lives

Aetiology and pathogenesis

The aetiology of PMS is unknown. Cyclical ovarian activity and the effects of oestrogen and progesterone on the neurotransmitters serotonin and GABA probably play a role. PMS does not occur before puberty, during pregnancy or after the menopause.

Clinical features

The most commonly reported symptoms of PMS are irritability, tension and dysphoria (unhappiness). The pattern of symptoms varies from woman to woman but is predictable across cycles for each individual.

- Physical symptoms include breast tenderness, bloating and headaches
- Behavioural symptoms include reduced visuospatial and cognitive ability and more frequent accidents
- Psychological symptoms include mood swings, irritability, depression and feeling out of control

Diagnostic approach

Symptoms should be present in multiple, consecutive cycles. Differential diagnoses to consider are psychiatric disorders, psychosexual problems, and menopause, as well as other causes of lethargy, tiredness and breast symptoms.

Premenstrual dysphoric disorder (PMDD) is a severe form of PMS affecting up to 2% of women. It is a repeating transitory cyclical disorder with clinical features similar to those of depression. Several antidepressants are effective in PMDD.

Investigations

A clear diagnosis is essential before treatment starts. A patient diary, in which symptoms are recorded across at least one menstrual cycle, establishes a lack of symptoms during the follicular phase.

Management

The aim of treatment is to relieve symptoms and improve function. Several drugs have shown promise in the treatment of PMS.

First-line drug therapy is with selective serotonin reuptake inhibitors, for example fluoxetine or sertraline, either during the luteal phase only or continuously across the menstrual cycle.

The use of the combined oral contraceptive pill, either continuously or with regular pill-free intervals (usually 7 days in every 28 days), is effective for many women.

Mild symptoms may respond to regular exercise and relaxation techniques. Some women find complementary/alternative therapies helpful. These include vitamin B6, agnus-castus and evening primrose oil. However, although such therapies are popular, there is little evidence for their effectiveness.

Menopause

Menopause is the permanent cessation of menstruation. In developed countries, the average age of menopause is 51 years, but it can also occur prematurely, for example in cases of primary ovarian dysfunction. Premature menopause is defined as menopause before the age of 40 years. Iatrogenic menopause is a consequence of surgical removal of the ovaries, pelvic radiotherapy or chemotherapy.

Clinical features

The extent of symptoms and the degree to which they affect quality of life varies between individuals. Symptoms relate to low oestrogen levels and include hot flushes, night sweats, vaginal dryness, mood changes and loss of libido.

Women going through the menopause frequently report low mood and anxiety. Menopause may bring about a sense of loss related to the end of fertility. In addition, the menopause transition years, the so-called 'perimenopause', often coincide with other life stressors, including:

- caring for, and/or the death of, elderly parents
- 'empty nest syndrome', when children leave home
- the birth of grandchildren, marking the start of old age and the end of middle age

The combination of hormonal changes and stressful life events makes the perimenopause an emotionally challenging time for many women.

It is also a challenging time for younger women experiencing premature menopause, particularly if they have not completed their families.

Diagnostic approach

Menopause is generally diagnosed on clinical grounds. It is confirmed by the absence of menstruation for at least 12 months, accompanied by persistently increased levels of LH and FSH.

Investigations

Increased serum concentrations of LH and FSH confirm the diagnosis. Levels vary from month to month in the perimenopause, so repeat testing is wise.

Management

Premature menopause is usually treated with HRT until the age of 50 years to maintain bone health. Oestrogen deficiency after the menopause is associated with a rapid fall in bone density due to an imbalance between bone resorption and new bone formation. Women who experience early menopause and do not take HRT are prone to osteoporosis and fractures in later life. If menopause is age-appropriate, treatment depends on the effect of symptoms on their quality of life.

Spontaneous ovarian function can return in premature ovarian dysfunction and women should be advised to continue with contraception if they do not wish to conceive.

Lifestyle changes

A healthy diet and regular exercise relieve mild symptoms. Diets high in natural phyto-oestrogens, such as soy, have been advocated for symptom control. However, there is little evidence for their effectiveness, and the theoretical risk of endometrial hyperplasia warrants caution.

Medication

Hormone replacement therapy with oestrogen is effective for vasomotor symptoms, i.e. hot flushes and night sweats; it also maintains bone health and improves mood disturbances (**Table 8.8**). HRT keeps the urogenital epithelium healthy and prevents vaginal dryness, vaginal atrophy and recurrent urinary tract infections, which are common manifestations of oestrogen deficiency after the menopause. It also reduces the symptoms of genital prolapse. However, various risks are associated with long-term HRT, so short courses (up to 5 years) are generally recommended for symptom control.

Combined HRT, which contains oestrogen and progestin, is prescribed for women with an intact uterus. Cyclical HRT is given to women with menopausal symptoms who are still menstruating. Continuous combined HRT is given to postmenopausal women. The oestrogen and progestin components of HRT are available in different preparations, including oral tablets, a transdermal patch, an implant and the levonorgestrel-releasing intrauterine system (coil). Transdermal patches are associated with the lowest rate of venous thromboembolic events. Vaginal oestrogen pessaries or creams are effective at improving symptoms associated with urogenital atrophy, and are safe even for women in whom systemic HRT is contraindicated. Adverse effects from vaginal oestrogen are rare because systemic absorption of the oestrogen is low. Testosterone supplementation improves sexual function for some women in whom HRT alone is insufficient.

Hormone replacement therapy: risks and benefits	
Benefits	**Risks**
Relief from vasomotor symptoms and vaginal atrophy	Increased incidence of thromboembolic disease and stroke
Reduced incidence of osteoporosis-induced fractures of the wrist, vertebral bodies and hip	Increased incidence of endometrial hyperplasia and cancer when unopposed oestrogen is used in women with an intact uterus
Reduced incidence of heart disease, colorectal cancer and Alzheimer's disease	Increased incidence of benign and malignant breast disease with prolonged use (> 10 years in women aged > 50 years)
	Increased incidence of ovarian cancer

Table 8.8 Risks and benefits of hormone replacement therapy

Prognosis

Premature (before the age of 40 years) or early menopause (before the age of 45 years) is associated with an increased risk of coronary heart disease and osteoporosis. Some women with primary ovarian dysfunction conceive naturally but pregnancy rates are very low. Fertility options include IVF with donated oocytes, donated embryos or adoption.

Answers to starter questions

1. The normal pubertal growth spurt is characterised by rapid growth of the long bones followed by fusion of the epiphyses, preventing further gains in height. In precocious puberty this growth spurt happens early and the epiphyses fuse prematurely. As a result, the child fails to achieve their full adult height potential. This is particularly troublesome if it occures at a very young age, e.g. 2 years of age.

2. Weight loss of approximately 10% below ideal body weight is associated with functional hypogonadotropic hypogonadism in which the normal release of hypothalamic gonadotropin-releasing hormone (GnRH) is lost. Consequently, the secretion of both FSH (which stimulates follicular development) and LH (which stimulates ovarian hormone production) is impaired, delaying puberty. This can be reversed with weight gain.

3. Prolactin is the primary hormone that stimulates milk production and in the non-pregnant/postnatal state prolactin secretion is inhibited by dopamine. Dopamine D2 receptor antagonists (e.g. haloperidol, metoclopramide, methyldopa) remove this inhibition and stimulate the production of milk by breast tissue, which is known as galactorrhoea in the non-pregnant/postnatal state.

Chapter 9
Fertility and contraception

Starter questions

Answers to the following questions are on page 279.

1. Why does the combined oral contraceptive pill prevent ovarian cancer?
2. Why is pregnancy less common in older women?
3. Why is obesity a contraindication to IVF treatment?
4. Can couples choose the sex of their child using assisted conception techniques?
5. What happens to surplus embryos created during IVF?

Introduction

Unintended pregnancy is common, affecting up to 5% of women of reproductive age. In the UK, for example, nearly half of all unintended pregnancies, more than one fifth of all pregnancies, are terminated every year. These statistics emphasise the need for freely available, effective methods of contraception. Many women are dissatisfied with their initial contraceptive choice and switch to a less effective method – or use no method at all. Long-acting reversible contraceptives appear to have lower discontinuation rates.

At the other end of the spectrum, one in seven couples experience an involuntary delay in achieving pregnancy. The prevalence of subfertility has not changed over the past 20 years, but the number of couples seeking investigation and treatment for difficulty conceiving has nearly trebled. Funding for subfertility services has become more widely available in recent years to help address the demand.

Case 9 Unwanted pregnancy

Presentation

Jane Hodgson, aged 22 years, visits her general practitioner in London, England, to request an abortion.

Initial interpretation

Termination of pregnancy is permitted in many countries in specific circumstances. In England, Wales and Scotland (but not in Northern Ireland) it is permitted if two physicians decide in good faith that one of the statutory grounds specified in the Abortion Act are met (**Table 9.1**). Jane presented in England so the rest of this discussion of her case is in the context of this legislation. Women may request an abortion for medical, social and other personal reasons; it is essential to maintain a supportive, caring and non-judgemental attitude, and any advice must be non-directive. Physicians who are ethically opposed to abortion have a duty of care to refer women to another provider without delay (**Table 9.2**).

Further history

Jane is referred to the termination of pregnancy clinic. She attends alone. She is due to get married next year to her long-term boyfriend, with whom she has never had sexual intercourse. She is horrified to find herself pregnant after a short-term relationship with another man.

She knows that if her fiancé and family find out, the consequences will be extreme. She is fearful that this will include violence against her. She cannot contemplate continuing with the pregnancy, hence her request for an abortion. She thinks her last period was about 8 weeks ago. She denies any previous sexual partners, sexually transmitted infections (STIs) or pregnancies. She is otherwise fit and well, with no significant medical history of note.

Examination

Jane is tearful and clearly upset. Abdominal examination is normal. Speculum examination shows a cream-coloured vaginal discharge. Pelvic examination finds a non-tender, bulky anteverted uterus with normal adnexae.

Interpretation of findings

Jane's emotional state and her situation mean that the pregnancy, if it were to continue, would be detrimental to her mental health.

Legal grounds for termination of pregnancy	
Before 24 weeks of pregnancy if continuing the pregnancy risks injury to either: ■ the woman's own physical or mental health or ■ the woman's existing child(ren)'s physical or mental health more so than terminating the pregnancy	At any time during the pregnancy (up to full term) if continuing the pregnancy risks grave permanent injury to: ■ the physical or mental health of the woman ■ the woman's life more so than terminating the pregnancy OR ■ if the baby were born it would suffer from severe permanent mental or physical abnormalities

Table 9.1 Legal grounds for termination in pregnancy. Based on The Abortion Act (1967, amended 1990) in England, Wales and Scotland

Case 9 *continued*

Standards of care for women requesting a termination of pregnancy	
Standard of care	Reason
Prompt referral to a provider of termination of pregnancy	To minimise delay
A non-judgemental, sensitive approach	To encourage women to seek help early
Female physician and/or interpreter, when needed	To provide equity of care
Screening for sexually transmitted infections	To allow treatment and contact tracing, if appropriate
Antibiotics to prevent infective complications	To minimise morbidity after the procedure
Rhesus prophylaxis	To prevent haemolytic disease of the newborn in subsequent pregnancies
Contraception after the termination	To prevent further unwanted pregnancies
Information provision	To provide advice regarding when and where to seek help after the procedure
Counselling after the termination	To prevent emotional and psychological sequelae of termination of pregnancy

Table 9.2 Standards of care for women undergoing termination of pregnancy

The history and examination findings suggest a pregnancy of 8–10 weeks' gestation. This is within the limit specified by the Abortion Act which permits termination of pregnancies after 24 weeks only in exceptional circumstances.

The cream-coloured vaginal discharge is normal in pregnacy and there is no evidence of bleeding or infection.

Investigations

A urinary pregnancy test result is positive. High vagina and *Chlamydia* swabs are negative for infection. Pelvic ultrasound confirms the presence of a viable intrauterine pregnancy of 8 weeks' gestation. The results of a group and screen, a test to determine blood group and rhesus status, show that Jane is rhesus-positive.

This means that she will not require prophylactic anti-D immunoglobulin at the time of her abortion, if she decides to go ahead with it.

Management

Jane is offered a termination under statutory ground C of the Abortion Act. She is given the choice between a surgical and medical termination and opts for the former, because she wants to 'get it over and done with as soon as possible'. Jane is provided with written information and advised that she may experience a range of emotions after the procedure. She is told where she can go for further psychological support, including the British Pregnancy Advisory Service (BPAS) and Marie Stopes.

Case 10 Failure to conceive

Presentation

Lucy and George Hamilton are referred to the subfertility clinic, because they have been trying to conceive for 4 years without success.

Initial interpretation

Fertility depends on ovulation, patent fallopian tubes and healthy sperm. A thorough assessment of both partners is necessary to identify the most likely cause, or causes, of their subfertility.

Further history

Lucy and George have been married for 6 years. They stopped using contraception 4 years ago, and have been actively trying to conceive for the past 2 years. They have sexual intercourse two or three times a week.

Lucy is 32 years old. She has never been pregnant. She started menstruating when she was 13 years old. She has regular menstrual cycles, bleeding for 5 days out of every 28. She has never had an STI or pelvic inflammatory disease. She is up to date with her cervical screening tests, and the results have always been normal.

She has no significant medical history of note and takes no regular medication. She works as a customer services manager. She does not smoke or take recreational drugs, and she drinks alcohol only occasionally.

George is 36 years old. He has never fathered a child. He has no history of testicular surgery, and reports no erectile or ejaculatory dysfunction. Apart from the presenting complaint, he is otherwise fit and well, with no medical history of note. He is an accountant. He stopped smoking 5 years ago and drinks about 28 units of alcohol per week.

Explaining IVF

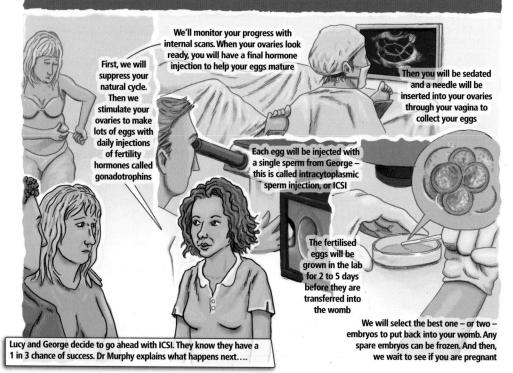

First, we will suppress your natural cycle. Then we stimulate your ovaries to make lots of eggs with daily injections of fertility hormones called gonadotrophins

We'll monitor your progress with internal scans. When your ovaries look ready, you will have a final hormone injection to help your eggs mature

Then you will be sedated and a needle will be inserted into your ovaries through your vagina to collect your eggs

Each egg will be injected with a single sperm from George – this is called intracytoplasmic sperm injection, or ICSI

The fertilised eggs will be grown in the lab for 2 to 5 days before they are transferred into the womb

We will select the best one – or two – embryos to put back into your womb. Any spare embryos can be frozen. And then, we wait to see if you are pregnant

Lucy and George decide to go ahead with ICSI. They know they have a 1 in 3 chance of success. Dr Murphy explains what happens next….

Examination

Lucy has a body mass index (BMI) of 27 kg/m². She has no physical signs of an endocrine disorder, such as excessive hair growth or goitre. Pelvic examination is normal. George has a BMI of 32 kg/m², normal male physical characteristics and external genitalia.

Interpretation of findings

This is a case of subfertility: failure to achieve a clinical pregnancy within 12 months despite regular unprotected sexual intercourse.

There is a decline in fertility with age, but couples in their early/mid thirties who are having regular unprotected sex without contraception will usually conceive within 12 to 24 months. The absence of previous STIs or pelvic inflammatory disease and the lack of symptoms that suggest endometriosis make tubal disease an unlikely cause of the couple's subfertility. This is an opportunity to promote healthy lifestyle choices; Lucy does not smoke, drink alcohol or take recreational drugs but she is overweight (BMI ≥ 25 kg/m²).

Fertility problems and weight gain are symptoms of polycystic ovary syndrome (PCOS) and some other endocrine disorders. However, there are no other signs or symptoms, such as menstrual irregularities, hirsutism or goitre, to indicate this possibility.

Male factor subfertility is more common in men with previous STIs, testicular surgery or chemotherapy, but George gives no history of these exposures. The frequency with which George and Lucy have sexual intercourse and George's lack of erectile or ejaculatory problems reduces the likelihood that sexual dysfunction is the cause of their subfertility.

George is obese (BMI ≥ 30 kg/m²). Obesity decreases serum SHBG levels, causing low serum total testosterone concentrations.

Some studies report that sperm count, motility and semen volume are inversely proportional to BMI. George's level of alcohol consumption is sufficiently high to impair fertility. The finding of normal male characteristics does not preclude a genetic cause of subfertility but these are uncommon.

Investigations

Regular menstruation suggests that Lucy is ovulating. This is confirmed by a serum progesterone concentration > 16 pmol/L on day 21 of her cycle, i.e. in the mid-luteal phase.

A follicle-stimulating hormone (FSH) concentration of 6 IU/L and a luteinising hormone (LH) concentration of 4 IU/L on day 4 of Lucy's menstrual cycle indicate that she has good ovarian reserve. This hormonal profile rules out PCOS as a cause of her subfertility.

Hysterosalpingography, an investigation in which radiopaque contrast agent is injected into the cervical canal, shows spill of the agent from both fallopian tubes. This normal result means that the tubes are not blocked, thereby excluding significant tubal disease.

George provides two semen samples for analysis, 3 months apart. Both show low sperm count (oligozoospermia), reduced sperm motility (asthenozoospermia) and an increased proportion of spermatozoa with abnormal morphology (teratozoospermia) (**Table 9.3**).

The results of further investigations, including measurement of testosterone, LH and FSH concentration, as well as routine karyotyping, are normal.

Diagnosis

The most likely cause of Lucy and George's failure to conceive is oligospermia (technically oligoasthenoteratozoospermia). Because George's clinical assessment and laboratory test results have all been

Case 10 *continued*

Semen analysis		
Term	Definition	Normal range
Oligozoospermia	Very low sperm count	>15 million sperm/mL
Asthenozoospermia	Reduced sperm motility	>40% sperm are motile
		>32% sperm are progressively motile
Teratozoospermia	Increased proportion of sperm with abnormal morphology	>4% sperm have normal morphology

Table 9.3 Semen analysis: interpretation of results

normal, a diagnosis of idiopathic oligo-spermia is made, although his high BMI and moderately high alcohol intake are undoubtedly contributing factors. Other causes of male factor subfertility are shown in **Table 9.4**.

After discussion, Lucy and George decide to try assisted conception using intra-cytoplasmic sperm injection (ICSI), which improves the chances of fertilisation in cases of poor semen quality.

Male factor subfertility: causes			
Category	Mechanism	Examples	Investigations
Pretesticular	Poor hormonal, nutritional and environmental support of the testes	Hypogonadism	Testosterone, LH and FSH tests
		Use of certain drugs (including steroids), excessive alcohol intake and smoking	Karyotyping and other genetic tests (e.g. cystic fibrosis gene, Y chromosome microdeletions)
		Strenuous bicycle or horse riding	
Testicular	Intrinsic testicular dysfunction	Age ≥ 70 years	Post-ejaculation urine test (to exclude retrograde ejaculation)
		Genetic abnormalities (e.g. Klinefelter's syndrome, Y chromosome microdeletions)	Semen fructose test (to exclude ejaculatory obstruction)
		Hydrocele or varicocele	
		Trauma or surgery	
		Infection (i.e mumps, malaria)	
		Tumour	
		Chemotherapy or radiotherapy	
Post-testicular	Outlet obstruction or failure to ejaculate	Absent or obstructed vas deferens (e.g. in cystic fibrosis)	
		Erectile dysfunction	
Idiopathic (unexplained)	Unknown	None	

FSH, follicle-stimulating hormone; LH, luteinising hormone.

Table 9.4 Causes of male factor subfertility

Contraception

Contraception (birth control), is the voluntary prevention of pregnancy. Many contraceptive methods are available. Each has its particular advantages and disadvantages, which must be weighed against each other when making a choice. Factors to consider are:

- effectiveness
- convenience
- duration of action
- reversibility
- adverse effects and risks
- non-contraceptive benefits
- cost
- availability

The main types of contraception are natural methods; hormonal, intrauterine and barrier contraceptives; and sterilisation. Of these options, only barrier contraceptives also offer protection from STIs ('safe sex').

Effectiveness

The failure rates of different contraceptive methods can be expressed as the percentage of women having an unintended pregnancy in the first year of use of a contraceptive method (**Table 9.5**). These rates are calculated using the Pearl index, which is based on the number of unintended pregnancies that occur for every 100 women using a particular method for 1 year. Effectiveness is expressed as both theoretical (perfect) effectiveness and actual (typical use) effectiveness. Typical use effectiveness takes into account inconsistent and incorrect use, for example forgetting to take the pill.

To address the problem of high failure rates with typical use of other methods of contraception, women can be encouraged to use long-acting, highly reliable, reversible contraceptives. The contraceptive injection and intrauterine

Failure rates for different contraceptive methods		
Type of contraception	Perfect use failure rate (%)*	Typical use failure rate (%)*
Natural		
Withdrawal method	4	22
Calendar method	0.4–5	24
Hormonal		
Combined hormonal contraceptives (pill, patch or ring)	0.3	9
Progestogen-only pill	0.3	9
Contraceptive injection	0.2	6
Contraceptive implant	0.05	0.05
Intrauterine		
Intrauterine device	0.8	0.8
Levonorgestrel-releasing intrauterine system	0.2	0.2
Barrier and other		
Male condom	2	18
Female condom	5	21
Diaphragm	6	12
Spermicide alone	18	28
*Percentage of women having an unintended pregnancy.		

Table 9.5 Pregnancy rate during first year of use of different contraceptive methods

devices are examples of such long-acting reversible contraceptives.

> **Contraceptive methods that minimise the opportunity for user error tend to be most effective.** Contraceptive pills may be forgotten or misplaced. Condoms must be available at the time of intercourse, when resolve to practise 'safe sex' and avoid pregnancy may be at its lowest. In contrast, long-acting reversible contraceptives do not rely on the user for their effectiveness, which helps explain why their typical and perfect use failure rates are identical.

Natural family planning

Some couples prefer to use less interventional methods of contraception for personal, religious or medical reasons. However, these natural methods have high failure rates with typical use.

- In the withdrawal method (coitus interruptus), the penis is withdrawn before ejaculation
- In the calendar method (fertility awareness or 'safe days'), intercourse is avoided or barrier contraception used during the 7–10 fertile days of the menstrual cycle; in women with regular periods, fertile times are predictable and can be calculated by counting days from the last menstrual period or by monitoring cervical mucus and body temperature changes across the cycle. This method is not suitable for women with irregular periods.

Hormonal contraceptives

Hormonal contraceptives prevent ovulation, thicken cervical mucus and reduce endometrial receptivity to implantation. Used correctly, they are highly effective.

Combined oral contraceptives

The combined oral contraceptive pill (COCP) contains both oestrogen and a progestogen. It is usually taken for 21 out of

every 28 days. A 'withdrawal bleed' occurs during the 7-day pill-free interval.

The COCP has numerous non-contraceptive benefits (**Table 9.6**). However, it is not suitable for all women; contraindications are listed in **Table 9.7**. At first prescription of the COCP, all women are informed that:

- COCP use is safe for most women but can be associated with rare but serious harms
  - there is a small increase in the risk of blood clots with COCP use
  - there is a very small increase in the risk of heart attack and stroke with COCP use
  - any increased risk of breast cancer is likely to be small and returns to no increased risk 10 years after stopping the COCP
  - there is a very small increase in the risk of cervical cancer that increases with duration of use
- the risk of ovarian and endometrial cancer is halved with COCP use, and protection lasts for ≥ 15 years after stopping

Adverse effects of the COCP include breakthrough bleeding, weight gain, breast pain, nausea, headache and hypertension.

Non-oral combined hormonal contraceptive options are the vaginal ring and transder-

Combined oral contraceptive pill: non-contraceptive benefits	
Condition	Benefits
Menstrual cycle disorders	Regular menstrual cycles
	Decreased menstrual blood loss
	Reduced dysmenorrhoea
	Reduced symptoms of premenstrual syndrome
Gynaecological disorders	Fewer benign ovarian cysts
	Reduced pelvic pain resulting from endometriosis
Disorders of androgenic excess	Less acne
	Reduced hirsutism
Cancer risk reduction	Reduced risk of ovarian, endometrial and colorectal cancer

Table 9.6 Non-contraceptive benefits of the combined oral contraceptive pill

Combined oral contraceptive pill: contraindications

Relative contraindications*	Absolute contraindications†
Age > 35 years and ex-smoker of < 1 year or current smoker of < 15 cigarettes/day	Age > 35 years and smoker of > 15 cigarettes/day
Obesity (BMI 30–39 kg/m²)	Obesity (BMI > 40 kg/m²)
Hypertension (blood pressure > 140/90 mmHg)	Multiple risk factors for cardiovascular disease (e.g. older age, smoking, diabetes, hypertension)
Migraine without aura, aged > 35 years	Hypertension (blood pressure > 160/95 mmHg)
Family history of venous thromboembolism in first-degree relative < 45 years of age	Previous stroke
Breast cancer > 5 years ago with no recurrence	Known ischaemic heart disease
Immobile (e.g. wheelchair-bound)	Migraine with aura
Mild cirrhosis of the liver	Personal history of venous thromboembolism
Use of drugs that induce liver enzymes (e.g. lamotrigine, carbamazepine, phenytoin, rifampicin)	Breast cancer
	Known thrombophilia
	Severe cirrhosis of the liver
	Hepatocellular adenoma or malignant hepatoma

BMI, body mass index; COCP, combined oral contraceptive pill.

*Risks generally outweigh benefits.

†Unacceptable risk precluding use.

Adapted from Combined hormonal contraception. Faculty of Sexual & Reproductive Healthcare. London, 2012.

Table 9.7 Contraindications for combined oral contraceptive pill use

mal patch, which are used for 3 out of every 4 weeks.

The risk of venous thromboembolic disease in COCP users is about two to three times higher than in non-users, and is greatest in the first few months of starting. The increased thrombotic risk is higher with certain progestins. Pills with levonorgestrel have the lowest risk of venous thromboembolism and are first choice for new prescriptions (**Table 9.8**).

> **Dianette contains oestrogen and an antiandrogen, cyproterone acetate, which has both progestagenic and antiandrogenic activity.** The antiandrogenic activity makes Dianette an effective treatment for women with acne and hirsutism. It is also an effective COCP, but it is not licensed solely for use as a contraceptive due to the increased risk of venous thromboembolism associated with its use.

Combined oral contraceptive pill: risk of venous thromboembolism

Scenario	Risk per 100,000 women-years
Women not using the COCP and not pregnant	5
Women using a norethisterone- or levonorgestrel-containing COCP (e.g. Microgynon)	15
Women using a desogestrel- or gestodene-containing COCP (e.g. Marvelon or Femodene)	25
In pregnancy	60

COCP, combined oral contraceptive pill.

Adapted from Combined hormonal contraception. Faculty of Sexual & Reproductive Healthcare. London, 2012.

Table 9.8 Risks of venous thromboembolism in users and non-users of the combined oral contraceptive pill

Progestogen-only pill

Taken every day, the progestogen-only pill is associated with vaginal spotting and irregular bleeding at first. With continued use, up to 50% of users have regular or no periods. It must be taken at the same time every day to maximise contraceptive effectiveness.

The lack of oestrogen makes the progestogen-only pill more broadly suitable than the COCP, because the oestrogen component of the COCP is contraindicated for certain women. Additional contraceptive precautions are needed to cover missed or forgotten pills.

> **Contraceptives can be prescribed for girls younger than 16 years without parental consent.** In the UK, the Fraser guidelines are used to determine the girl's competence to consent to treatment in the context of contraception (see page 383). It is important to consider the risk of harm without treatment and the girl's ability to understand the implications of sexual activity and contraceptive treatment. Girls should be encouraged to talk to their parents.

Contraceptive injection

Long-acting medroxyprogesterone (e.g. Depo-provera) is given by subdermal injection in the arm or buttock every 12 weeks. Adverse effects include irregular vaginal bleeding, amenorrhoea, weight gain, alopecia, depression and reduced libido. Fertility can be slow to return after discontinuation. Long-term use is associated with osteopenia.

Contraceptive implant

This is a small plastic rod containing the progestagen etonogestrel; it is implanted subdermally in the upper arm (**Figure 9.1**). It is a long-acting reversible contraceptive that lasts for 3 years. Its effectiveness rates are high.

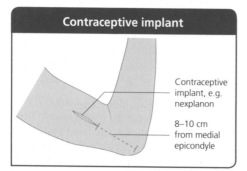

Contraceptive implant

Contraceptive implant, e.g. nexplanon

8–10 cm from medial epicondyle

Figure 9.1 Contraceptive implant, a small progestagen-containing plastic rod placed subdermally in the upper arm.

The adverse effects of implants can be complicated and uncomfortable if the implant has migrated or fibrosis has occurred.

Intrauterine contraceptives

Intrauterine devices, or coils, prevent fertilisation and implantation by inducing a non-infective inflammatory reaction that is hostile to ova, sperm and zygotes.

Intrauterine device

This is a copper-containing device that can be inserted at any time of the menstrual cycle once pregnancy has been excluded. It is left in situ for 5–10 years. There is a small risk of uterine perforation (< 1%), infection or expulsion (5%). Adverse effects, which include heavy periods and dysmenorrhoea, limit its acceptability.

There is a six-fold increased risk of pelvic inflammatory disease in the 20 days after insertion of an intrauterine device, after which infection rates decrease to baseline levels. A sexual history is taken at the initial assessment, and high-risk women are tested for chlamydia and gonorrhoea.

> **Emergency equipment including atropine must be available at the time of fitting or removal of an intrauterine device.** Occasionally, patients experience a vasovagal response characterised by syncope or presyncope, bradycardia, hypotension and nausea. Stopping the procedure is sufficient to resolve symptoms for most women.

Levonorgestrel-releasing intrauterine system

A intrauterine system is a framed T-shaped device with a progestagen-releasing sleeve around its stem (**Figure 9.2**). The slowly released levonorgestrel causes endometrial atrophy and thickening of the cervical mucus. It is a highly effective long-acting reversible contraceptive that can remain in situ for 5 years. Irregular bleeding or spotting is common for the first 6–9 months, after which time most women benefit from reduced menstrual blood flow (see page 290).

Levonorgestrel-releasing intrauterine system

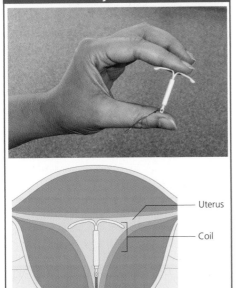

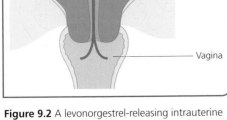

Figure 9.2 A levonorgestrel-releasing intrauterine system (e.g. Mirena coil): progestogen-laden device is inserted into the uterine cavity through the cervical os.

Because of differences between brands, prescribing is done by brand name to avoid inadvertent switching.

> On reaching the menopause, contraception should be continued for 2 years after the last period if the woman is younger than 50 years and for 1 year afterwards if she is older than 50 years. If a woman is taking hormonal contraceptives that mask her natural cycles, persistently increased serum FSH concentrations confirm menopause. Oestrogen-containing contraceptives should be stopped before measurement of FSH.

Barrier contraceptives

These work on the principle of preventing sperm from gaining access to the female upper genital tract. They also reduce the risk of STIs.

Barrier contraceptives include male and female condoms, cervical caps and diaphragms. They must be used before penetration. Diaphragms and caps need to be fitted by a specialist, because several sizes are available, and should be used with spermicide.

Spermicides are available in tablet, cream or foam form. They are inserted into the vagina before penetration to kill sperm. They are effective for 6–8 h.

Emergency contraception

Emergency contraception is used to prevent implantation of an early blastocyst after unprotected sexual intercourse. The intrauterine device is the most effective method of emergency contraception, and should be inserted within 120 h of unprotected intercourse or up to 5 days after the earliest predicted time of ovulation.

Oral emergency contraception

Two types of emergency contraceptive pill are available: levonorgestrel and ulipristal. Adverse effects include nausea and vomiting.

Levonorgestrel
This progestagen can be used up to 72 h after unprotected intercourse. Its effectiveness decreases with time since unprotected intercourse; the pregnancy rate is 5% if it is taken in the first 24 h but increases to 58% at 72 h. It can be taken more than once in a single menstrual cycle. In the UK, some pharmacies dispense it without the need for a prescription.

Ulipristal acetate
This is a selective progesterone receptor modulator. It can be used up to 120 h after unprotected intercourse, and up to this point the pregnancy rate is 1–2%. It can be taken only once in a menstrual cycle and is available only on prescription.

Sterilisation

Sterilisation is considered a permanent form of contraception, so other long-acting reversible methods of contraception are offered first. Reversal procedures are available, but their success rates vary.

Female sterilisation

Tubal occlusion is usually achieved laparoscopically by applying Filshie clips to the isthmic part of both fallopian tubes (**Figure 9.3**). Alternatively, the fallopian tubes are divided or removed during open surgery, for example caesarean section, for other indications. Tubal occlusion can also be achieved hysteroscopically by inserting small coils into the tubes; these cause scarring and luminal obstruction. Female sterilisation has a failure rate of 1 in 200.

Male sterilisation

Vasectomy is the occlusion or interruption of the vas deferens (**Figure 9.4**). It is usually carried out under local anaesthestic. The procedure does not carry the risks associated with achieving the pneumoperitoneum necessary for female sterilisation. However, 12–52% of patients report chronic testicular pain.

Male sterilisation has a 1 in 2000 failure rate. Semen samples taken after 16 weeks, and at least 24 ejaculations, are recommended before clearance to stop contraception is given. Two negative tests (when semen analysis shows no sperm) are required.

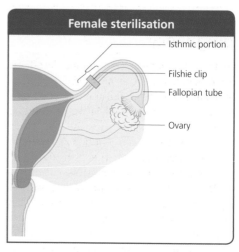

Figure 9.3 Female sterilisation: Filshie clips are used to occlude both fallopian tubes to prevent sperm reaching and fertilising the oocyte.

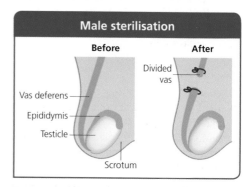

Figure 9.4 Male sterilisation: the vas deferens is divided on each side to prevent sperm reaching the ejaculate.

Termination of pregnancy

Legislation relating to termination of pregnancy varies from country to country, but in England, Scotland and Wales (not Northern Ireland), a legally sanctioned termination must be justified under one or more of the approved statutory grounds according to two physicians (see **Table 9.1**).

A fetus has no rights in UK law, because it is not considered a legal person until after birth. If there is a conflict between the interests of the mother and those of the fetus, the mother's interests are deemed to take precedence. Ensure you understand the law regarding fetal rights in the country you practice in.

Medical termination of pregnancy

In the UK, medical termination is offered for pregnancies up to 24 weeks' gestation, and sometimes later, but the risk of complications increases beyond 14 weeks. Medical termination is relatively safe. The main risk is failure, which occurs in 1 in 1000 procedures. Failure necessitates a further procedure.

Regimens of oral mifepristone, an antiprogesterone, followed 48 h later by misoprostol, a prostaglandin analogue, can be used safely and effectively to terminate a pregnancy at any week of gestation. Misoprostol is administered orally or vaginally in repeated doses until termination is achieved. Gastrointestinal adverse effects are common.

Surgical evacuation of the uterus is indicated if medical termination of pregnancy is complicated by uncontrollable bleeding or if the procedure fails.

Prognosis

There are no proven associations between medical termination of pregnancy and subsequent ectopic pregnancy, placenta praevia or subfertility. Women experience a range of emotions after the procedure; these may include grief, regret and relief.

Surgical termination of pregnancy

Surgical termination is offered for pregnancies of up to 14 weeks' gestation. There is an increased risk of failure if it is carried out before 7 weeks. In exceptional circumstances, surgical termination can be done up to 20 weeks, but the risks of bleeding and uterine perforation are increased.

> The World Health Organization calls safe, legal abortion 'a fundamental right of women, irrespective of where they live'. It also states that 'ending the silent pandemic of unsafe abortion is an urgent public-health and human-rights imperative.'

In some countries, vacuum aspiration is considered the method of choice, because it is associated with reduced blood loss and shorter operating times than with sharp curettage. Surgical termination of pregnancy is generally done with the patient under general anaesthesia. The main risks are bleeding, infection, failure and uterine perforation.

Before surgery, nulliparous women require cervical preparation with prostaglandins, for example misoprostol or gemeprost, to reduce the risk of cervical trauma.

Prognosis

Surgical termination of pregnancy has not been proved to be associated with subsequent ectopic pregnancy, placenta praevia or subfertility, and different women experience different emotions afterwards.

Subfertility

In the general population, > 80% of couples conceive within 12 months and 90% within 2 years of having regular unprotected sexual intercourse. Subfertility is defined as an involuntary delay in achieving a pregnancy.

Epidemiology

Between 10 and 15% of British couples are affected by subfertility. The probability of conceiving every month, known as fecundity, reduces significantly with the age of the woman.

Some reproductive health disorders are more common in specific ethnic groups. For example, PCOS is more prevalent in South-Asian women.

Aetiology

Subfertility is defined as primary, in cases of no previous pregnancy, or secondary, in cases of one or more previous pregnancies. Causes of subfertility are categorised as follows:

- Female factors
  - anovulation (a factor in 25% of cases) (Table 9.9)
  - tubal disease, i.e. blockage or damage to the fallopian tubes (20% or cases)
- uterine or peritoneal disease (10% of cases)
- Male factors (30% of cases) (Table 9.10)
- Unexplained (25% of cases)

Many couples present with both male and female factors.

Anovulatory disorders				
Category	Presenting features	Investigation results	Aetiology	Treatment
WHO I: hypogonadotrophic hypo-oestrogenic	Amenorrhoea May also present with: low body weight galactorrhoea	Low FSH Low LH Low oestradiol High serum prolactin	Hypothalamic dysfunction Pituitary disease (e.g. tumour) and associated radiotherapy Hyperprolactinaemia Low body fat (anorexia, excessive exercise)	Treatment of underlying cause Encouragement of weight gain and reduction of exercise, as appropriate Ovulation induction Treatment of prolactinoma with dopamine agonist (e.g. bromocriptine)
WHO II: normogonadotrophic normo-oestrogenic	Oligomenorrhoea or amenorrhoea May also present with: high body weight acne hirsutism	Gonadotrophins in normal range High LH:FSH ratio High testosterone Low sex hormone–binding globulin High free androgen index Polycystic ovaries on ultrasound	PCOS Occasionally seen without PCOS in women with high BMI	Weight loss (target BMI, < 30 kg/m²) Ovulation induction (e.g. clomifene citrate with or without metformin, letrozole, gonadotrophins) Ovarian drilling (see page 250)
WHO III: hypergonadotrophic hypo-oestrogenic	Amenorrhoea May also present with hot flushes	Low oestradiol High FSH High LH Low antimüllerian hormone High TSH and low T4 (hypothyroidism) Abnormal karyotye, e.g. 45XO (Turner's syndrome), XX gonadal dysgenesis Fragile X mutation carrier	Genetic Immunological Idiopathic	HRT recommended for osteoprotection Donor oocytes needed if patient has fertility treatment

BMI, body mass index; FSH, follicle-stimulating hormone; HRT, hormone replacement therapy; LH, luteinising hormone; PCOS, polycystic ovary syndrome; WHO, World Health Organization.

Table 9.9 World Health Organization classification of anovulatory disorders

Male factor subfertility	
Aetiology	Investigation result(s)
Chromosomal abnormality (e.g. Klinefelter's syndrome)	Positive test result (e.g. XXY karyotype for Klinefelter's syndrome)
Hypothalamic or pituitary disease	Low FSH, low LH
Testicular failure	High FSH, high LH
Congenital absence of vas deferens	Positive test result for cystic fibrosis gene
Idiopathic (60% of cases)	Diagnosis of exclusion
FSH, follicle-stimulating hormone; LH, luteinising hormone.	

Table 9.10 Male factor subfertility

Clinical features

If the subfertility is a symptom of a specific disease, clinical features consistent with the underlying cause are present.

Diagnostic approach

Because subfertility can result from male factors, female factors or a combination of both, each of the partners is assessed. Both must be asked about previous pregnancies as well as medical, surgical, medication and family history. Female partners are asked about their menstrual cycle and previous gynaecological disease. Male partners are asked about previous testicular surgery.

Assessment at the subfertility clinic is an ideal opportunity to offer preconception advice on:

■ stopping smoking, limiting alcohol intake and maintaining or achieving a healthy BMI (19–29 kg/m^2)

■ checking rubella immunity (pre-pregnancy is the perfect time for rubella immunisation if the woman is not immune)

■ changing certain medications that are not safe for use in pregnancy

■ ensuring cervical screening tests are up to date (because screening is less effective during pregnancy)

■ starting daily folic acid for 3 months before and 3 months after conception (to prevent fetal neural tube defects)

Investigations

Investigations are required for both partners.

■ Investigations for the female partner are carried out to ensure that she is ovulating regularly and has patent Fallopian tubes
■ Investigations for the male partner are done to ensure that his semen is of sufficient quality to achieve a pregnancy

Blood and urine tests (female partner)

A mid-luteal phase (day 21) progesterone concentration > 16 pmol/L confirms ovulation. An endocrine profile (day 2–5 FSH, LH, oestradiol, testosterone, sex hormone-binding globulin and prolactin concentration, and thyroid function tests) establishes the cause of irregular or infrequent menstrual cycles (see **Table 9.9**). High testosterone and LH:FSH ratios are present in PCOS. High FSH (> 10 IU/L) and low antimüllerian hormone (< 5 pmol/L) indicate low ovarian reserve.

A urine sample is collected to test for chlamydia, which is a common cause of tubal disease.

Imaging (female partner)

Ultrasound of the female genital tract is used to diagnose abnormalities of the ovaries, for example PCOS; the uterus, for example fibroids, polyps or septum; and the Fallopian tubes, for example hydrosalpinx.

Tubal patency must be confirmed before embarking on ovulation induction regimens.

■ In low-risk women, i.e. those with no history of pelvic infection or abdominal surgery, tubal patency is established by hysterosalpingography (Figure 2.15) or hysterosalpingo-contrast sonography
■ In high-risk women, i.e. those with previous pelvic infection or abdominal surgery, a laparoscopy and dye test is the first-line investigation

Hysteroscopy is indicated if uterine abnormalities are suspected or found on ultrasound.

Semen analysis

The male partner provides a semen sample after 3–4 days of abstinence from ejaculation. Normal values are defined by World Health Organization criteria (2010) as follows.

- Volume: 1.5 mL (95% confidence interval, 1.4–1.7 mL)
- Semen concentration: 15×10^6/mL (95% confidence interval, $12–16 \times 10^6$/mL)
- Progressive motility: 32% (95% confidence interval, 31–34%)
- Morphology: 4% (95% confidence interval, 3–4%)

A reduction in any of these variables necessitates a repeat sample after 3 months to exclude temporary intercurrent illness. Azoospermia, the absence of sperm in the ejaculate, prompts investigation into the cause (see **Table 9.10**). In two thirds of cases, no cause is identified.

Management

Couples with subfertility are advised to have sexual intercourse every 2–3 days throughout the menstrual cycle to maximise their chances of pregnancy. The detrimental effects of smoking and excessive alcohol intake are emphasised.

Women whose BMI is $< 18 \text{ kg/m}^2$ or $> 30 \text{ kg/m}^2$ are advised to gain or lose weight, respectively, because normalising body weight often re-establishes ovulatory cycles. Obesity (BMI $> 30 \text{ kg/m}^2$) in either partner is associated with subfertility and a lower chance of a successful outcome with treatment.

Couples are provided with written information to help them make informed decisions regarding treatment. They are offered counselling and made aware of organisations offering support, such as Infertility Network UK.

It is unclear whether or not stress reduces a couple's chances of conceiving. However, stress is experienced by many couples undergoing investigations and treatment for subfertility. They may need help to develop strategies to cope with potentially overwhelming feelings of anxiety and depression.

Medication

Ovulation induction agents are tried if semen analysis is normal, tubal patency has been confirmed, and the female partner has a BMI $< 30 \text{ kg/m}^2$. If she is amenorrhoeic, a withdrawal bleed is induced by treatment with a progestagen, for example norethisterone, for 7–10 days before embarking on ovulation induction.

Table 9.11 lists ovulation induction agents. Clomifene citrate is used alone or in conjunction with metformin, letrozole, human menopausal gonadotrophin (hMG) and recombinant FSH. The response to therapy is monitored by ultrasound. Intercourse is avoided if too many follicles develop, so as to avoid higher order multiple pregnancies, i.e. triplets or more. Monitoring is also necessary so that treatment can be adjusted to avoid ovarian hyperstimulation syndrome (see page 278).

The success rate for ovulation induction agents is highest in the first few months. Pregnancy is unlikely after six failed cycles.

Surgery

Tubal surgery is offered only to women under the age of 37 with mild tubal disease. Hysteroscopic tubal cannulation restores tubal patency in cases of isolated cornual occlusion. Reversal of sterilisation procedures can also be effective, particularly in younger women.

Women with moderate or severe tubal disease are referred for assisted conception. Hydrosalpinges are removed first, because this has been shown to improve success rates.

In women with endometriosis, laparoscopic ablation of endometriotic deposits improves conception rates, albeit for a short period of time. Endometriomas > 4 cm in diameter are removed, usually laparoscopically, because this also increases the likelihood of pregnancy.

Uterine abnormalities are treated surgically. For example, uterine polyps and submucosal fibroids are removed hysteroscopically. Uterine septa and adhesions are also treated hysteroscopically in women who wish to conceive.

Ovulation induction agents		
Agent	**Type of agent**	**Mechanism of action**
Clomifene citrate	Antioestrogen	Blocks negative feedback of oestradiol to pituitary gland, thereby increasing FSH secretion and subsequent folliculogenesis
Metformin	Insulin sensitiser	Reduces insulin levels Reduces androgen levels Increases ovulation rates when combined with clomifene citrate
Letrozole	Aromatase inhibitor	Reduces oestrogen production by ovarian granulosa cells, thereby reducing negative feedback to the pituitary gland and increasing FSH secretion and subsequent folliculogenesis
hMG or FSH and LH	Gonadotrophins	Stimulates folliculogenesis
Ovarian drilling	Diathermy 'stabs' to ovary at time of surgery	Interrupts intraovarian hormonal environment, possibly by reducing levels of antimüllerian hormone, thereby enabling spontaneous ovulation

FSH, follicle-stimulating hormone; hMG, human menopausal gonadotrophin.

Table 9.11 Ovulation induction agents

Prognosis

Pregnancy rates depend on the underlying cause and the patient's response to treatment. Couples with unexplained subfertility have the highest rates of natural conception after referral for assessment and treatment.

Assisted conception

Assisted conception is the manipulation of oocytes, sperm or embryos outside the body. Almost 2% of all babies born in the UK are the result of assisted conception treatment. Assisted conception is an option for single people or same-sex couples who wish to have children. Assisted conception is regulated in the UK by the Human Fertilisation and Embryology Authority, in accordance with the Human Fertilisation and Embryology Act.

Intrauterine insemination

In intrauterine insemination (IUI), fast moving spermatozoa are separated from sluggish ones and injected directly into the uterus shortly after ovulation. It is used when donor spermatozoa are required, for example in cases of oligozoospermia, surrogacy or when there is no male partner.

In vitro fertilisation

In vitro fertilisation (Latin: in vitro, 'in glass') is the direct manipulation of oocytes and sperm to optimise fertilisation and pregnancy rates. The single most important predictor of IVF success is the woman's age. Most centres in the UK restrict IVF treatment to women younger than 43 years. However, the use of donated oocytes and cryopreserved embryos has enabled postmenopausal women to achieve pregnancy in some settings (e.g. in women who have undergone premature menopause).

In vitro fertilisation treatment is carried out in the following stages:

1. Ovarian hyperstimulation
2. Oocyte recovery
3. Insemination
4. Embryo culture and transfer
5. Luteal phase support

Ovarian hyperstimulation

In the long agonist protocol, a gonadotrophin-releasing hormone agonist is used first to achieve pituitary down-regulation and thereby prevent premature ovulation. This is followed by daily FSH or hMG injections to stimulate follicular growth and development.

On day 8, and every 2 days thereafter, pelvic ultrasound is done. When a lead follicle of 18 mm and two further follicles of ≥ 16 mm are visible, an injection of β-human chorionic gonadotrophin (hCG) is given. The effects of this artificial LH replicate those of the LH surge: ovulation is triggered.

In the short antagonist protocol, the woman receives daily FSH or hMG injections from day 2 of the menstrual cycle. After 4–6 days, daily injections with a gonadotrophin-releasing hormone antagonist are added to prevent premature ovulation. Ultrasound monitoring is then carried out from day 8, as per the long agonist protocol.

Oocyte recovery

Ultrasound-guided transvaginal oocyte recovery is carried out 34–36 h after hCG administration. This is done with the patient under conscious sedation.

Insemination

On the day of oocyte recovery, the male partner produces a semen sample. The sample is prepared and 25,000–50,000 spermatozoa are added to each Petri dish containing a single oocyte. By 18 h later, 50–70% of the oocytes have fertilised.

Embryo culture and transfer

Fertilised oocytes are examined daily by the embryologist, who selects one or two embryos for transfer (**Figure 9.5**). Selection criteria include the number of cells formed by cleavage of the fertilised egg (blastomeres), symmetry and degree of fragmentation. Supernumerary embryos of sufficient quality are cryopreserved. Between days 3 and 5, a fine catheter

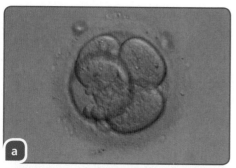
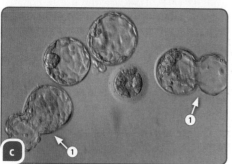
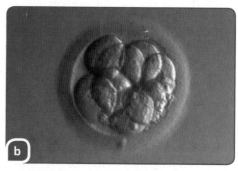

Figure 9.5 Photomicrographs showing (a) Day 2 embryo with four cells. (b) Day 3 embryo with six to eight cells. (c) Day 5–6 embryos: four blastocysts, with two starting to hatch out of the zona pellucida ①. Not to the same scale. Courtesy of Diane Critchlow.

is used to transfer one or two embryos to the uterus under ultrasound guidance.

The procedure is generally painless, and the woman can return to normal activity afterwards. A maximum of two embryos are transferred, except in exceptional circumstances. This is to maximise the chances of pregnancy while minimising the possibility of multiple pregnancy.

Luteal phase support

Progesterone supplementation is used to support the pregnancy until 10 weeks of gestation, when the placenta starts to make progesterone itself. This luteal phase support increases success rates.

> In the UK, individuals who donate their sperm or oocytes to help others conceive do not have the right to remain anonymous. When a child conceived using a donated gamete reaches 18 years of age, they have the right to find out the identity of the donor. The removal of the right to anonymity has been criticised by some, who worry that this decision has deterred potential donors.

Intracytoplasmic sperm injection

The procedure for intracytoplasmic sperm injection (ICSI) is the same as that for standard IVF, except that fertilisation is achieved by injecting a single sperm into each mature oocyte (**Figure 9.6**), rather than the mixing of sperm with oocytes. ICSI is used if the semen is of poor quality in terms of concentration, motility or morphology of sperm, or if fertilisation has failed previously. In other circumstances, it does not improve success rates and should not be used because the sperm selected by the embryologist may not be of high quality. ICSI is used in about half of IVF cycles.

> The experience of undergoing IVF and other fertility treatments is emotionally challenging. It is commonly described as 'an emotional rollercoaster'.

Preimplantation genetic diagnosis

In preimplantation genetic diagnosis, one or two cells are removed from each embryo for use in tests for specific genetic mutations and aneuploidy. The technique is used to screen embryos for potentially lethal or severely disabling genetic abnormalities, such as sickle cell disease and Von Hippel-Lindau disease; only healthy embryos are selected for embryo transfer.

Oocyte, sperm and embryo donation

Donated gametes may be required if one partner cannot produce their own. A couple may also choose to use donated gametes or embryos to avoid passing on a genetic condition.

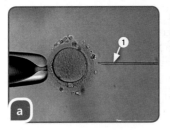 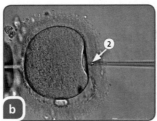 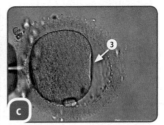

Figure 9.6 In intracytoplasmic sperm injection, a single sperm is selected and injected into each mature oocyte. (a) A single sperm ① inside the needle is lined up alongside the oocyte, which is held steady by the embryologist. (b) The sperm ② is injected into the oocyte. (c) A clear indentation ('funnel') in the plasma membrane of the oocyte marks the site of sperm injection ③. Courtesy of Ruth Arneson.

In Europe, European Union rules ensure that an individual cannot be paid for gamete or embryo donation, but they can receive a compensation fee. The fee is higher for women, because oocyte donation requires them to undergo invasive and potentially harmful procedures.

For the significant proportion of couples for whom fertility treatment fails, the realisation that they will never have a biological child of their own can be devastating. An empathic approach is essential, because infertility can be very isolating, with many couples feeling unable to disclose their predicament to friends and family members. Some couples who prefer not to undergo fertility treatment, or for whom treatment has been unsuccessful, apply to adopt a child. For those facing an involuntarily childless future there are patient organisations offering information and support, for example, More to Life, an initiative of Infertility Network UK.

Surrogacy

Surrogacy is a rare treatment used when a woman has had a hysterectomy, has an underlying medical condition that prohibits pregnancy or has a poor obstetric history. The oocytes used come from the intended mother, the surrogate herself, or from a donor. The surrogate is the legal mother, and she cannot hand over legal parental responsibility until the child is 6 weeks old.

Risks of IVF and ICSI

Assisted reproduction is associated with risks to the mother and the fetus.

Risks to the mother

Ovarian hyperstimulation syndrome is the most significant risk of IVF and ICSI. It affects 7% of patients overall, and 1% develop severe OHSS. The main risk factors for OHSS are low BMI, younger age and PCOS. It is caused by excessive ovarian stimulation and generally presents 2–3 days after oocyte recovery.

Late onset OHSS occurs after 7–10 days and is associated with an ongoing pregnancy. The syndrome is associated with capillary leakage resulting in pleural effusion, pericardial effusion, ascites and intravascular volume depletion. Treatment is supportive, with fluid replacement, thromboprophylaxis and drainage of fluid collections.

Risks to the fetus

With IVF and ICSI, there is an increased risk of multiple pregnancy and the associated risks of fetal growth restriction, premature birth and other poor outcomes. The Human Fertilisation and Embryology Authority has stipulated that no more than 10% of IVF cycles should result in multiple pregnancy.

It is unclear whether or not ICSI is associated with an increased fetal abnormality rate. Long-term follow-up studies are required.

Prognosis

Factors associated with a high pregnancy rate with IVF and ICSI include younger age of the female partner (< 30 years), BMI 19–29 kg/m^2, previous pregnancies and short duration of subfertility. Poor prognostic factors are advanced age (> 35 years) for the female partner and low ovarian reserve.

The success rate for IVF is about 25% when all attempts are considered, and 32% for women younger than 35 years.

Answers to starter questions

1. It is thought that the combined oral contraceptive pill (COCP) prevents ovarian cancer because the progestin in the COCP helps damaged ovarian cells to die by apoptosis, rather than become cancerous. Woman who take the COCP for 5 years or more reduce their risk of ovarian cancer by up to 50%. The effect is higher the longer they take the pill and lasts for at least 20 years after stopping.

2. Ovarian function peaks in a woman's mid-twenties and declines sharply after 37 years of age. An older woman's ovaries are less responsive to gonadotrophins; there are fewer oocytes; chromosomal abnormalities are more common in the oocytes that remain; miscarriage rates are higher, even for genetically normal conceptuses; an older woman is more likely to have medical co-morbidities that impact on/prohibit pregnancy; IVF is less likely to be successful; and pregnancy is more likely to be high risk.

3. Women undergoing IVF should have a BMI <29 kg/m². Obese women respond poorly to ovulation induction and require higher doses of gonadotrophins. Oocyte harvest and embryo transfer is technically more difficult and fewer oocytes are retrieved. Fertilisation rates are poorer and embryo quality is impaired. These factors mean that the pregnancy rate is lower and there is an increased risk of early pregnancy loss.

4. Sex selection is possible, either through preimplantation genetic diagnosis (PGD), a process by which embryos are selected on the basis of sex for replacement in the uterus, or by sorting a semen sample into male and female subgroups. In many parts of the world, sex selection is available on demand. Current UK law prohibits parents from choosing the sex of their child except to avoid X-linked diseases, such as haemophilia and muscular dystrophy.

5. The creation of surplus embryos is common and are usually cryopreserved for future use by the couple. In the UK, both partners must give their consent for the future use or storage of surplus embryos, which are stored for up to 10 years, after which the couple must decide what to do with them. Choices include donating them to another couple, donating them to research or destroying them.

Chapter 10
Abnormal vaginal bleeding

Starter questions

Answers to the following questions are on page 296.

1. Why are hysterectomy rates falling?
2. Why are periods painful?
3. Why do non-steroidal anti-inflammatory drugs reduce menstrual blood loss?

Introduction

The average woman of reproductive age experiences monthly menstrual bleeds that last about 5 days. Abnormal vaginal bleeding is classified as:

- absence or infrequency of menstrual periods, not explained by pregnancy, lactation, hysterectomy or menopause (amenorrhoea and oligomenorrhoea, respectively)
- heavy menstrual bleeding
- menstruation associated with pain that significantly reduces quality of life (dysmenorrhoea)
- bleeding between periods (intermenstrual bleeding), after intercourse (postcoital bleeding) or after menopause (postmenopausal bleeding)

Cancers of the endometrium, cervix, vagina and vulva all present with abnormal vaginal bleeding: it is a 'red flag' symptom that warrants urgent assessment. Amenorrhoea is a hallmark of anatomical, endocrine and chromosomal abnormalities with sometimes catastrophic consequences for reproductive function and fertility: specialist referral, investigations and treatment are required for the few patients who have serious underlying pathology, while reassurance and symptomatic relief are provided for the vast majority who do not.

Case 11 Heavy, painful periods

Presentation

Sarah Bannister, a music teacher aged 44 years, presents to the gynaecology outpatient clinic complaining of heavy, painful periods.

Initial interpretation

It is first necessary to establish the amount of bleeding, the nature and severity of the pain, and the effects of these symptoms on Sarah's quality of life. A thorough history and examination will establish the likely cause.

History

Sarah has had heavy, painful periods for about 5 years. She has to change her sanitary protection hourly for the first 2 days of her period, after which the blood loss slows. She regularly passes clots. Although she wears both tampons and sanitary towels to cope with the flow, blood soaks through to her clothes and bed sheets.

She has tried tranexamic acid and mefenamic acid, prescribed by her general practitioner, but these have been ineffective. Her periods last 10 days and are regular, every 28 days, with no bleeding between periods or after sex.

Sarah lives with her husband and three children. The children were born by uncomplicated vaginal delivery and are now aged 10, 7 and 5 years. Her periods became heavy after the birth of her last child, but she has been too busy raising her young family to worry about her symptoms. Now that her youngest child is at school and she has returned to work, she has decided to do something about the bleeding. She feels tired and a little breathless when she climbs the stairs.

Bleeding post-hysterectomy

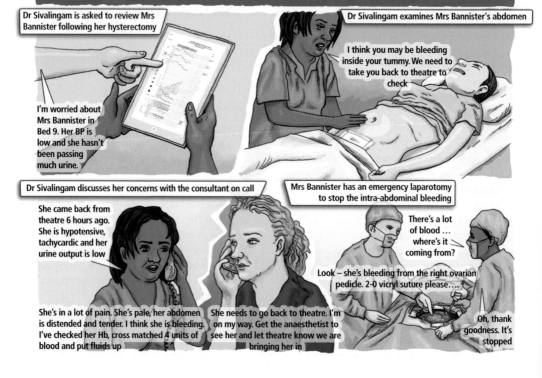

Case 11 *continued*

The first 2 days of her period are painful. She has cramping pain in her lower abdomen, particularly when passing clots and when the flow is greatest. It is bad enough for her to take painkillers and occasionally stops her from going to work or getting on with her daily routine. She avoids sexual intercourse throughout the menstrual cycle because it is uncomfortable.

Sarah is otherwise fit and well, with no medical history of note. She has no urinary or bowel symptoms. Her cervical screening tests are up to date, and the results have always been normal. She does not bleed excessively if she cuts herself. She does not smoke cigarettes or drink alcohol.

Interpretation of history

Sarah's description of heavy periods with the passage of blood clots, having to change pads hourly, flooding (soaking through pads) and the need for double protection (wearing both pads and tampax) indicates heavy menstrual bleeding. The associated tiredness and breathlessness suggest iron deficiency anaemia. The symptoms are having a significant negative effect on Sarah's quality of life and activities of daily living by stopping her from going to work on occasion. They may also be affecting her relationship with her husband given her avoidance of sexual intercourse due to discomfort.

Tranexamic acid is prescribed to reduce or stop heavy bleeding, and mefenamic acid to relieve pain. They are prescribed by general practitioners for the management of heavy menstrual bleeding and dysmenorrhoea but have not resulted in any benefit for Sarah. This is why she has been referred to secondary care to discuss further options for relieving her symptoms.

The regularity of the periods, and the absence of bleeding between them or after sexual intercourse, exclude intermenstrual bleeding and postcoital bleeding.

The development of heavy menstrual bleeding in later life, as described here, is more likely to be due to underlying pathological causes, such as fibroids and endometriosis, than heavy periods that have been present since menarche. Many women put off seeing their doctor about their symptoms as they ascribe them to a normal change in menstrual pattern after childbirth, believing that they are something that has to be put up with.

Following repeated caesarean sections, the myometrium becomes thin at the site of the uterine incision. Endometrial ablation is relatively contraindicated in these circumstances as there is a higher risk of uterine perforation. This is not a concern for Sarah who had all her children vaginally.

Her description of crampy, lower abdominal pain only with her period is characteristic of dysmenorrhoea. It is caused by the release of prostaglandins from endometrial cells during menstruation, causing contraction of the uterine muscles and temporary oxygen deprivation to tissues as a result. Dysmenorrhoea can be idiopathic in origin, though it can also be caused by fibroids, endometriosis and pelvic inflammatory disease; these diagnoses need excluding. The associated dyspareunia may indicate pelvic pathology.

The absence of urinary or bowel symptoms makes alternative causes of Sarah's lower abdominal pain, such as urinary tract infection or inflammatory bowel disease, less likely. Her recent cervical screening result makes cervical cancer a remote possibility.

Nothing in the history suggests underlying endocrine disease, for example hypothyroidism; this presents with lethargy, constipation, feeling cold and hair thinning.

The absence of excessive bleeding when cut makes coagulopathy, a clotting disorder such as von Willebrand's disease, less

Case 11 *continued*

likely. Liver disease, for example alcohol-induced cirrhosis, can cause abdominal pain and a tendency to bleed more easily but Sarah does not drink.

Examination

Sarah is pale. Her body mass index is 24 kg/m². Abdominal examination finds a firm abdominopelvic swelling to three fingers' breadth below the umbilicus, which is mildly tender to palpation.

Speculum examination fails to locate the cervix, which is displaced behind the pelvic mass. Digital vaginal examination is uncomfortable but confirms the presence of a large uterine mass, which is smooth, regular and firm to palpation. The cervix is very posterior but feels normal in consistency and texture.

Interpretation of findings

In the context of heavy menstrual bleeding, the uterine mass is likely to be a fibroid. However, pregnancy must always be excluded, and pelvic ultrasound is indicated to rule out ovarian pathology, such as a benign cyst or malignant tumour. A large pelvic mass can cause dyspareunia, urinary or bowel symptoms because of pressure effect.

Investigations

A full blood count shows a microcytic (abnormally small red blood cells) picture: haemoglobin concentration, 100 g/dL and mean corpuscular volume, 69 fL. These results are consistent with iron deficiency anaemia.

Pelvic ultrasound confirms the presence of a fibroid uterus which is equivalent in size to a 20-week gestation pregnancy. There are no suspicious features such as mixed echogenic parts or central necrosis. Both ovaries are small and appear normal.

Diagnosis

The diagnosis is heavy menstrual bleeding secondary to uterine fibroids and associated with iron deficiency anaemia. Medical treatments for heavy menstrual bleeding are often ineffective in women with large fibroids. The alternative treatment is surgery. She is counselled about the risks of this option, which include bleeding, infection, thrombosis, injury to surrounding structures and surgical menopause, if she also chooses to have her ovaries removed, with its attendant vasomotor symptoms, such as hot flushes, and risk of osteoporosis. These risks can be reduced by the use of HRT.

After discussion of the treatment options, Sarah is keen to have a hysterectomy as she does not wish to have any more children and other treatments are less effective when fibroids are the cause of heavy menstrual bleeding.

Amenorrhoea

Amenorrhoea is defined as:

- Absence of menstruation by the age of 16 years
- In over-16s, absence of menstruation for ≥ 6 months that is not explained by pregnancy, lactation, hysterectomy or menopause

Epidemiology

Physiological amenorrhoea occurs in prepubescence, during pregnancy and lactation, and after menopause. Pathological amenorrhoea occurs in 3–4% of women of reproductive age.

Aetiology

Menstruation depends on pelvic anatomy and normal endocrine function. Disorders of pelvic anatomy are inherited or acquired. The most common inherited causes of amenorrhoea are:

- müllerian agenesis, also called Mayer-Rokitansky-Küster-Hauser syndrome is the congenital absence of all or part of the uterus and vagina (1 in 5000 female births)
- imperforate hymen (1 in 2000 women) or transverse vaginal septum (1 in 70,000 women), which obstructs menstrual blood flow (**Figure 10.1**)

The most common acquired causes are:

- intrauterine adhesions (Asherman's syndrome) or intrauterine scarring caused by over-vigorous endometrial curettage in early pregnancy (e.g. during surgical management of an early miscarriage or termination of pregnancy)
- cervical stenosis resulting from previous cone biopsy, cervical dilation and curettage, or infection

The most common endocrine disorders that cause amenorrhoea are:

- premature ovarian failure, for example as a result of Turner's syndrome (45XO karyotype; see page 251)
- polycystic ovary syndrome
- primary hypothalamic-pituitary dysfunction, for example caused by anorexia, excessive weight loss, depression, brain tumour, prolactinoma or chronic illness (see page 251)

Another endocrine cause of amenorrhoea is suppression of normal reproductive hormone activity, for example by long-term treatment with the contraceptive injection or gonadotrophin-releasing hormone analogues. The latter are used in patients with endometriosis to alleviate their symptoms of pelvic pain.

Clinical features

Amenorrhoea caused by outflow obstruction is associated with cyclical pelvic pain. Absence of the external cervical os on speculum examination, together with the presence of a bulky uterus filled with debris, is typical of cervical stenosis. A bluish vaginal bulge is visible on inspection of the vulva when the hymen is imperforate and menstrual blood is trapped behind it.

Endocrine disorders usually have non-reproductive signs and symptoms, for example

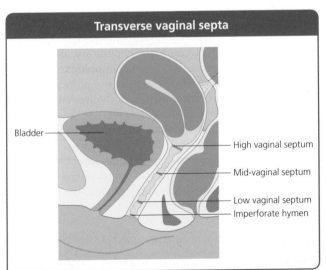

Transverse vaginal septa

Bladder

High vaginal septum

Mid-vaginal septum

Low vaginal septum
Imperforate hymen

Figure 10.1 Transverse vaginal septa can be high, midway or low in the vagina and are a cause of obstruction to menstrual blood flow.

the typical phenotype of Turner's syndrome (see page 251). These help in diagnosis.

Diagnostic approach

Evaluation requires a systematic approach to diagnosis, with primary (never had a period) and secondary (previously had periods) amenorrhoea needing different investigative pathways due to their differing underlying pathology (**Figure 10.2**).

Investigations

Investigations for amenorrhea are blood tests, imaging and karyotyping.

Blood tests

Pregnancy must be excluded either by checking the serum beta-human chorionic gonadotrophin level or by performing a urinary pregnancy test. Measurement of serum luteinising hormone, follicle-stimulating hormone, oestradiol, testosterone and prolactin concentration, and thyroid function tests, are used to identify endocrine disorders. In cases of amenorrhoea caused by an endocrine disorder, the critical distinction is between hypogonadotropic hypogonadism and hypergonadotropic hypogonadism, for which the primary abnormality is dysfunction of the hypothalamic-pituitary axis and the ovary, respectively (see page 251).

Imaging

Pelvic ultrasound is used to confirm the presence or absence of normal pelvic anatomy, and to identify the likely site of any obstruction, i.e. the cervix or vagina. Hysteroscopy is necessary to diagnose and treat intrauterine adhesions. If the primary abnormality is suspected to be hypothalamic-pituitary dysfunction, magnetic resonance imaging (MRI) of the head is required to exclude a pituitary or hypothalamic mass lesion.

Karyotyping

This is used to identify underlying chromosomal abnormalities, including Turner's syndrome (45XO; see page 251) and disorders of

sexual designation (e.g. androgen insensitivity syndrome, see page 247).

> **If a structural or chromosomal abnormality is detected, psychological support is an essential part of the management of amenorrhoea.** Girls and women whose symptoms arise from such abnormalities may never be able to bear children, and those with a disorder of sexual designation will need to develop strategies to cope with the disparity between their genotype and phenotype.

Management

The aim of treatment is to restore normal reproductive function and fertility, if possible, and in accordance with the patient's fertility intentions. If the patient is younger than 50 years and does not wish to become pregnant, hormone replacement therapy (HRT) is recommended to prevent oestrogen deficiency-associated osteoporosis.

Counselling and psychiatric treatment

Referral for counselling, psychiatric assessment or both is required for stress-related causes of amenorrhoea, including depression and eating disorders.

Medication

Premature ovarian failure is treated with HRT. Hypothalamic-pituitary dysfunction is treated with gonadotrophins, if fertility is desired. Management of polycystic ovary syndrome depends on the woman's fertility intentions (see page 250).

Prolactinomas are treated with a dopamine agonist drug, for example bromocriptine or cabergoline. Iatrogenic causes of hyperprolactinaemia respond to drug cessation, treatment with metoclopramide or both.

Surgery

This is needed to correct outflow obstruction, for example in cases of imperforate hymen.

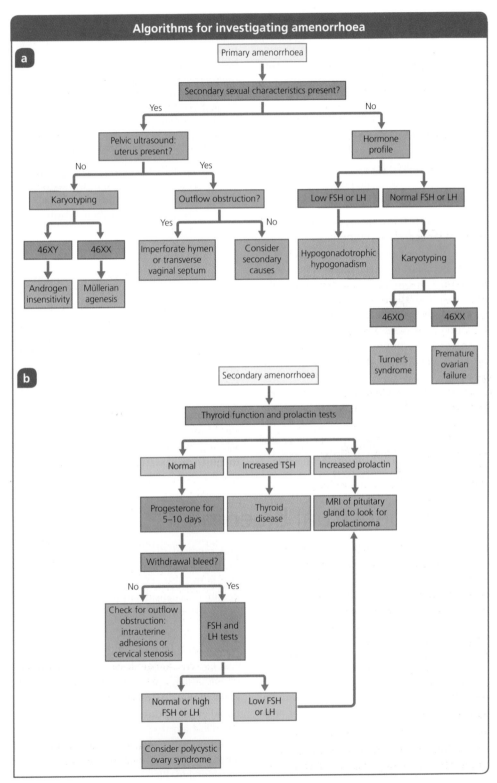

Figure 10.2 Investigating primary (a) and secondary amenorrhoea (b). FSH, follicle-stimulating hormone; LH, luteinising hormone; TSH, thyroid-stimulating hormone.

In cases of congenital absence of the lower genital tract, graduated vaginal dilators are used to create a neovagina. If this is unsuccessful, a neovagina is created by plastic surgery, for example by using a bowel graft.

Intracranial tumours require neurosurgery. Patients who are phenotypically female with non-functioning gonads, either ovaries or testes, have these organs removed because of the high risk of malignancy if they are left in situ.

Oligomenorrhoea

Oligomenorrhoea is menstruation with abnormally long intervals (> 35 days) between periods.

Aetiology

Oligomenorrhoea occurs in adolescent girls and menopausal women, where it is associated with failed ovulation. If ovulation fails, oestrogenic stimulation of the endometrium continues unopposed by progesterone until the tissue outgrows its blood supply and sheds in an irregular, unpredictable pattern. This is called anovulatory dysfunctional uterine bleeding.

Other common causes of oligomenorrhoea include:

- endocrine dysfunction, for example polycystic ovary syndrome, hyperthyroidism or hyperprolactinaemia
- stress, weight loss or excessive exercise
- iatrogenic causes, for example the use of contraceptives and hormones used to treat menstrual or fertility disorders, including the contraceptive injection and gonadotrophin-releasing hormone analogues

Management

Management is directed towards the underlying cause: amenorrhoea (see page 286), polycystic ovary syndrome (see page 250) or prolactinoma (see page 255). In patients with anovulatory dysfunctional uterine bleeding, the combined oral contraceptive pill can be used to impose regular endometrial shedding or withdrawal bleeds. Patients are advised that their irregular bleeding is likely to return on cessation of treatment.

Heavy menstrual bleeding

Heavy menstrual bleeding is excessive menstrual blood loss that interferes with a woman's physical, emotional, social or material quality of life. It occurs either alone or in combination with other symptoms.

Epidemiology

The condition affects up to a third of women during their lifetime. It is a common cause for referral to a gynaecologist, with 5% of women aged 30–45 years seeking professional help for heavy menstrual bleeding.

Aetiology

Heavy menstrual bleeding is caused by pelvic pathology as well as certain endocrine and medical disorders, but no underlying cause is found in a large proportion of cases (**Table 10.1**). Heavy menstrual bleeding without obvious causal pathology is referred to as dysfunctional uterine bleeding.

Clinical features

Women with heavy menstrual bleeding usually experience pain, bloating, mood changes and tiredness, all of which restrict their functional capacity during this time. Between 20 and 60% have iron deficiency anaemia.

The negative impact of heavy menstrual bleeding on a woman's quality of life can be considerable. Bleeding interferes with sexual activity, and absenteeism from school or work is a problem.

Heavy menstrual bleeding: causes

Category	Examples
Idiopathic (40–60% of cases)	None (no cause identified)
Uterine abnormalities	Uterine polyp, fibroids, endometrial hyperplasia or cancer
Cervical abnormalities	Cervical polyp, cervical cancer
Inflammatory disorders	Endometriosis, adenomyosis
Infection	Pelvic inflammatory disease, cervicitis
Endocrine disorders	Polycystic ovary syndrome, hypothyroidism
Blood dyscrasias	Von Willebrand's disease, prothrombin deficiency, platelet disorders, leukaemia
Systemic disease	Cirrhosis, kidney disease
Use of certain drugs	Use of intrauterine contraceptive device (coil), progesterone-only contraceptives, warfarin

Table 10.1 Causes of heavy menstrual bleeding

Blood loss chart

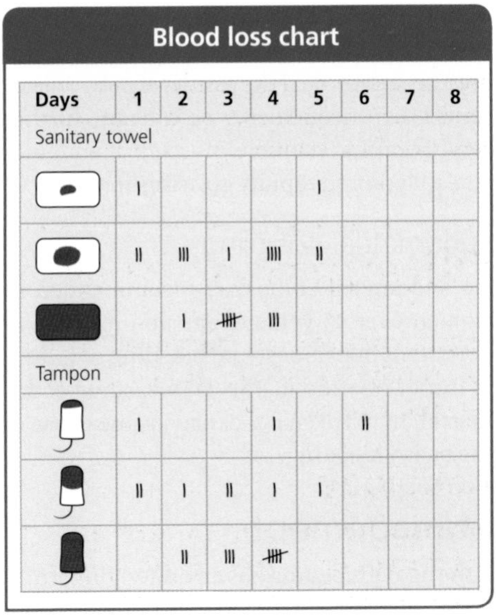

Figure 10.3 Patient diary for recording blood loss in the assessment of heavy menstrual bleeding.

Diagnostic approach

A thorough history and examination are essential to exclude underlying pathology (see **Table 10.1**). Associated dysmenorrhoea is typical of endometriosis and adenomyosis. A history of bleeding during dental extractions or after minor surgery suggests a coagulation disorder. Fibroids are palpable on abdominal examination, pelvic examination or both. Speculum and pelvic examinations in most cases exclude sinister causes of heavy menstrual bleeding.

> **Ruling out pregnancy-related complications is the first priority** in all women of reproductive age who present with abnormal vaginal bleeding.

Investigations

Investigations are needed to assess the extent of bleeding and exclude an underlying treatable cause.

Assessment of blood loss

Direct measurement of blood loss is not practical or recommended. A menstrual diary is helpful to define the bleeding pattern (**Figure 10.3**).

> **The amount of blood lost during menstruation is subjective and difficult to quantify.** On heavy days, i.e. days 1–3 of the menstrual cycle, it is normal to change sanitary protection every 2–3 h. If a woman needs to change her pad hourly, regularly passes clots and finds that blood has soaked through to her clothes ('flooding'), she has heavy menstrual bleeding.

Blood tests

A full blood count is necessary to diagnose anaemia. Thyroid function tests are carried out if hypothyroidism is suspected. A family history of bleeding disorders prompts testing for a coagulopathy. Liver function tests are needed if cirrhosis of the liver is the suspected cause.

Imaging

Pelvic ultrasound is indicated if pelvic examination is abnormal. This is the first-line test to diagnose fibroids as the cause of heavy menstrual bleeding. Hysteroscopy, MRI or both are required if the results of pelvic ultrasound are inconclusive or warrant further evaluation for example in cases of endometrial polyps and rapidly growing fibroids.

Endometrial sampling

An endometrial biopsy is recommended in women over 45 years of age and in cases of persistent intermenstrual bleeding or failure of initial treatment. This is to exclude endometrial hyperplasia or cancer as the cause of the heavy bleeding.

Management

If the heavy bleeding has an underlying structural, histological or endocrine cause, the aim of treatment is to address this. For example, heavy menstrual bleeding associated with fibroids is managed by a range of medical treatments as well as surgical procedures (see page 317). However, no underlying aetiology can be identified in about half of women presenting with heavy menstrual bleeding, in which case the following treatments are tried in the order in which they are presented here.

Medication

Drugs that reduce or prevent menstrual blood loss are effective in 90% of women with heavy menstrual bleeding.

Levonorgestrel-releasing intrauterine system

The first-line treatment for heavy menstrual bleeding is the levonorgestrel-releasing intrauterine system (Mirena coil). For women in whom underlying pathology is unlikely, it can be tried in the primary care setting without the need for pelvic imaging or specialist referral. It successfully reduces blood loss in four out of five women with heavy menstrual bleeding.

Antifibrinolytic agents

Tranexamic acid is an antifibrinolytic agent that reduces menstrual blood loss by about 50%.

Non-steroidal anti-inflammatory drugs

These drugs, for example mefenamic acid, are used alone or in combination with tranexamic acid to reduce menstrual blood loss. They are particularly useful in cases of heavy menstrual bleeding without coexisting dysmenorrhoea.

Combined oral contraceptive pill

This is effective in reducing menstrual blood loss. It is particularly useful in younger, nulliparous women who also want contraception.

Other medications

Other hormonal treatments can be tried, for example cyclical norethisterone (5 mg three times a day on days 5–26 of the menstrual cycle) or the contraceptive injection. Gonadotrophin-releasing hormone analogues are very effective. However, they are expensive, they cause menopausal symptoms, and heavy menstrual bleeding usually recurs on cessation of the drug.

Gonadotrophin-releasing hormone analogues are commonly used to shrink fibroids, and therefore reduce intraoperative blood loss, before surgery.

Surgery

If medical management fails, surgery is appropriate for the treatment of heavy menstrual bleeding.

Endometrial ablation or resection

The endometrium that bleeds excessively can be destroyed or removed by endometrial ablation or resection, respectively; the damaged tissue is then replaced with fibrous tissue during healing. This option is suitable only for women who do not want to bear children and have completed their families.

Ablation is carried out by:

- microwave
- fluid-filled thermal balloon (**Figure 10.4**)
- impedance-controlled bipolar radiofrequency

Transcervical resection of the endometrium is useful if submucous fibroids are present, but it has largely been superseded by ablative techniques. Endometrial ablation reduces blood loss in four out of five women with heavy menstrual bleeding.

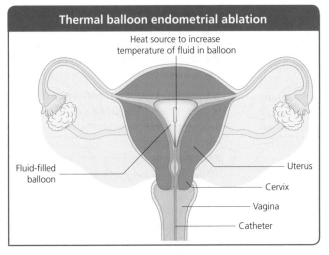

Thermal balloon endometrial ablation

Heat source to increase temperature of fluid in balloon

Fluid-filled balloon

Uterus

Cervix

Vagina

Catheter

Figure 10.4 Fluid-filled thermal balloon endometrial ablation destroys the endometrium and thereby reduces heavy menstrual bleeding.

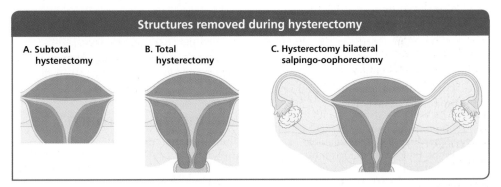

Structures removed during hysterectomy

A. Subtotal hysterectomy

B. Total hysterectomy

C. Hysterectomy bilateral salpingo-oophorectomy

Figure 10.5 Organs removed during hysterectomy. It is (a) subtotal, (b) total or (c) combined with salpingo-oophorectomy to remove the ovaries and fallopian tubes as well. The procedure is carried out abdominally through an open wound, vaginally, laparoscopically or robotically. Conservation of the cervix, ovaries or both is appropriate in some situations.

Hysterectomy

If more conservative treatments fail, hysterectomy is a long-term solution for many women (**Figure 10.5**). Vaginal or laparoscopic hysterectomy has a shorter postoperative recovery period than abdominal hysterectomy. Decisions regarding ovarian conservation are made on an individual basis, taking into account the patient's age, history and risk factors.

Dysmenorrhoea

Dysmenorrhoea, or painful periods, is pain during menstruation that interferes with daily activities. It is classified as primary or secondary, depending on the cause.

The condition affects up to a quarter of women. It is most common in adolescents and young women. Prevalence decreases with age.

Aetiology

Primary dysmenorrhoea is not associated with pelvic pathology. It is thought to be caused by excessive secretion of prostaglandin by the uterus.

Secondary dysmenorrhoea is caused by underlying pathology (**Table 10.2**). The most common cause is endometriosis, which affects up to 70% of women with dysmenorrhoea (page 301). Other causes are:

- adenomyosis (condition in which endometrial cells are found in the myometrium)
- fibroids
- pelvic inflammatory disease

Clinical features

Women with dysmenorrhoea describe midline cramping pain in the suprapubic or lower abdominal area that precedes or coincides with menstruation and is most severe at the time of maximal flow.

> **Dysmenorrhoea has a considerable impact on the quality of life for many women.** It is a common cause of absenteeism from school and time off work with potential negative effects on examination success and career progression.

Pelvic examination is normal in women with primary dysmenorrhoea. In contrast, women with secondary dysmenorrhoea may have signs of underlying pathology (see **Table 10.2**), for example:

- nodularity, thickening or tenderness of the uterosacral ligaments and a fixed retroverted uterus are signs of endometriosis
- mucopurulent discharge and acute tenderness on palpation of the cervix are signs of pelvic inflammatory disease

> **Pain associated with menstruation should be differentiated from other types of pelvic pain.** Some causes of pelvic pain, for example irritable bowel syndrome, are non-gynaecological. Clinical assessment is facilitated by asking the patient to keep a menstrual calendar noting the timing of her symptoms in relation to menstruation.

Diagnostic approach

The aims of diagnostic evaluation are threefold:

- to establish the presence or absence of underlying pathology
- to assess the effects of symptoms on the woman's quality of life

Dysmenorrhoea: causes		
Underlying abnormality	Features	Examination findings
Primary dysmenorrhoea (no organic cause identified)	Pain precedes and accompanies menstruation Onset with or shortly after menarche	Normal examination and investigations
Endometriosis	Associated with heavy periods and dyspareunia	Uterosacral nodularity and/or tenderness Fixed retroverted uterus
Adenomyosis	Associated with prolonged, heavy periods	Bulky uterus
Fibroids	Pain, the result of pressure effects on adjacent organs or fibroid degeneration	Pelvic mass
Chronic pelvic inflammatory disease	History of sexually transmitted infection Pain not limited to menstruation	Mucopurulent discharge Cervicitis Pelvic mass

Table 10.2 Causes of dysmenorrhoea

- to determine what treatments have been tried and the degree to which they relieved symptoms

Investigations

Investigations are required if clinical features suggest underlying pathology, i.e. secondary dysmenorrhea.

Imaging

Ultrasound of the pelvis is useful when an anatomical abnormality is suspected on clinical examination. It is used to identify fibroids, hydrosalpinges (dilated, fluid-filled fallopian tubes) and ovarian cysts, including endometriomas, but is only moderately successful at detecting adenomyosis.

Laparoscopy

Diagnostic laparoscopy is required to investigate dysmenorrhoea when endometriosis is suspected.

Management

Primary dysmenorrhea is managed medically. Surgery is frequently needed to treat secondary dysmenorrhoea.

Medication

Non-steroidal anti-inflammatory drugs (NSAIDs) and hormonal contraceptives are the mainstays of drug therapy for dysmenorrhoea. No trials have compared the efficacy of NSAIDs against that of hormonal contraceptives for the relief of primary dysmenorrhoea. If either is ineffective, a 3-month trial with the other is recommended. Combination therapy is also an option.

Surgery

For women with secondary dysmenorrhoea in whom pain medication is insufficient, surgery is considered. The type of surgery depends on the underlying pathology and is described in other chapters: endometriosis (see page 303), or fibroids (see page 318).

Prognosis

Primary dysmenorrhoea improves with age and often after childbearing.

Intermenstrual and postcoital bleeding

Bleeding between periods (intermenstrual bleeding) and bleeding after sexual intercourse (postcoital bleeding) are common and usually have a benign cause.

Aetiology

Intermenstrual bleeding and postcoital bleeding are caused by:

- physiological changes, such as mid-cycle bleeding as a consequence of the oestradiol surge, or cervical ectopy
- hormonal imbalance, for example with the use of hormonal contraceptives, particularly in cases of poor adherence to treatment
- infection, for example chlamydia or trichomoniasis
- drug use, for example in cases of drug interaction with the combined oral contraceptive pill
- benign tumours, such as endometrial or cervical polyps (**Figure 10.6**)
- malignant tumours, such as endometrial, cervical, vaginal or vulval tumours

Clinical features

Intermenstrual bleeding and postcoital bleeding are 'red flag' symptoms that raise suspicion of gynaecological cancer. The role of the clinician is to exclude serious underlying pathology and reassure the majority of women, whose symptoms have a benign cause.

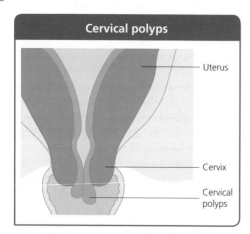

Cervical polyps

Uterus

Cervix

Cervical polyps

Figure 10.6 Cervical polyps cause intermenstrual and postcoital bleeding. They are visible on speculum examination.

Diagnostic approach

All patients presenting with abnormal vaginal bleeding require examination. The examination findings, together with a thorough history, establish the patient's age, menstrual history, sexual history, use of exogenous hormones, coexisting medical conditions and drug history, as well as the presence or absence of associated vaginal discharge, pelvic pain and fever. Inspection of the vulva, vagina and cervix, followed by bimanual pelvic examination, is essential to determine the source of the bleeding.

> **Patients may find intimate examinations embarrassing and uncomfortable, so their dignity must be respected at all times.** Informed consent for intimate examinations is essential, and they are conducted in a private area of the clinic and, whenever possible, in the presence of a chaperone.

Investigations

Investigations are carried out to exclude pregnancy as well as sinister causes of intermenstrual or postcoital bleeding.

Initial tests

A pregnancy test is indicated in all women of reproductive age. Cervical cytology is taken for screening, if it is due. Triple swabs are taken from the top of the vagina (high vaginal swabs) and the endocervix; microbiological investigation of the samples obtained this way will identify most infective causes.

Imaging

Colposcopy (see page 378) is indicated if the findings of cervical examination are suspicious. Transvaginal ultrasound identifies endometrial polyps. Hysteroscopy and endometrial biopsy is done to exclude endometrial hyperplasia or cancer in women over 45 years of age.

Management

Management is based on treating the underlying cause, if one is found.

- Adjustment of hormonal imbalance is achieved by ensuring adherence with hormonal contraceptive treatment, avoiding drug interactions or switching to a higher dose of oestrogen
- Removal of an intrauterine contraceptive device is considered if the bleeding is suspected to be the result of endometritis
- Women with lower genital tract infections are referred to a genitourinary medicine clinic for further investigation, treatment, test of cure and contact tracing
- Physiological mid-cycle bleeding does not require treatment

Cryocautery

This procedure is used to freeze the ectocervical cells and thereby reduce postcoital bleeding caused by cervical ectopy. It is carried out only if the patient's cervical screening tests are up to date and the result of the most recent test was negative.

Polypectomy

Cervical and endometrial polyps are removed to reduce symptoms and exclude malignancy.

Postmenopausal bleeding

Postmenopausal bleeding is defined as vaginal bleeding ≥ 12 months after the last menstrual period.

> **Most clinicians attribute postmenopausal bleeding to uterine bleeding, but it may be non-uterine.** Bleeding may arise from any part of the genital tract, i.e. the endometrium, cervix, vagina or vulva. It may also be non-genital in origin, from the bladder, urethra, bowel or anus. A thorough history followed by inspection of the external genitalia, and speculum and pelvic examinations, help distinguish genital tract bleeding from non-genital tract bleeding.

Aetiology

Although postmenopausal bleeding is a 'red flag' symptom for gynaecological cancer, most cases are the result of atrophic changes in the genital tract or unscheduled bleeding on HRT. Only 10% of cases are caused by malignancy.

Postmenopausal bleeding is caused by:

- atrophic vaginitis
- unscheduled bleeding on HRT
- endometrial or cervical polyps
- cancer of the endometrium, cervix, vagina or vulva

Clinical features

Ongoing or heavy bleeding is more alarming to patients, but any degree of postmenopausal bleeding must be treated as suspicious for gynaecological cancer. A thorough history will elicit the following risk factors:

- Obesity, diabetes, nulliparity, oestrogen-only HRT and tamoxifen use are risk factors for endometrial cancer
- Non-attendance for cervical screening tests or previously abnormal test results, smoking and multiparity are risk factors for cervical cancer

Examination may find the source of the bleeding.

Diagnostic approach

Postmenopausal bleeding is investigated as a matter of urgency. Most gynaecological departments offer a dedicated service with direct referral access to general practitioners. A 'one-stop' clinic allows patients to be seen and investigations carried out on the same day, with the result that most patients can be reassured and discharged as soon as possible.

Investigations

The aim of investigations is to exclude gynaecological cancer as the cause of postmenopausal bleeding.

Ultrasound

The endometrium is normally atrophic in postmenopausal women. If the endometrial thickness is ≥ 5 mm on transvaginal ultrasound (**Figure 10.7**), endometrial biopsy is carried out to exclude hyperplasia or cancer.

Hysteroscopy

This can usually be done as an outpatient procedure. It allows targeted biopsies of suspicious lesions and removal of endometrial polyps (**Figure 10.8**).

Biopsy

An endometrial biopsy is taken blindly with a Pipelle endometrial sampler (**Figure 10.9**)

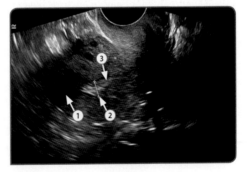

Figure 10.7 Transvaginal ultrasound scan showing a thickened endometrium of 8.4 mm in a postmenopausal woman. ① Uterus, ② callipers measuring endometrial thickness, ③ endometrium.

or under direct vision at the time of hysteroscopy. Any suspicious vulval, vaginal or cervical lesions are biopsied to exclude malignancy.

Management

The aim of management is to treat the cause of the postmenopausal bleeding.

- Vaginal atrophy is treated with topical oestrogen cream or pessaries
- Benign endometrial and cervical polyps are removed
- Malignant disease is managed by a specialist according to the type, stage and grade of tumour (see Chapter 12)

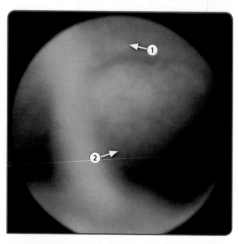

Figure 10.8 Hysteroscopic photograph showing an intrauterine polyp. ① Uterine wall. ② Intrauterine polyp.

Figure 10.9 Pipelle device used to sample the endometrium and exclude endometrial pathology.

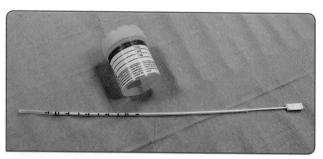

Answers to starter questions

1. The most common indications for hysterectomy are fibroids, endometriosis, prolapse and menstrual disorders. The development of effective non-surgical treatments for heavy menstrual bleeding, such as endometrial ablation and the levonorgestrel-releasing system (Mirena coil), have led to a reduction in the number of hysterectomies being performed. Nevertheless, 1 in 5 British women can expect to have a hysterectomy by the time they are 55 years of age.

2. During menstruation, prostaglandins and inflammatory mediators are released from the endometrium, causing the uterus to contract. When it does, the blood supply to the endometrium is compromised and the cells are unable to compensate. They die and are sloughed off. The blood supply to the myometrium is also compromised and this causes the cramping pains experienced during menstruation.

3. Non-steroidal anti-inflammatory drugs (NSAIDs) reduce the volume of menstrual blood loss by 20–50% in most women with heavy menstrual bleeding. They work by reducing the synthesis of prostaglandins PGE2 and PGF2-α by the endometrium. This causes local vasoconstriction and reduced bleeding. NSAIDs are less effective than the levonorgestrel-releasing system (Mirena coil) and tranexamic acid at reducing menstrual blood loss, but they do also reduce dysmenorrhoea.

Chapter 11
Inflammatory and infective disorders

Starter questions

Answers to the following questions are on page 310.

1. What causes endometriosis?
2. Why does endometriosis cause subfertility?
3. Could HPV vaccination benefit boys?

Introduction

Inflammatory and infective disorders affect either the internal or external female genitalia. Disorders affecting the external genitalia cause vulval skin conditions, while those affecting the internal genitalia cause:

- chronic pelvic pain
- dyspaureunia
- subfertility
- menstrual dysfunction

Chronic pelvic pain

Pelvic pain present for more than 6 months is referred to as chronic; it accounts for 10% of all gynaecological referrals. The most common causes are endometriosis and chronic pelvic inflammatory disease (PID), which are described in this chapter. The correlation between the severity of pain and the extent of pelvic pathology is poor. For example, some women with severe scarring resulting from endometriosis are asymptomatic, while some women with little scarring experience severe pain. This contradiction can be frustrating for patients, particularly when managing their pain is difficult.

Other causes of pelvic pain include fibroids (see page 316), adhesions and primary dysmenorrhoea (see page 291). The last of these is not associated with any pelvic pathology; it may result from excessive prostaglandin secretion.

No cause can be identified at laparoscopy in up to a third of women with chronic pelvic pain.

Case 12 Painful periods

Presentation

Jane Evans, aged 32 years, presents to the gynaecology clinic with a 2-year history of period pain.

Initial interpretation

Period pain, i.e. dysmenorrhoea, is classified as primary if no underlying cause can be identified, and secondary if it is a consequence of pelvic pathology.

The aims of clinical assessment are to establish the severity of symptoms, identify any underlying cause and determine fertility intentions, because these affect a patient's treatment options.

Further history

Jane started her periods when she was 11 years old. They were normal until 2 years ago, when they became increasingly painful. The pain starts 3 days before the onset of bleeding. She describes it as a cramping or burning sensation in her lower abdomen that builds in intensity. Once the bleeding starts, the pain begins to settle and is gone by the third or fourth day of her period.

Sometimes the pain is incapacitating, in which case Jane has to take time off from her work as a laboratory scientist and go to bed. Her work has started to suffer, and she is worried that her contract will not be renewed.

Jane's long-term boyfriend, Steve, is supportive. However, there are tensions between them because she finds sex unbearably painful. They have talked about getting married and having children when the time is right. She has not told her family and friends how bad her symptoms are, because she worries that they will think she is exaggerating.

Endometriosis: impact on life

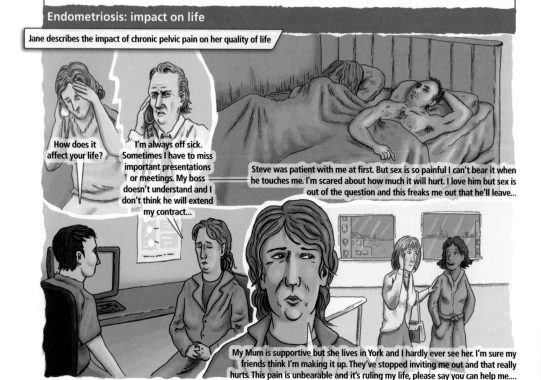

Jane describes the impact of chronic pelvic pain on her quality of life

How does it affect your life?

I'm always off sick. Sometimes I have to miss important presentations or meetings. My boss doesn't understand and I don't think he will extend my contract...

Steve was patient with me at first. But sex is so painful I can't bear it when he touches me. I'm scared about how much it will hurt. I love him but sex is out of the question and this freaks me out that he'll leave...

My Mum is supportive but she lives in York and I hardly ever see her. I'm sure my friends think I'm making it up. They've stopped inviting me out and that really hurts. This pain is unbearable and it's ruling my life, please say you can help me....

Jane's periods are regular. They last for 7 days on average and are heavy for the first 2 days. There is no bleeding between periods or after sex. Her cervical screening tests are up to date, and the results have been normal. On the rare occasions when she is able to have sex, she uses condoms for contraception. She is otherwise fit and well, takes no regular medications and has no medical history of note. She drinks alcohol infrequently and does not smoke.

Examination

Jane is slim, with a body mass index (BMI) of 22 kg/m². Her abdomen is mildly tender to palpation suprapubically. Speculum examination is normal but not tolerated well. Pelvic examination finds a fixed bulky retroverted uterus that is tender to palpation.

Interpretation of findings

Jane's history of cramping pelvic pain that precedes menstruation and subsides several days after the onset of bleeding is typical for endometriosis. Deep dyspareunia is another common symptom. The absence of bleeding between periods or after sex makes pelvic inflammatory disease less likely as a diagnosis.

Jane has not tried hormonal contraceptives previously; this information is important as relief of symptoms with hormonal treatment occurs in endometriosis. The examination findings of discomfort during speculum examination and a fixed, bulky, retroverted uterus that is tender to palpate also support a diagnosis of endometriosis. The latter is due to scarring caused by endometriosis pulling the uterus backwards.

Endometriosis can significantly reduce a woman's quality of life. Its chronic and debilitating symptoms can interfere with her ability to fulfil work commitments and affect her relationships with others. Emotional difficulties and dyspareunia can cause problems between her and her partner, and she is more likely to experience subfertility.

Imaging and a diagnostic laparoscopy are required in order to investigate Jane's symptoms; laparoscopy is needed to confirm a diagnosis of endometriosis and to establish the extent of disease. Ultrasound excludes other differential diagnoses, such as fibroids, but may not be informative in all cases of endometriosis if the disease does not cause anatomical distortion. Jane's normal BMI makes performing these investigations easier.

Investigations

Transvaginal ultrasound shows bilateral haemorrhagic ovarian cysts characteristic of endometriomas (see page 319).

Diagnostic laparoscopy confirms the presence of the bilateral ovarian cysts, which are lodged in the rectouterine pouch. The uterus is fixed in a retroverted position by dense adhesions. Endometriotic nodules are present in the uterovesical pouch.

A nodule is sent for histological review, and the results confirm endometriosis.

Diagnosis

The findings at laparoscopy of ectopic endometrial tissue confirm a diagnosis of endometriosis. Jane is relieved that her symptoms have been taken seriously and a diagnosis reached. She knew that something was wrong but was worried about being thought of as a hypochondriac. The impact of her endometriosis has been considerable, but both her and her doctor are hopeful that, with treatment, her symptoms and quality of life will start to improve.

Case 13 Vaginal discharge

Presentation

Penny Burton, who is 20 years old, presents to her general practitioner (GP) complaining of smelly vaginal discharge.

Initial interpretation

Vaginal discharge is a common complaint with many physiological and pathological causes (see **Table 11.4**). It is important to take a detailed sexual and contraceptive history, to carry out a speculum and pelvic examination and to take swabs for microbiological investigations to determine the cause of the discharge.

Physiological causes of vaginal discharge include pregnancy, use of the combined oral contraceptive pill, and cervical ectopy (see page 24). Infection is the most common pathological cause of vaginal discharge in young women, but other, more sinister causes are always considered, including cervical cancer.

Further history

Penny has noticed the discharge for a couple of weeks. She has had no associated pelvic pain, dyspareunia or abnormal bleeding. Her periods are normal.

Penny has had several sexual partners over the past few months. She is on the combined oral contraceptive pill but often forgets to take it. She does not always use condoms with a new partner. She has never been diagnosed with a sexually transmitted infection (STI) or been pregnant.

She is a university student, smokes 15 cigarettes per day and drinks 'too much' alcohol at weekends.

Apart from the discharge, she is fit and well and has no medical history of note.

Examination

Penny is slim, with a BMI of 24 kg/m². Abdominal examination is normal. Inspection of the external genitalia reveals no abnormality. Speculum examination shows cervical ectopy and a copious, offensive grey vaginal discharge. Pelvic examination finds a non-tender mobile anteverted uterus with normal adnexa.

Interpretation of findings

Given the history of unprotected sexual intercourse with different partners, an infective cause for the vaginal discharge is most likely. There are no signs of PID necessitating emergency gynaecological referral, such as fever, vomiting or significant lower abdominal pain requiring parenteral analgesia.

Cervical ectopy is a common finding in women taking the combined oral contraceptive pill. This can cause postcoital or irregular vaginal bleeding, and cream-coloured watery vaginal discharge.

Microbiological swabs need to be taken from the endocervix and vagina to identify the organism causing her discharge and to establish antibiotic sensitivities.

Investigations

Penny's GP takes various swabs for tests and contacts her with the results a few days later. The endocervical swab sample is negative for gonorrhoea. Her chlamydia screen is negative.

The sample of discharge from the high vaginal swab gives a positive result with the potassium hydroxide 'whiff' test, has a pH > 4.5 and has large numbers of clue cells. These findings are consistent with a diagnosis of bacterial vaginosis.

Diagnosis

The diagnosis is bacterial vaginosis, so Penny is started on antibiotic treatment.

Her GP offers sexual health advice. She suggests that Penny considers switching

Case 13 *continued*

to long-acting reversible contraception, for example the contraceptive injection, and advises always using condoms with new partners. She invites Penny to attend an STI screen at the local sexual health clinic.

The GP also uses the opportunity to offer general health advice to stop smoking, reduce alcohol intake and avoid binge drinking.

Endometriosis

Endometriosis is the presence of endometrial glands and stroma (supportive tissue) outside the uterine cavity.

Epidemiology

The prevalence of endometriosis is 5–10% of women in the reproductive age group, 40% of women with subfertility and 80% of women with chronic pelvic pain.

Aetiology

The cause of endometriosis remains unknown. The most widely accepted theory is that retrograde menstruation allows seeding of endometrial tissue in the pelvis (**Table 11.1**).

Because aetiology of endometriosis is unknown, there is no proven prevention strategy. However prevalence is lower in women using hormonal contraception, suggesting hormones may be involved in the aetiology. Hormonal contraceptives do not eradicate it, but they can suppress symptoms whilst they are being taken.

Pathogenesis

The ectopic endometrium responds to the hormones that regulate the menstrual cycle. The resultant cyclical bleeding of this tissue causes peritoneal irritation, which in turn causes scarring and distortion of pelvic anatomy.

Clinical features

Endometriosis causes cyclical pelvic pain, deep dyspareunia and subfertility. In severe cases, examination findings include a fixed retroverted uterus, nodular uterosacral ligaments and tender enlarged adnexae (**Table 11.2**).

Endometriosis can be mild, affecting few areas (**Figure 11.1**), or widespread and associated with severe adhesions and fibrosis. The severity of symptoms does not correlate well with the extent of the disease, as determined at laparoscopy.

Diagnostic approach

Clinical findings support the diagnosis of endometriosis. Investigations are used to

Aetiology of endometriosis: theories	
Theory	Description
Retrograde menstruation	Endometrial cells reflux through the fallopian tubes during menstruation and implant in the pelvis
Coelomic metaplasia	Coelomic epithelium in the peritoneal cavity is stimulated to transform into endometrial cells
Vascular dissemination	Endometrial cells are transported to disseminated sites via the blood
Autoimmune disease	A disorder of immune surveillance allows ectopic endometrial implants to grow

Table 11.1 Theories on the aetiology of endometriosis

confirm the diagnosis and assess the extent of the disease.

> **Pelvic pain is a common symptom with many different causes.** The relationship of the pain to menstruation and bowel and urinary function can distinguish the likely cause. Gynaecological causes must be considered for every female, especially those of reproductive age.

Investigations

Ultrasound of the pelvis shows endometriomas, i.e. blood-filled 'chocolate' ovarian cysts. Endometriomas are present in 20–40% of women with endometriosis. Neither ultrasound nor magnetic resonance imaging (MRI) can be used to identify superficial disease, but the latter may be useful to assess the depth of infiltrating endometriosis.

Laparoscopy is the gold standard diagnostic technique for endometriosis. Visual

Endometriosis: symptoms and signs	
Symptoms	**Signs**
Cyclical pelvic pain	Tenderness in posterior or lateral vaginal fornices
Deep dyspareunia (pelvic pain during penetrative sexual intercourse)	Pain on movement of the uterus
Subfertility	Tender adnexal mass
Heavy menstrual bleeding	Lateral displacement of the cervix as a result of asymmetrical involvement of one uterosacral ligament
Ovulatory pain	
Fatigue	
Depression	Palpable tender nodules in the rectouterine pouch, uterosacral ligaments or rectovaginal septum
Symptoms suggesting irritable bowel syndrome	
Dysuria (pain during micturition)	Fixation of adnexa or uterus in a retroverted position
Dyschezia (pain on defecation)	
Cyclical bleeding from other organs (rare)	

Table 11.2 Symptoms and signs of endometriosis

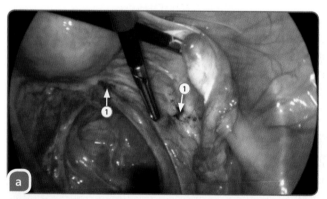

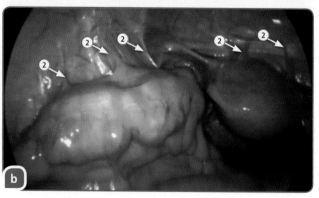

Figure 11.1 Laparoscopic appearance of endometriosis. (a) ①, typical small, flat, dark patches or flecks of blue–black ('powder burns') in the right ovarian fossa and on the right uterosacral ligament. (b) ②, fine adhesions between the sigmoid colon and the left pelvic sidewall, and between the anterior surface of the uterus and the anterior abdominal wall. Courtesy of Andrew Pickersgill.

assessment of the peritoneal cavity establishes the sites and extent of disease (**Table 11.3**). The clinical appearances of endometriosis are many and varied, and histological confirmation is recommended.

> **Endometriosis is associated with an increased risk of certain epithelial ovarian cancers, notably endometrioid, clear cell and low-grade serous ovarian cancers.** This may be because endometriosis cells are transformed into cancer cells. Alternatively, risk factors or antecedent mechanisms, including genetic predisposition, immune dysregulation, and environmental factors, may be common to both conditions.

Management

Management depends on a woman's fertility intentions. There is no role for medical management of endometriosis in women trying to conceive.

Medication

The aim of medical management is to suppress ovulation and induce amenorrhoea. It includes the use of the combined oral contraceptive pill, progestogen-only pills, the contraceptive injection or implants, or the levonorgesterol-releasing intrauterine system. Gonadotrophin-releasing hormone analogues with add-back (supplementary) hormone replacement therapy simulate the menopausal state without the associated symptoms of hot flushes, night sweats, mood alterations, vaginal dryness, etc. Symptomatic management with analgesics such as non-steroidal anti-inflammatory drugs is useful in women whose symptoms are not completely resolved by hormonal treatments.

Symptom recurrence is normal after cessation of treatment.

Surgery

The aim of surgery is to excise or ablate deposits of ectopic endometrial tissue,

Endometriosis: laparoscopic appearances	
Laparoscopic finding	Appearance or stage of disease
Superficial or deep implants	'Powder burns'
	Flame lesions
	Vesicular lesions
	White glands
	Nodular disease
Adhesions	Filmy or dense
Rectouterine pouch	Complete obliteration
Lesions visible during surgery*	Minimal (stage 1)
	Mild (stage 2)
	Moderate (stage 3)
	Severe (stage 4)

*Scoring of lesions used to grade endometriosis according to the American Fertility Society classification system.

Table 11.3 Laparoscopic appearances of endometriosis

divide adhesions and restore pelvic anatomy. Removal of endometriomas of ≥ 6 cm improves fertility rates. Recurrence rates of 20–40% have been reported after conservative surgery. Intractable symptoms may warrant hysterectomy and even bowel resection, depending on their severity and the sites of disease.

Prognosis

Endometriosis resolves spontaneously in one third of women without active treatment, but in general it is a chronic, progressive disease with significant morbidity. Patient support groups, provide much needed support and information to help women cope with the disease (e.g. Endometriosis UK). Typically, symptoms improve after the menopause as lesions become quiescent due to the lower levels of circulating oestrogen.

Lower genital tract infections

Lower genital tract infections (infections of the cervix, vulva and vagina) are common in young, sexually active women. Risk factors include multiple sexual partners, non-barrier methods of contraception, smoking, antibiotic use and immunosupression. Infections can be asymptomatic or present with offensive, unusually coloured discharge. Management is based on identification of the underlying cause and appropriate antibiotic or antifungal treatment.

Sexually transmitted infections are conditions transmitted by genital, anogenital or orogenital contact. They may be bacterial, viral, spirochaetal or protozoan. Coinfection with more than one STI is common. Changes in sexual behaviour, including having a greater number of sexual partners and reduced use of barrier contraception, have made STIs more common.

Syphilis, HIV and hepatitis B and C cause symptoms that affect organs outside of the reproductive tract. These infections use the reproductive tract as a site of entry and travel via the circulation to the tissues and cells that they later infect.

Vulvovaginitis

Vulvovaginitis is caused by infection of the vulva and vagina, and is the most common gynaecological problem for which women seek treatment. Symptoms include vaginal discharge, odour and itch. The most common infective causes are bacterial vaginitis, vaginal thrush and trichomoniasis (**Table 11.4**).

> In contrast to oral infections, vulvovaginal thrush is not an opportunistic infection, and unlike *Trichomonas vaginalis* infections, it is not considered sexually transmitted. Sporadic attacks occur without an identifiable precipitating factor. However, recurrent vulvovaginal thrush is associated with type 2 diabetes mellitus, use of broad spectrum antibiotics, immunosuppression and increased oestrogen levels, such as in pregnancy and with use of the combined oral contraceptive pill.

Chlamydia

Chlamydia is the most common STI in high-income countries. The causative organism is *Chlamydia trachomatis*, an obligate intracellular bacterial that infects columnar epithelial cells, including endocervical cells. Symptoms include purulent discharge and postcoital bleeding. However, many women

Vulvovaginitis: common infective causes				
Condition	Aetiology	Symptoms	Diagnosis	Treatment
Bacterial vaginosis	Overgrowth of anaerobic bacteria	Vaginal discharge Fishy odour (Asymptomatic in 50% of cases)	At least 3 of the following; ■ positive potassium hydroxide 'whiff' test result ■ pH > 4.5 ■ > 20% clue cells on wet mount ■ grey discharge	Antianaerobic antibiotics (e.g. metronidazole)
Vaginal thrush	*Candida albicans* (fungus)	Itch Erythema	Hyphae on wet mount Fungal growth on culture	Antifungal cream, pessary or tablet (e.g. clotrimazole, fluconazole)
Trichomoniasis	*Trichomonas vaginalis* (protozoan)	Offensive vaginal discharge Postcoital bleeding Erythema	Trichomonads on wet mount pH > 4.5 White blood cells	Oral metronidazole

Table 11.4 Common infective causes of vulvovaginitis

are asymptomatic and the diagnosis follows partner notification. About 30% of women with gonorrhoea have coinfections with chlamydia.

Diagnosis is by testing a sample obtained by endocervical swab, or a sample of urine, by fluorescent monoclonal antibody test, polymerase chain reaction or nucleic acid amplification test. Treatment is with tetracycline and macrolide antibiotics such as doxycycline or azithromycin.

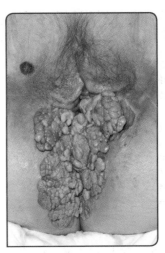

Figure 11.2
Extensive vulval warts in an immunocompromised woman.

> **Chlamydia is common in young women, and although most infections are asymptomatic, about 10% of patients develop PID.** Urine testing to screen women aged 18–25 years for chlamydia has been shown to reduce the prevalence of PID and associated morbidity, which includes chronic pelvic pain, tubal factor infertility and ectopic pregnancy.

Gonorrhoea

Gonorrhoea is caused by *Neisseria gonorrhoeae*, a Gram-negative diplococcus. The most common symptom of infection is vaginal discharge, and 10–20% of patients develop PID.

Gonorrhoea is also a cause of Bartholin's abscess (abscess of the Bartholin's gland), neonatal conjunctivitis (ophthalmia neonatorum) and seronegative arthropathy (joint disease). The rectum, urethra and oropharynx can also be infected. Some women have asymptomatic infection.

Treatment is with ceftriaxone and azithromycin in order to prevent drug resistance.

Genital warts

Genital warts, i.e. condyloma acuminata, are caused by human papillomavirus (HPV) and spread by skin-to-skin contact. They are the most common viral STI (**Figure 11.2**).

Immunosuppression and pregnancy are risk factors. Diagnosis is usually on clinical grounds. Treatment includes topical podophyllotoxin, topical imiquimod, cryotherapy or surgery, but recurrence is common.

> **The incidence of genital warts may decrease in countries where prophylactic HPV vaccination is offered to adolescent girls, as in the UK.** The quadrivalent HPV vaccine protects against HPV types 16 and 18, which are high-risk types associated with cervical cancer, as well as HPV types 6 and 11, which are low-risk types that cause genital warts.

Genital herpes

Herpes simplex virus (HSV) infection causes painful vulval ulceration (**Figure 11.3**). HSV type 1 is responsible for 15% of cases of genital herpes, and HSV type 2 for 85%.

Genital herpes infections are spread through intimate sexual contact and the incubation period is about 7 days. Once the ulcers have appeared, they take up to 14 days to scab over and heal. The infection lies dormant in the dorsal root ganglia, and infection can recur throughout the woman's life.

First-episode primary HSV is characterised by malaise and fever. The first episode is usually the worst, and ulcers can be so painful that they cause urinary retention. Subsequent episodes are less painful and shorter lasting. Treatment is with oral aciclovir, which shortens the attack but is not curative.

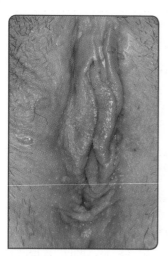

Figure 11.3 Genital herpes.

Syphilis

Syphilis is caused by the spirochaete *Treponema pallidum*. Primary infection is characterised by a painless solitary ulcer at the site of infection. Untreated, this can lead to secondary syphilis, which commonly presents with malaise, a generalised rash affecting the palms and soles but not the face, lymphadenopathy (enlarged lymph nodes) and condylomata lata (warty lesions on the genitals specifically due to syphilis infections).

Latent syphilis is the term given to *T. pallidum* infection with no signs or symptoms and diagnosed on serological testing. Late syphilis may affect the central nervous system, causing tabes dorsalis (degeneration of nerve fibres in the spinal cord causing unsteadiness of gait, lightning pains and urinary incontinence) or dementia, or the cardiovascular system, causing aortitis (inflammation of the aorta). There may be progressive destructive lesions or gummata (soft tissue swellings in the liver, brain and heart).

Diagnosis is based on the results of serological tests: the Venereal Disease Research Laboratory (VDRL) test, rapid plasma reagin test, *T. pallidum* particle heamagglutination assay (TPHA) and enzyme immunoassay (EIA). Treatment is with intramuscular benzathine benzylpenicillin.

HIV

Human immunodeficiency virus is a retrovirus transmitted by:

- unprotected sex
- exposure to infected blood and other bodily fluids
- vertical transmission from mother to child through childbirth or breastfeeding

Transmission rates vary according to type of exposure. For example, the per-act risk of transmission is 5 per 10,000 with penetrative vaginal intercourse but 50 per 10,000 with anal intercourse (figures for receptive partner). The number of new heterosexually acquired HIV infections now equal those acquired by men who have sex with men. Vertical transmission and intravenous drug abuse are uncommon routes of transmission in countries with a low background prevalence of HIV, e.g. the UK.

Antibodies develop within 4–8 weeks after exposure. The initial seroconversion period can be asymptomatic or associated with a mild flu-like illness. Treatment with antiretroviral medications can defer the development of AIDS.

> **Acute HIV infection presents with non-specific symptoms including fever, lymphadenopathy, sore throat, rash, arthralgia (painful joints) and headache.** Diagnosing acute HIV infection is essential from a public health perspective, because individuals who know they are HIV-positive are less likely to engage in unsafe sex and needle sharing. In addition, prompt initiation of antiretroviral therapy reduces viral load and thereby lessens the risk of transmission to others.

Hepatitis B and C

Hepatitis B and C can be transmitted sexually by exposure to contaminated blood or blood products or vertically from mother to baby during pregnancy and delivery. Hepatitis B vaccination is offered to high-risk individuals, including health care professionals, sex workers and people with liver disease.

Pelvic inflammatory disease

Pelvic inflammatory disease (PID) is an ascending infection of the upper female genital tract. It is the most common complication of lower genital tract infections, such as chlamydia or gonorrhoea. There is very little data regarding the incidence of PID worldwide due to poor reporting and variations in the criteria used to define it. In developed countries, however, it is estimated that 1 in 20 women will be treated for PID in their lifetime.

Aetiology

Chlamydia trachomatis and *Neisseria gonorrhoeae* are the most common causative organisms. Others include *Mycoplasma genitalium*, *Gardnerella vaginalis* and mixed anaerobes. Risk factors include age < 25 years, multiple sexual partners, unprotected sexual intercourse and recent insertion of a copper intrauterine contraceptive device.

Prevention

The risk of PID is reduced by the use of barrier contraception and antibiotic prophylaxis for women at high risk of sexually transmitted infections prior to insertion of intrauterine devices.

Pathogenesis

Ascending genital tract infection causes cervicitis (inflammation of the cervix), endometritis (inflammation of the endometrium), salpingitis (inflammation of the fallopian tubes) and in severe cases the development of tubo-ovarian abscesses.

Clinical features

Typical symptoms of acute PID are severe lower abdominal pain, abnormal vaginal bleeding (intermenstrual or postcoital), offensive vaginal discharge and fever.

Common examination findings are pyrexia, lower abdominal tenderness, mucopurulent or blood-stained vaginal discharge, cervical excitation (pain on cervical movement), adnexal tenderness and swelling.

Diagnostic approach

Clinical suspicion is necessary, because PID may present with non-specific symptoms. The presence of unusual vaginal discharge, bilateral lower abdominal pain and a recent change in sexual partner should prompt investigation for PID. Investigations are used to confirm the diagnosis, assess the extent of disease and guide treatment.

Investigations

Pregnancy should be excluded, because some of the antibiotics used to treat PID are teratogenic. Appropriate blood tests include a white cell count and C-reactive protein test. Microbiological investigation includes an nucleic acid amplification test for chlamydia and gonorrhoea, and for those patients at high risk of infection, serological investigation for HIV, using samples obtained by high vaginal and endocervical swabs.

Imaging

Transvaginal ultrasound or MRI can show dilated fallopian tubes or a tubo-ovarian mass (**Figure 11.4**). Free fluid may be visible in the rectouterine pouch.

Laparoscopy

Diagnostic laparoscopy is useful to obtain fluid for culture, assess complicated or unresolved infection and drain an inflammatory mass. Perihepatic adhesions suggest Fitz-Hugh-Curtis syndrome, a rare complication of PID often caused by chlamydia.

Management

Pelvic inflammatory disease is a polymicrobial infection requiring broad spectrum antibiotic therapy covering both aerobic and anaerobic bacteria. Empirical antibiotic treatment is started without waiting for microbiology results because a negative microbiological screen does not rule out an infection. Prompt treatment reduces the risk of chronic PID, pelvic pain and infertility.

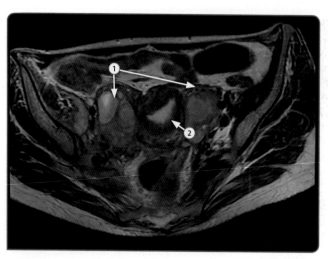

Figure 11.4 A tubo-ovarian mass can be a magnetic resonance imaging finding in pelvic inflammatory disease. ①, bilateral tubo-ovarian abscess. ②, uterus.

Outpatient treatment is usually possible. However, in-patient care is necessary if the patient is clinically unwell.

Medication

Antibiotic regimens simultaneously cover chlamydia, gonorrhoea and anaerobic organisms. Ceftriaxone, doxycycline and metronidazole are commonly used in combination to treat patients with PID.

Different hospitals advise different antibiotic regimens for PID. The choice of antibiotics depends on the most common causative organisms in the local area and their sensitivity to specific antibiotics.

Surgery

This may be necessary to drain pelvic abscesses that continue to enlarge and cause pain and pyrexia despite antibiotics. Seventy-five per cent of pelvic abscesses respond to antibiotics alone.

Prognosis

The prognosis following an episode of acute PID is generally good as long as prompt antibiotic treatment is received. The longer treatment is delayed, the higher the likelihood of long term sequelae. The long-term sequelae of acute PID are chronic pelvic pain, pelvic adhesions, ectopic pregnancy and subfertility or infertility.

Vulval skin disorders

Skin disorders may affect the vulva in isolation or be one manifestation of a systemic disease such as Crohn's disease, psoriasis or eczema. The aim of management is symptom control and maintenance of sexual function. Vulval skin disorders have various causes (**Table 11.5**).

Epidemiology

Up to one fifth of women are affected by a vulval skin disorder during their lifetime, typically after the menopause.

Clinical features

The most common symptoms are itching and irritation. Some disorders have characteristic appearances (**Figure 11.5**; see also **Table 11.5**), but these can be highly variable. Most vulval skin disorders are chronic conditions that tend to relapse after periods of good symptom control.

Vulval skin disorders: aetiology		
Condition	Description	Signs
Lichen sclerosus	Autoimmune disease with 5–10% risk of vulval cancer during follow-up	Whitened skin in figure-of-eight distribution Loss of vulval architecture
Vulval intraepithelial neoplasia	Intraepithelial neoplasia Associated with high-risk human papillomavirus infection, immunosuppression and smoking 5–10% risk of vulval cancer during follow-up	Variable clinical appearance: white, red or pigmented nodules or patches most common May coexist with an invasive vulval cancer
Extramammary Paget's disease	Intraepithelial neoplasia Associated with vulval cancer (10% of cases) or underlying cancer of the breast, colon or genitourinary tract (up to 30% of cases)	Red plaques with white 'cake icing' effect
Chronic vulval dermatitis	Allergy or hypersensitivity disorder	Reddened vulval skin in 'nappy distribution'

Table 11.5 Aetiology of vulval skin disorders

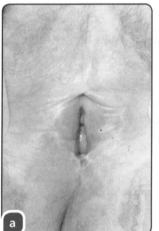 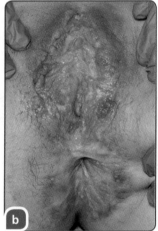 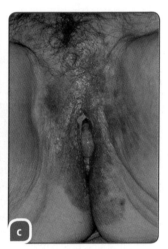

Figure 11.5 Premalignant vulval skin disorders: (a) lichen sclerosus, (b) vulval intraepithelial neoplasia and (c) vulval extramammary Paget's disease. The vulval appearances are highly variable and can mimic benign conditions. Courtesy of Jennifer Yell.

Diagnostic approach

A detailed history is required to exclude medical conditions that affect the vulva, including Crohn's disease, psoriasis and eczema. A history of diabetes suggests candidiasis (see page 304) or an autoimmune disorder, and factors such as a change of washing powder, changes to personal hygiene routine and allergy may be relevant. Examination includes inspection of all mucosal and skin surfaces.

Investigations

Many vulval disorders can be recognised clinically and a 6-week course of treatment started empirically. If symptoms do not improve, and in ambiguous cases, a vulval biopsy is essential for histological diagnosis. This is vital when vulval cancer is suspected. Autoimmune conditions prompt exclusion of diabetes and thyroid disease.

Indications for vulval biopsy are:

- clinically suspicious lesions, i.e. those showing rapid change, with bleeding or an irregular border, and non-healing ulcers
- inability to confidently diagnose a benign condition by visual inspection
- unsuccessful empirical topical treatment
- patient concern

> **Most cases of vulval cancer present late.** Physicians may be reluctant to examine because of time pressures, lack of a chaperone or embarrassment, and patients may be reluctant to be examined, mainly because of embarrassment. It is essential to examine every patient with vulval symptoms, because failure to do so can lead to delayed diagnosis and a fatal outcome.

Management

General advice for vulval skin care is relevant for all conditions.

- Avoid potential irritants that may exacerbate symptoms, such as soap, perfumed products, synthetic fabrics and preservatives in topical treatments
- Use soap substitutes such as an emollient

Vulval manifestations of systemic disorders are managed accordingly. Topical corticosteroids can relieve symptoms in patients with lichen sclerosus, lichen planus and vulval intraepithelial neoplasia. Surgical excision is effective but disfiguring, so it is reserved for women with unbearable symptoms and cases in which cancer is suspected.

Prognosis

Lichen sclerosus, lichen planus and vulval intraepithelial neoplasia are all premalignant conditions that carry a 5–10% risk of progression to cancer. Annual check-ups are required to exclude malignant disease. Patients are also encouraged to inspect their vulva regularly and report any concerns.

Answers to starter questions

1. The aetiology of endometriosis is unknown although several theories exist. The most widely held view is that reflux of endometrial cells through the Fallopian tubes occurs during menstruation. In some women, these cells become attached to peritoneal surfaces where they invade and grow in response to ovarian hormonal stimulation. It is unclear why this occurs in some but not all women. The amount of menstrual blood that refluxes through the tubes may be important, as well as altered or deficient immunological mechanisms that fail to 'mop up' endometrial cells in the peritoneal cavity. This theory does not explain distant endometriotic deposits, such as those found outside the pelvis.

2. Endometriosis is the cause of subfertility in 5–15% of couples. Minimal or mild endometriosis causes an overproduction of prostaglandins, cytokines and chemokines that impair ovarian, tubal, endometrial and peritoneal function. Moderate or severe endometriosis causes pelvic adhesions that distort pelvic anatomy and therefore interfere with oocyte release, tubal pickup and fertilisation.

3. Adolescent girls are offered HPV vaccination at 12–13 years of age, to prevent cervical cancer in many countries. In 2013, Australia became the first country to introduce HPV vaccination for boys aged 12–13 years of age. There is evidence that herd immunity against HPV could develop if enough girls are vaccinated, which will afford boys some degree of protection against infection with HPV 6, 11, 16 and 18. For example, in young men in countries where HPV vaccination of girls is widespread there has been a decline in new cases of genital warts, which are caused by HPV 6 and 11.

Chapter 12
Gynaecological tumours

Starter questions

Answers to the following questions are on page 334.

1. Why is ovarian cancer known as the 'silent killer'?
2. Why does removing the fallopian tubes reduce the risk of ovarian cancer?
3. Why is endometrial cancer becoming more common?
4. How does cervical screening prevent cancer?

Introduction

Much of gynaecological practice is directed towards excluding cancer as a cause of a patient's symptoms. The four main gynaecological cancers – ovarian, endometrial, cervical and vulval – present in very different ways.

■ Ovarian cancer, the most deadly of the four, presents late with non-specific abdominal symptoms when it has reached a stage at which surgical cure is unlikely
■ Endometrial cancer presents early following the onset of postmenopausal bleeding and has an excellent prognosis
■ Cervical cancer presents with abnormal bleeding but its incidence is decreasing due to the success of screening and is

expected to fall further as a result of the introduction of HPV vaccination
■ Vulval cancer occurs in older women and presents with pain and/or bleeding from a vulval lump or ulcer

A tumour is a mass of cells: in benign tumours the cells lack the ability to invade neighbouring tissues, in malignant tumours the cells undergo faster turnover and are able to invade into adjacent tissues and metastasise. They often present similarly and pre-operative differentiation is difficult. Removal and pathological examination is the only way to accurately tell them apart.

Case 14 Bloating and abdominal pain

Presentation

Margaret Turner, aged 57 years, is referred to the rapid access gynaecology clinic with bloating and abdominal pain.

Initial interpretation

These non-specific symptoms are typical for ovarian cancer, however, they can also be present in many other conditions, including irritable bowel syndrome, diverticulitis and gastroesophageal reflux disease. Bloating, abdominal pain and irregular bowel habit in a postmenopausal woman are 'red flag' symptoms for ovarian cancer, particularly if they are persistent or frequent. Imaging, including ultrasound and CT scans, make the diagnosis by finding a pelvic mass, with or without metastatic spread to other pelvic and abdominal organs, and exclude other conditions.

Further history

Mrs Turner has been feeling bloated for several months. Her bowel habit has been erratic, fluctuating between constipation and diarrhoea. She also has abdominal discomfort that varies in intensity. Her appetite is poor, but she must have gained weight because her trousers are tighter around the waist. She easily becomes out of breath on exertion. Until now, she has always been fit and healthy, and she has no family history of note.

Examination

Mrs Turner is pale. She becomes breathless when undressing.

Abdominal examination finds a symmetrically distended abdomen. There is flank dullness on percussion. Her abdomen is mildly tender all over. Pelvic examination finds a fixed hard swelling in the rectouterine pouch (pouch of Douglas). There is stony dullness to percussion and reduced air entry on the left side of the chest.

Interpretation of findings

These clinical findings are consistent with a diagnosis of ovarian cancer.

Mrs Turner has reported an increase in abdominal girth, consistent with an expanding pelvic mass or large volume ascites (accumulation of fluid in the peritoneal cavity). A change in bowel habit and abdominal pain are other symptoms of a pelvic mass or ascites. Loss of appetite is common in ovarian cancer, but cachexia is rare.

Mrs Turner's breathlessness indicates diaphragmatic splinting (inhibition of movement) as a result of increased intra-abdominal pressure, or pleural effusions. Other potential causes of breathlessness include anaemia (which would be diagnosed on the basis of a low haemaglobin concentration on a full blood count), a pulmonary embolus (excluded by CTPA) or pulmonary metastases. The findings of stony dullness to percussion and reduced air entry on the left side of the chest are consistent with the presence of fluid as a pleural effusion. Pulmonary metastases are a late event in ovarian cancer and are diagnosed by chest imaging (either X-ray or CT). Pallor is a sign of anaemia and is due to blood loss or the presence of a chronic disease, such as cancer.

The symmetrical distension of the abdomen described here is characteristic of ascites. Assymmetrical distension occurs in large abdominal and pelvic masses. The presence of flank dullness is also consistent with ascites; fluid accumulates in dependent areas so that when the abdomen is percussed, the usual tympanic sound of gas in the bowel is lost at the sides. If the patient is rolled away from the examiner,

Case 14 *continued*

the boundary between the tympanic and dull sounds moves as the fluid redistributes; this characteristic is known as shifting dullness. The generalised tenderness is caused by distension of the abdomen due to accumulating ascites. Abdominal symptoms of ovarian cancer are subtle until the disease is advanced.

In cases of ovarian cancer, a pelvic mass is often palpable on vaginal examination, abdominal examination or both. Fixed hard masses are more likely to be malignant than soft, mobile ones.

Given the symptoms and signs described, a diagnosis of ovarian cancer is highly likely. Imaging, by CT scan, is required to confirm the diagnosis and to assess the extent of disease. This will guide subsequent management.

Investigations

A CT scan of Mrs Turner's abdomen and pelvis shows a suspicious pelvic mass, moderate volume ascites and an omental cake (an abnormal thickening of the greater omentum) (**Figure 12.1**). These findings warrant a blood test to measure the concentration of CA125, a protein commonly raised in the presence of ovarian cancers. The CA125 level is grossly elevated at 3250 IU/mL.

A chest radiograph shows a left-sided pleural effusion but no obvious pulmonary metastases (**Figure 12.2**). The results of ultrasound-guided omental biopsy show high-grade serous adenocarcinoma, most likely of primary female genital tract origin.

Diagnosis

The histology of the omental biopsy has confirmed a diagnosis of ovarian cancer. The CT scan and chest X-ray have established that the disease is advanced as it is affecting other abdominal organs and has potentially spread to the chest because of the finding of a pleural effusion, although

Ovarian cancer: breaking bad news

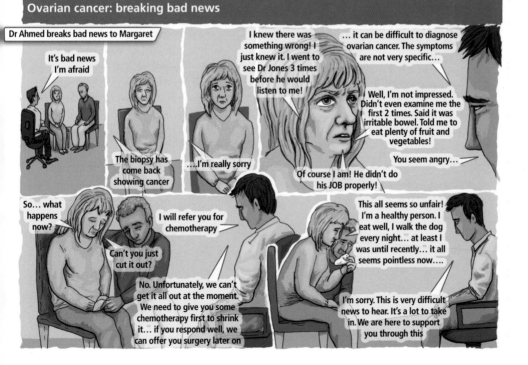

Case 14 *continued*

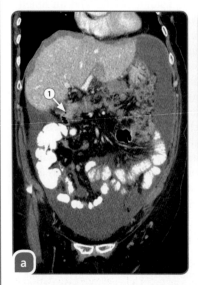

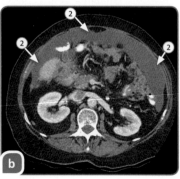

Figure 12.1 Imaging findings consistent with advanced ovarian cancer. (a) CT scan showing pelvic mass. ①, omental cake. (b) CT scan showing moderate ascites ②. Courtesy of Rishi Sethi.

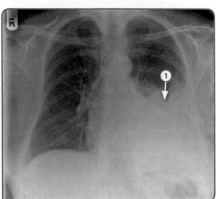

Figure 12.2 Erect chest radiograph showing a large right pleural effusion ①. Courtesy of Rishi Sethi.

no pulmonary metastases have been seen.

A management plan consisting of neo-adjuvant (before surgery) chemotherapy followed by interval debulking surgery (surgery after chemotherapy to remove all remaining tumour deposits) is decided at the gynaecological oncology multidisciplinary team meeting.

Mrs Turner is invited back to clinic to receive the diagnosis. She is clearly devastated. She is seen by a gynaecological cancer specialist nurse, who provides her with written information about ovarian cancer and contact details for sources of support through this difficult time.

Case 15 Postmenopausal bleeding

Presentation

Hilary Swanton, who is 65 years old, presents to her general practitioner with postmenopausal vaginal bleeding and is urgently referred to the postmenopausal bleeding clinic.

Initial interpretation

Postmenopausal bleeding is a 'red flag' symptom for gynaecological cancer. It is also caused by benign conditions, such as atrophic vaginitis, but more serious pathology must always be excluded first. The most important differential diagnoses to rule out are cancers of the endometrium and cervix, both of which present with abnormal vaginal bleeding.

Further history

Mrs Swanton has had several episodes of painless vaginal bleeding over the past few months. She has one daughter, born by normal delivery, but she struggled to become pregnant because she had polycystic ovary disease. She went through the menopause at 56 years of age and has never taken hormone replacement therapy. She is up to date with her cervical screening tests, and the results have always been normal.

She has type 2 diabetes mellitus, hypertension and ischaemic heart disease. She is not very mobile and walks with a stick. She does not smoke. She drinks one to two glasses of wine most nights and lives alone, having recently been widowed.

Examination

Mrs Swanton's body mass index is 47 kg/m². Abdominal and pelvic examinations are unhelpful in view of her body habitus. Speculum examination finds a healthy cervix and confirms the presence of blood in the vagina. The vulva and vagina appear healthy.

Interpretation of findings

The clinical picture is suspicious for a diagnosis of endometrial cancer. She has several risk factors for the disease, including polycystic ovary disease, late menopause (after 55 years), type 2 diabetes, hypertension and morbid obesity.

Mrs Swanton's history of normal results from cervical screening tests makes cervical cancer less likely.

In a slim woman, it is occassionally possible to feel a bulky uterus full of tumour, but the real value of vaginal examination is to exclude other pathology and assess the amount of vaginal bleeding. In Mrs Swanton's case, inspection of the vulva, vagina and cervix has been reassuring, thus excluding cancer of the lower genital tract as a diagnosis, and there is minimal active vaginal bleeding.

Based on these findings, it is important to perform an ultrasound to assess the thickness of the endometrial lining. Endometrial cancer is rare if the lining of the uterus is thin (<5 mm thick). If thickened, a biopsy is needed to make a diagnosis.

Investigations

Transvaginal ultrasound shows a bulky anteverted uterus with an endometrial mass.

Mrs Swanton attends for hysteroscopy as an outpatient. An endometrial polyp with features that suggest malignancy is found.

Endometrial biopsy shows a well-differentiated endometrioid adenocarcinoma. An MRI scan shows a large endometrial tumour, but there is minimal invasion of the myometrium (**Figure 12.3**).

Case 15 *continued*

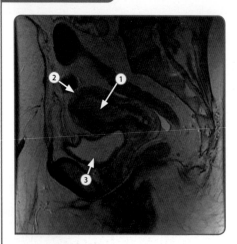

Figure 12.3 An MRI scan of the pelvis, showing a large mass distending the uterine cavity. Myometrial invasion is minimal, which is consistent with stage IA endometrial cancer. ①, endometrial cancer; ②, uterus; ③, bladder. Courtesy of Rishi Sethi.

Diagnosis

The histology from the endometrial biopsy has confirmed the diagnosis of endometrial cancer. The cancer is classified as stage IA, based on the MRI finding of minimal myometrial invasion and the absence of spread to lymph nodes or other organs.

The case is discussed at the gynaecological oncology multidisciplinary team meeting, at which hysterectomy and removal of the fallopian tubes and ovaries are recommended. Because Mrs Swanton has several medical comorbidities, including obesity, she is referred to the anaesthetist to assess her fitness for surgery.

Fibroids

Uterine leiomyomas or fibroids are benign tumours of smooth muscle; they develop in the muscular middle layer of the wall of the uterus (the myometrium). They are extremely common, affecting up to 50% of women.

Aetiology and pathogenesis

Fibroids are benign monoclonal tumors arising from the smooth muscle cells of the myometrium. It is unclear what causes fibroids to start growing but once they have grown, they are responsive to oestrogen and progesterone; they usually grow during pregnancy and shrink after the menopause.

They are usually multiple and range from microscopic to > 20 cm in diameter. They are classified according to their anatomical location:

- Intramural fibroids (commonest type) develop within the myometrium
- Subserosal fibroids are beneath the peritoneal surface of the uterus. If they grow outwards they can develop a stalk and become pedunculated
- Submucosal fibroids develop beneath the endometrium and distort the uterine cavity
- Cervical fibroids lie in the cervix

Intraligamentary fibroids are found in supporting structures of the uterus such as the broad ligaments (**Figures 12.4** and **12.5**).

Clinical features

Most fibroids are asymptomatic. Others present with a range of clinical features:

- heavy menstrual bleeding
- pressure symptoms affecting the bladder and bowel
- abdominal pain
- subfertility or recurrent miscarriage

Large fibroids are palpable on abdominal examination, bimanual pelvic examination or both.

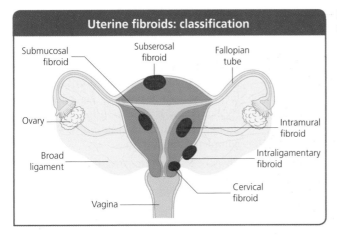

Figure 12.4 Classification of uterine fibroids.

Uterine fibroids: classification

Submucosal fibroid

Subserosal fibroid

Fallopian tube

Ovary

Broad ligament

Vagina

Intramural fibroid

Intraligamentary fibroid

Cervical fibroid

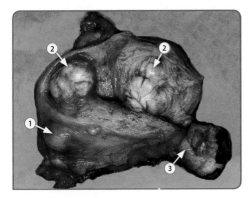

Figure 12.5 Bisected uterus, showing intramural, subserosal ① and submucous fibroids ②. ③, cervix. Courtesy of Richard Slade.

> Fibroids can grow so large and fast that they outgrow their own blood supply. Their subsequent degeneration is a common cause of abdominal pain in mid pregnancy.

Diagnostic approach

Fibroids are suspected on clinical grounds and confirmed on imaging.

Most are incidental findings during imaging for other indications. When fibroids are suspected, pelvic ultrasound is the initial investigation of choice. Hysteroscopy is used to identify submucous fibroids and facilitate their removal through hysteroscopic resection.

> Rapid growth of a uterine mass is a concerning feature, particularly in a postmenopausal woman, because it raises suspicion of a uterine sarcoma. Uterine sarcomas are aggressive malignant tumours with a poor prognosis (see page 326). Most arise de novo within the myometrium. The risk of a fibroid undergoing sarcomatous change is just 0.2%.

Management

Many patients do not require treatment because they are asymptomatic. Indications for treatment are:

- excessive menstrual loss
- significant pressure symptoms
- distortion of the uterine cavity, leading to subfertility or recurrent miscarriage
- rapid growth of the uterus suggesting possible sarcomatous change

If symptoms are not controlled with medication or the patient wishes definitive treatment then radiological or surgical management is offered.

Medication

Heavy bleeding is reduced with the combined oral contraceptive pill, the levonorgestrel-releasing intrauterine system (coil) or oral progestins. A gonadotrophin-releasing hormone analogue, e.g. goserelin, given for

6 months shrinks the fibroids before surgical resection.

Interventional radiology

Uterine artery embolisation is an alternative to surgery. It reduces blood flow to the fibroids, which causes them to shrink. However, the procedure is painful and up to one third of women require a repeat intervention within 5 years.

Surgery

Hysteroscopic or laparoscopic myomectomy is the first-line treatment for women who wish to retain their fertility. Fibroids are occasionally so large or plentiful that myomectomy is only possible via laparotomy. Hysterectomy is an option for women who do not want to have children or who have completed their families.

Benign ovarian cysts

Ovarian cysts are fluid filled sacs in the ovary. There are several different types of cyst based on their aetiology. Between 5 and 10% of women have surgery for an ovarian cyst during their lifetime.

Aetiology and pathogenesis

Normal physiological processes occurring during the ovarian cycle cause functional cysts including follicular or corpus luteal cysts. Follicular cysts form if ovulation does not occur and the follicle does not release its egg, instead it grows to form a cyst. Corpus luteal cysts form if the corpus luteum does not break down as usual in the absence of a pregnancy forming and instead expands with blood or fluid. Endometriomas originate from endometrial tissue (endometriosis) growing within the ovary. Mature teratomas or dermoid cysts are germ cell tumours that contain elements of all three germ layers (ectoderm, endoderm and mesoderm). These common cysts may become very large and typically contain bone, teeth, hair and sebum (**Table 12.1**).

Diagnostic approach

Ovarian cysts are detected incidentally during imaging for other indications (**Figure 12.6**). Endometriomas are common in women with endometriosis, who present with chronic pelvic pain, dyspareunia and subfertility.

Large ovarian masses are palpable on abdominal examination. Smaller cysts are discovered on pelvic examination.

The challenge is differentiating between benign and malignant ovarian masses (see page 322). Several risk-scoring tools are used for this. They include the risk of malignancy index (RMI), which determines a woman's risk of ovarian cancer as high, intermediate or low, depending on menopausal status, CA125 level and ultrasound findings.

Management

The principles of management are:

- to promote conservative management of benign cysts, when appropriate, to avoid the risks associated with surgery
- to promote laparoscopic removal of benign cysts, when possible, because postoperative recovery is better with laparoscopic procedures than with open surgery
- to ensure timely referral to gynaecological oncology if malignancy is suspected

Conservative management

Simple cysts < 5 cm in size are monitored by serial ultrasound scans. They do not always require treatment.

Benign ovarian cysts: characteristics		
Diagnosis	Origin	Features
Functional ovarian cyst ■ Follicular cyst ■ Corpus luteal cyst	Physiological	Common Small, fluid-filled cyst Generally asymptomatic Resolves spontaneously
Endometrioma ('chocolate cyst')	Endometrium within the ovary (endometriosis)	Common Cyst filled with altered blood at different stages of clot formation and break down May present with pelvic pain
Mature teratoma ('dermoid cyst')	Germ cell tumour	Very common Thick capsule May contain fat, hair, bone, cartilage Can be very large 10% are bilateral
Cystadenoma ■ Mucinous ■ Serous	Ovarian epithelium	Common May grow very large Can be complex and multilocular and filled with thin clear (serous) or thick mucoid (mucinous) fluid 10–15% are bilateral
Fibroma	Fibrous tissue	Relatively uncommon
Thecoma	Hormone-secreting stromal cells	Relatively uncommon Solid and cystic components Secrete oestrogen May present with abnormal vaginal bleeding 20% have associated endometrial pathology
Borderline ovarian tumours	Ovarian epithelium	Cells are mitotically active but there is no stromal invasion Can be serous or mucinous Extraovarian disease (implants) may be found in the peritoneal cavity 30% are bilateral Associated with pseudomyxoma peritonei in 10% of cases Excellent prognosis but can recur

Table 12.1 Characteristics of benign ovarian cysts

Ultrasound surveillance is appropriate for the management of many non-suspicious ovarian cysts, particularly in premenopausal women. Repeat scans 3–4 months apart are used to assess 'interval change' as an indicator of malignancy. If the cyst has a stable appearance over time, and particularly if the CA125 level is also static, women are reassured that that the cyst is almost certainly benign.

Surgery

This is necessary for symptomatic cysts and in cases in which malignancy cannot be excluded. Endometriomas > 6 cm in size are removed before assisted reproduction, because this improves pregnancy rates.

Prognosis

Ovarian cysts can undergo rupture, bleeding or torsion. These so-called cyst accidents present with acute abdominal pain. A torted ovarian cyst is untorted urgently to preserve ovarian viability.

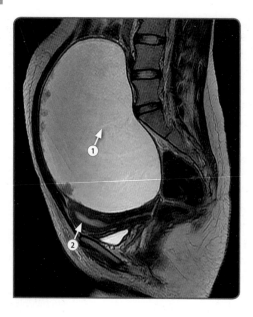

Figure 12.6 An MRI scan of the pelvis, showing a large complex adnexal mass ① pressing on the uterus ②. Courtesy of Rishi Sethi.

Ovarian cancer

Ovarian cancer is the deadliest gynaecological cancer in many developed countries, including the UK. In these countries, it is responsible for more deaths than all the other gynaecological cancers combined. Median age at diagnosis is 60 years.

Aetiology

The great majority of ovarian cancers are epithelial in origin; germ cell tumours and sex cord-stromal tumours are much less common (**Table 12.2**).

Most ovarian cancer is sporadic, but hereditary factors account for 10–15% of cases. The majority of hereditary ovarian cancers are associated with mutations in two genes: the breast cancer type 1 and type 2 susceptibility genes (BRCA1 and BRCA2, respectively). BRCA1 and BRCA2 mutations are inherited in an autosomal dominant pattern and increase a woman's lifetime risk of breast cancer by 50–85%, and that of ovarian cancer by 15–40%.

Risk factors for ovarian cancer are shown in **Table 12.3**.

Prevention

The combined oral contraceptive pill decreases the risk of ovarian cancer by up to 50%, depending on duration of use. Other protective factors are shown in **Table 12.3**.

Prophylactic removal of both ovaries and fallopian tubes reduces the risk of ovarian cancer by 90% and the risk of premenopausal breast cancer by 50%. It is recommended for women who carry the BRCA mutation and are older than 35 years, unless they wish to retain their fertility.

> Although prophylactic removal of the fallopian tubes and ovaries reduces the risk of ovarian cancer, a woman with a BRCA mutation still has a 3–5% risk of developing primary peritoneal cancer during her lifetime. This cancer originates in the peritoneum and behaves similarly to high-grade serous ovarian cancer.

Ovarian cancer: classification		
Cellular origin	**Type**	**Features**
Epithelial ovarian (90% of cases)	Serous tumour	> 50% of ovarian tumours
		High-grade (aggressive) or low-grade (indolent) tumours
		Increased CA125 levels in 90% of advanced and 50% of early stage tumours
		Associated with BRCA mutations
	Mucinous tumour	5–10% of ovarian tumours
		Associated with mucinous ascites
		Pseudomyxoma peritonei is a primary appendiceal neoplasm that may present with ovarian metastases
	Clear cell carcinoma	6% of ovarian tumours
		Associated with endometriosis
	Endometrioid carcinoma	8% of ovarian tumours
		40% have concurrent endometrial cancer
	Transitional cell carcinoma	Very rare
Sex cord–stromal (< 5% of cases)	Granulosa–stromal cell tumour	2% of ovarian tumours
		Slow-growing tumour
		Produces oestrogen
		Presents with irregular or heavy vaginal bleeding
		Increased inhibin levels
	Sertoli–stromal cell tumour	Produces testosterone
		Leads to defeminisation and then progressive masculinisation
		Presents with anovulation or oligomenorrhoea
		Later stages present with hirsutism, deep voice, clitoromegaly
Ovarian germ cell (< 5% of cases)	Choriocarcinoma	Rare aggressive tumour
		Placental trophoblastic tumour
		Presents with irregular bleeding, abdominal pain, nausea and vomiting
		Young girls may present with precocious puberty
		Increased hCG levels
	Dysgerminoma	Rare
		Increased α-fetoprotein, hCG, CA125 and inhibin A and B levels
	Immature teratoma	Rare
Metastatic tumour	Krukenberg's tumour	Metastatic spread from breast or gastrointestinal tumours
		Mucin-secreting signet ring cells are pathognomic

hCG, β-human chorionic gonadotrophin.

Table 12.2 Classification of ovarian cancer

Pathogenesis

The incessant ovulation theory is the most widely accepted explanation for ovarian carcinogenesis. According to this theory, ovarian cancer is a consequence of the repeated damage and repair to the epithelial surface of the ovary that occurs during ovulation. It is now thought that some ovarian cancers, e.g. high grade serous adenocarcinomas, actually originate in the fallopian tube.

Ovarian cancer: risk and protective factors	
Risk factors	**Protective factors**
Nulliparity	Pregnancy
Infertility	Breastfeeding
Endometriosis	Combined oral contraceptive pill use
Hormone replacement therapy	Tubal ligation
Previous benign ovarian cysts	Hysterectomy
Personal history of breast cancer	Risk-reducing prophylactic removal of both fallopian tubes and ovaries
Family history of ovarian cancer	Normal body mass index and regular physical activity
Obesity	
Tall stature	
Talc exposure	

Table 12.3 Risk factors and protective factors for ovarian cancer

Prophylactic bilateral salpingectomy with delayed oophorectomy has been suggested as a risk-reducing strategy for young BRCA mutation carriers, avoiding premature menopause. However, this has not yet been tested so its efficacy is unknown, although opportunistic salpingectomy at hysterectomy for benign indications is known to reduce ovarian cancer risk in women who are not BRCA carriers.

Clinical features

Ovarian cancer presents at an advanced stage. Symptoms are vague and non-specific, so are often overlooked by patients and physicians. Typical symptoms are abdominal pain, bloating, fluctuating bowel habit and urinary symptoms. Examination may find a pelvic mass, free fluid (ascites) or both.

Diagnostic approach

The key to early diagnosis is a high index of clinical suspicion. Clinical features that raise suspicion are investigated early with tumour markers and pelvic ultrasound scans.

Poor survival has stimulated research into screening and detection of early-stage ovarian cancer. Surgical cure is more likely in early asymptomatic disease, however it is not yet known if screening will save more lives.

Investigations

Investigations include serum tumour markers, imaging and histopathology.

Blood tests

Tumour markers are measured to aid diagnosis and indicate response to treatment if monitored over time. CA125 is high in 90% of advanced and 50% of early stage ovarian cancers. A steep CA125 increase over time is more indicative of malignancy than a single or static high level.

Imaging

Transvaginal ultrasound is used to characterise ovarian masses. Certain features raise suspicion of malignancy:

- bilateral cysts
- septations
- papillary projections
- solid components
- ascitic fluid
- lymphadenopathy

Malignant-looking ovarian masses are usually further assessed by CT scan (of the thorax, abdomen and pelvis), MRI scan or both to determine extraovarian spread and operability, based on proximity to and likely invasion of the bowel, bowel mesentery, liver and other organs.

Staging

Ovarian cancer is surgically staged according to the International Federation of Gynaecology and Obstetrics (FIGO) system (**Table 12.4**).

Management

The management of ovarian cancer depends on the stage of disease.

FIGO staging for ovarian cancer		
Stage	Description	5-year survival rate (%)
I	Tumour limited to one (IA) or both (IB) ovaries	80–90
II	Tumour extends to adjacent pelvic structures	65–70
III	Tumour extends to peritoneal surfaces outside pelvis and/or involves lymph nodes	30–50
IV	Distant metastases	15

Table 12.4 International Federation of Gynaecology and Obstetrics (FIGO) staging system for ovarian cancer

Early stage disease

This is treated by midline laparotomy, hysterectomy, removal of the fallopian tubes and ovaries, peritoneal washings, peritoneal biopsies, omentectomy, and pelvic and para-aortic lymphadenectomy. This allows true stage IA disease, i.e. cancer confined within the ovary, to be differentiated from more advanced disease. Women with true stage IA disease do not need adjuvant chemotherapy.

Staging is the process of determining the extent to which a cancer has spread. It takes into account the size of the tumour, invasion of adjacent organs and whether local lymph nodes or distant sites are involved. It is used in making decisions about treatment and determines prognosis.

Advanced disease

The standard treatment for patients with advanced ovarian cancer is complete surgical debulking combined with six cycles of chemotherapy. Debulking is the removal of all macroscopic disease, as detailed above, as well as bowel resection and removal of other intra-abdominal tumour deposits, as necessary. The order in which patients receive surgery and chemotherapy does not appear to affect survival.

Chemotherapeutic agents commonly used to treat ovarian cancer include the following.

- Platinum, for example carboplatin, inhibits DNA replication and repair, thereby leading to apoptosis; adverse effects include vomiting, myelosuppression, nephrotoxicity and peripheral neuropathy
- Taxanes, for example paclitaxel, stabilise microtubules and inhibit mitosis; adverse effects include hair loss, myelosuppression and neurotoxicity
- Monoclonal antibodies against vascular endothelial growth factor, for example bevacizumab, which inhibit angiogenesis; adverse effects include hypertension, delayed wound healing, gastrointestinal perforation and arterial thromboembolic events

Prognosis

Prognostic factors for ovarian cancer include age, stage (see **Table 12.4**), performance status, volume of ascites and extent of residual disease after surgery. There is no international consensus as to whether resectability primarily reflects surgical effort or the inherent biological characteristics of the tumour.

Endometrial cancer

Endometrial cancer presents at an early stage with postmenopausal bleeding. Its overall 5-year survival rate is excellent. Median age at diagnosis is 60 years.

Epidemiology

Endometrial cancer is the most common gynaecological cancer in Europe, North America and Australasia. Its incidence is increasing, and there are also more deaths from the disease despite improvements in overall survival.

Classification

Endometrial cancer is divided into two types: type 1, i.e. endometrioid, tumours (80% of cases) and type 2, i.e. non-endometrioid, tumours (20% of cases) (**Table 12.5**).

- Type 1 tumours are associated with exposure to unopposed oestrogen (**Table 12.6**); they are preceded by a premalignant precursor called atypical endometrial hyperplasia
- Type 2 tumours are a heterogenous group of biologically more aggressive tumours that develop via different pathways

Simple hyperplasia of the endometrium is a consequence of oestrogenic stimulation. It is not considered premalignant. In contrast, atypical endometrial hyperplasia progresses to invasive endometrial cancer in 50% of cases. Hysterectomy specimens from women with atypical hyperplasia often show coexisting endometrial cancer that had not been detected beforehand.

Aetiology and pathogenesis

Type 1 endometrial cancer is caused by obesity. The aromatisation of androgens to oestrogen by adipose tissue creates a state of oestrogenic excess 'unopposed' by progesterone in women who are anovulatory due

Endometrial tumours: classification			
Type 1	**Characteristics**	**Type 2**	**Characteristics**
Endometrioid	Associated with unopposed oestrogenic stimulation of the endometrium	Clear cell	Not associated with oestrogenic stimulation
	Atypical endometrial hyperplasia is precursor lesion	Serous	Arise in atrophic endometrium
		Carcinosarcoma	No precursor lesion
	Tend to be well-differentiated tumours with excellent prognosis		High-grade tumours with poor prognosis

Table 12.5 Classification of endometrial tumours

Endometrial cancer: risk and protective factors	
Risk factors	**Protective factors**
Unopposed oestrogenic stimulation of endometrium (relative oestrogen excess and/or progesterone deficiency): ■ Obesity ■ Polycystic ovary syndrome ■ Tamoxifen use in breast cancer survivors ■ Oestrogen-only hormone replacement therapy ■ Early menarche or late menopause ■ Oestrogen-secreting ovarian tumour ■ Nulliparity	Hysterectomy Combined oral contraceptive pill use Levonorgestrel-releasing intrauterine system (Mirena coil) Lifestyle measures to reduce weight and increase physical activity Pregnancy
Insulin resistance: ■ Type 2 diabetes mellitus ■ Metabolic syndrome	
Hereditary: Lynch syndrome (hereditary non-polyposis colorectal cancer, HNPCC; see text)	
Hypertension	
Increasing age	

Table 12.6 Risk factors and protective factors for endometrial cancer

to PCOS and in postmenopausal women. Oestrogen activates the PI3K-AKT-mTOR pro-proliferative oncogenic signalling pathway, causing the endometrium to grow. This process is further stimulated by insulin, insulin-like growth factor and the obesity-associated pro-inflammatory cytokine milieu. Disordered proliferation predisposes the endometrium to tumorigenesis.

Lynch syndrome is an autosomal dominant cancer susceptibility syndrome caused by a germline mutation in one allele of a DNA mismatch repair gene. If the second allele is inactivated by mutation, loss of heterozygosity, or epigenetic silencing by promoter hypermethylation, the cell is unable to correct the natural mistakes that occur during normal DNA replication, leading to genomic instability and subsequent tumorigenesis. Lifetime risk of endometrial cancer is 40–60%.

The cause of other type 2 endometrial cancers is not known.

> **Patients with Lynch syndrome are at increased risk of colorectal, endometrial and other cancers.** Screening by colonoscopy is recommended from 25 years of age, and transvaginal ultrasound scan/CA125 testing from 35 years of age.

Prevention

Hysterectomy is offered to women with Lynch syndrome if they have completed their families or do not want children. Other interventions that reduce endometrial cancer risk while preserving fertility are shown in **Table 12.6**.

Clinical features

The most common presenting complaint is postmenopausal bleeding. Premenopausal women present with heavy, prolonged or intermenstrual bleeding. Endometrial cancer may be diagnosed after an incidental finding of 'abnormal endometrial cells' on a routine cervical screening test.

Diagnostic approach

Postmenopausal bleeding warrants an urgent gynaecological referral. Most hospitals have 'one stop' clinics dedicated to the investigation of postmenopausal bleeding. These allow ultrasound, hysteroscopy and endometrial biopsy to be performed in one visit, decreasing the time interval between symptoms and diagnosis and increasing patient satisfaction.

Investigations

Abnormal bleeding is investigated by transvaginal ultrasound, hysteroscopy and endometrial biopsy.

Imaging

Transvaginal ultrasound is used to measure endometrial thickness. Postmenopausal women should have a thin, regular endometrial stripe of ≤ 4 mm. Abnormal findings, for example irregular or thickened endometrium, or polyps, prompt visualisation of the uterine cavity by hysteroscopy, endometrial sampling or both.

Histology

Endometrial biopsy is needed to confirm the diagnosis. The biopsy is taken blindly by using an endometrial sampling device, or during direct visualisation at hysteroscopy. The grade of endometrial cancer is based on tumour architecture. In grade 1 (well-differentiated) tumours, <5% of the tumour is solid (non-gland forming), in grade 2 (moderately differentiated) <50% of the tumour is solid and in grade 3 (poorly differentiated) >50% of the tumour is solid.

Staging

Endometrial cancer is surgically staged according to the FIGO system (**Table 12.7**).

Management

Management is predominately surgical and is curative in the majority of women. Alternative treatment options include radiotherapy and hormonal treatment for women unfit for surgery or who decline it.

Surgery

Standard treatment for endometrial cancer is total hysterectomy and removal of the fallopian tubes and ovaries. There is no

FIGO staging for endometrial cancer		
Stage	Description	5-year survival rate (%)
I	Tumour confined to uterus with superficial (<50%, IA) or deep (>50%, IB) myometrial invasion	75–80
II	Tumour extends into cervical stroma only	70
III	Tumour extends to serosal surface of uterus, ovaries or vagina and/or involves lymph nodes	45–60
IV	Tumour invades bladder or bowel, or distant metastases	15

Table 12.7 International Federation of Gynaecology and Obstetrics staging system for endometrial cancer

international consensus as to whether systematic pelvic and para-aortic lymphadenectomy should be carried out routinely for staging, therapeutic purposes or both. Laparoscopic or robotic-assisted hysterectomy is recommended when resources and skills permit, because postoperative recovery times are shorter than with open surgery.

Adjuvant therapy

Postoperative vaginal brachytherapy is recommended for intermediate-risk disease, i.e. stage IA, grade 3, and stage IB, grade 1 or 2.

High-risk disease, i.e. stage IB, grade 3 and above, is generally treated with both adjuvant chemotherapy and radiotherapy.

> **Many patients with endometrial cancer are morbidly obese.** This makes surgery technically challenging and dangerous for the patient, who is at risk of bleeding, injury to adjacent organs, thrombosis, infection, wound complications and prolonged hospital stay. Laparoscopic hysterectomy is considered for obese patients, because the associated perioperative complication rate is lower than that for open surgery.

Hormone therapy

Some women are unfit for surgery, and others wish to preserve their fertility. In these circumstances, progesterone is an alternative to hysterectomy. It is given either orally, for example as high-dose medroxyprogesterone acetate, or via a levonorgesterol-releasing intrauterine system (Mirena coil). Hormonal treatment is unlikely to cure endometrial cancer, and there is a high risk of recurrence on its discontinuation.

Prognosis

This depends on stage at diagnosis (see **Table 12.7**). Early stage disease is cured by hysterectomy, but advanced disease has a poor prognosis.

Leiomyosarcoma

Leiomyosarcomas are rare tumours arising from the myometrium (**Figure 12.7**). They have a peak incidence at age 40–60 years, often recur after removal and frequently metastasise. They sometimes arise in pre-existing fibroids (0.2–1% of fibroids develop into sarcomas) but more commonly arise de novo. Most uterine leiomyosarcomas are sporadic. Previous radiotherapy for pelvic malignancy is a risk factor.

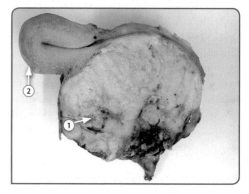

Figure 12.7 Large uterine sarcoma ① arising from the posterior aspect of the uterus ②. Courtesy of Godfrey Wilson.

Cervical cancer

Cervical cancer is the second leading cause of cancer-related deaths among women worldwide. Its incidence has decreased in many high-income countries because of the success of cervical screening, which enables precancerous lesions to be identified and treated, thereby reducing the risk of invasive disease (see page 375). The relatively recent introduction of human papillomavirus (HPV) vaccination for adolescents is likely to further reduce the incidence of cervical cancer.

Cervical cancer arises either in the squamous epithelium lining the ectocervix (squamous cell carcinoma) or in the glandular epithelium lining the endocervix (adenocarcinoma). Other rarer types of cervical cancer include neuroendocrine, clear cell and small cell tumours; they have a poor prognosis.

Aetiology

Risk factors for cervical cancer are shown in **Table 12.8**. Squamous cell carcinoma is the most common diagnosis (75–80% of cases). Adenocarcinoma (20–25% of cases) arises from the endocervix and is less likely to be detected by cytology in its precancerous stage stage.

Cervical cancer is caused by persistent infection with certain types of HPV, a small double-stranded DNA virus. There are more than 100 different types of HPV, which are classified as high risk or low risk depending on their oncogenic potential. Thirteen high-risk types have been linked with cervical cancer, including HPV types 16 (55% of all cervical cancers), 18 (15%), 31, 33 and 45.

Pathogenesis

Genital HPV infection is extremely common in young, sexually active women but most infections are self limiting and clear spontaneously. However, in some women, HPV persists and becomes a chronic infection. This is more likely in smokers and women who are immunocompromised. Persistent infection interferes with the normal function of cellular tumour suppressor gene products p53 and Rb. As a result, cellular turnover increases and apoptosis is suppressed. This is observed histologically as the precancerous lesion cervical intraepithelial neoplasia (CIN) 1, 2 or 3, depending on the extent of abnormality observed (see page 379). HPV becomes integrated into the cellular genome, mutations occur but are not corrected and these allow the cell to invade the epithelial basement membrane and metastasise.

Prevention

Women between the ages of 25 and 65 should be offered screening for cervical cancer every 3–5 years. In countries with a programme of regular screening, 50% of cervical cancers diagnoses are made in women who do not attend for screening, or who do so infrequently. Cervical cancer takes at least 10 years to develop; if a woman has three cervical screening tests during this time (as in the UK), this gives ample opportunity for a premalignant lesion to be detected and treated. A single test is unlikely to significantly decrease a woman's chances of developing cervical cancer, but regular tests will.

Population-based immunisation of adolescent girls with the bivalent or quadrivalent

Cervical cancer: risk and protective factors	
Risk factors	**Protective factors**
Early onset sexual activity	Regular cervical screening
Multiple sexual partners	Human papillomavirus vaccination
Sexually transmitted infections	Monogamy or abstinence
Low socioeconomic status	Barrier contraception
High parity	Male circumcision for sexual partners
Smoking	
Immunosuppression	

Table 12.8 Risk factors and protective factors for cervical cancer

HPV vaccine is likely to reduce the incidence of cervical cancer over the next 10–20 years. Vaccination must occur before sexual debut because it generates an antibody response to HPV that prevents, but cannot clear, an established infection.

> The UK's vaccination programme is offered by school and practice nurses to girls aged 12–13 years using Gardasil, a recombinant HPV vaccine that protects against:
>
> - HPV types 16 and 18, which are responsible for 70% of cervical cancers
> - HPV types 6 and 11, which cause benign genital warts
>
> Vaccination is given as two doses over 6–24 months. Take up is 75–85% of eligible girls. Vaccinated girls still require cervical screening tests when they reach eligible age, because 30% of cervical cancers are caused by HPV types not covered by the vaccine, e.g. types 31, 33 and 45.

Clinical features

A high proportion of cervical cancers are detected in asymptomatic women through cervical screening (50% in the UK). Symptoms of cervical cancer include postcoital, intermenstrual, irregular or persistent vaginal bleeding. Advanced disease presents with pelvic pain, urinary or faecal leakage, back pain or weight loss.

Examination is normal in early disease. A visible tumour is ulcerated or exophytic (outward growing) and tends to bleed on contact. A palpable cervical tumour is often hard, irregular, craggy and asymmetrical. Involvement of the parametrium, bladder or rectum can be assessed properly only by examination under anaesthesia.

Investigations

Investigations are needed to make the diagnosis and determine the most appropriate treatment.

Histology

Cervical cancer is diagnosed based on the results of examination of tissue obtained by punch biopsy at colposcopy, an investigation required when cervical cytology findings are abnormal. Biopsy of a larger tissue sample, for example obtained by knife cone biopsy or large loop excision of the transformation zone, is needed to confirm the diagnosis and determine the dimensions of the tumour.

Imaging

An MRI scan is carried out to determine the size of the tumour and to assess spread and involvement of lymph nodes (**Figure 12.8**).

Staging

Cervical cancer is clinically staged according to the FIGO system (**Table 12.9**). This requires a formal examination under anaesthetic, cystoscopy, proctoscopy and chest X-ray; the latter if advanced disease is suspected.

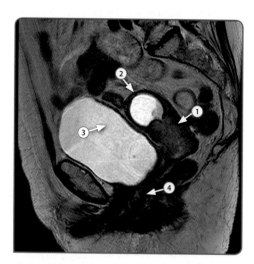

Figure 12.8 An MRI scan of the pelvis, showing a large cervical tumour ①. ②, Uterus. The uterine cavity is distended due to the accumulation of fluid following obstruction of the endocervical canal by the tumour; ③, bladder; ④, vagina. Courtesy of Rishi Sethi.

Management

Management of pre-cancerous cervical intraepithelial neoplasia detected during screening is discussed in pages 378–380. Management of cervical cancer depends on the stage of the disease and the patient's desire for future fertility.

Surgery

Early stage disease is treated surgically (Table 12.10). Adjuvant chemoradiotherapy is recommended when surgical margins are involved with tumour, or when lymph nodes are positive for metastatic disease.

Chemoradiotherapy

Primary radical chemoradiotherapy with curative intent is used to treat all stages of disease not suitable for surgical treatment. The standard regimen is weekly cisplatin plus pelvic external beam radiotherapy followed by brachytherapy, in which radioactive implants are placed into the cervix.

Chemoradiotherapy is used for early stage (stage 1) disease with equal efficacy, but compared with surgery it carries an increased risk of toxicity to the bladder or bowel. Toxicity is acute or chronic, and can reduce quality of life in long-term survivors of

FIGO staging for cervical cancer		
Stage	Description	5-year survival rate (%)
I	Tumour confined to cervix	80–90
II	Tumour extends to adjacent pelvic structures but not to pelvic sidewall or lower third vagina	60
III	Tumour invades pelvic sidewall or lower third of vagina, causes hydronephrosis and/or involves regional lymph nodes	35
IV	Tumour involves bladder or bowel mucosa or extends beyond true pelvis	15

Table 12.9 International Federation of Gynaecology and Obstetrics (FIGO) staging system for cervical cancer

Cervical cancer: surgical management				
Stage of disease	Standard treatment	What is removed	Fertility-sparing alternative	What is removed and what is spared
Microscopic stage I (max 7 mm width x 3 mm depth)	Cone biopsy	Cervical tumour and margin of healthy cervical tissue	Cone biopsy	Removed: cervical tumour and margin of healthy cervical tissue Spared: bulk of cervix, uterus, ovaries and fallopian tubes
	Simple hysterectomy	Cervix and uterus Optional: fallopian tubes and ovaries		
Small volume stage I (max dimension 4 cm)	Radical hysterectomy and bilateral pelvic lymph node dissection	Cervix Vaginal cuff Uterus Paracervical tissue Uterosacral ligaments Common iliac, external iliac, internal iliac and obturator lymph nodes Optional: fallopian tubes and ovaries	Radical trachelectomy and bilateral pelvic lymph node dissection	Removed: cervix; vaginal cuff; paracervical tissue; common iliac, external iliac, internal iliac and obturator lymph nodes Spared: uterus, ovaries and fallopian tubes

Table 12.10 Surgical management of cervical cancer

cervical cancer by causing urinary frequency, diarrhoea or incontinence of bowel or bladder.

> Improvements in early diagnosis and treatment mean that more women than ever are surviving cervical cancer. The long-term morbidity of radical treatment and its effects on quality of life are now important considerations. 'Survivorship', is concerned with optimisation of physical, psychosocial and sexual functioning in cancer survivors.

Recurrent disease

Radiotherapy-naive patients are treated with chemoradiotherapy if their cancer recurs. Pelvic exenteration, i.e. hysterectomy plus removal of the bladder and/or bowel and surrounding structures, is the only curative option for postradiation central pelvic recurrence.

Prognosis

This depends the stage. Five-year survival rates are given in **Table 12.9**. Progressive cervical cancer causes intractable bone or nerve pain; vesicovaginal or rectovaginal fistulas; and ureteric obstruction and subsequent renal failure, unless urine flow is diverted.

Vulval cancer

Vulval cancer is rare, accounting for 5% of all gynaecological malignancies. It is a disease of elderly women who present late because of reluctance to tell their physician about their symptoms. Squamous cell carcinoma is the most common type (90% of cases) with malignant melanoma (5% of cases), adenocarcinoma and basal cell carcinoma occurring less frequently. In recent years, vulval cancer has become more common in women in their thirties and forties as a consequence of exposure to high-risk HPV.

Aetiology

In younger women, persistent infection with high-risk HPV, especially type 16, is the likely cause. Risk factors for HPV infection include cigarette smoking and immunosuppression. Vulval cancer may be preceded by vulval intraepithelial neoplasia (see page 309).

In older age groups, lichen sclerosus and chronic inflammation may contribute to vulval carcinogenesis. Extramammary Paget's disease is a rare premalignant condition of the vulva (see page 309).

Prevention

There is no screening programme for vulval cancer, but women with premalignant conditions, including vulval intraepithelial neoplasia and lichen sclerosus, are reviewed regularly and taught self-examination to increase the likelihood of early detection of malignant disease. The widespread introduction of prophylactic HPV vaccination for adolescent girls will decrease the future incidence of vulval cancer.

Clinical features

Vulval cancer presents as a lump or ulcer, with associated pain, itch, bleeding or discharge (**Figure 12.9**).

Investigations

Investigations are needed to make the diagnosis and determine the most appropriate treatment.

Histology

Vulval biopsy confirms the diagnosis. Small lesions (< 1–2 cm) that would be effectively excised by biopsy are usually photographed first to guide future management. If extensive tumours impinge on important anatomical structures, such as the urethra and anus, examination under anaesthetic may be required to determine whether resection would compromise urinary or faecal continence.

Imaging

A CT or MRI scan is useful in advanced disease to exclude groin lymph node metastases, but staging is surgical and retrospective.

Staging

Vulval cancer is surgically staged according to the FIGO system. Tumours are either:

- Stage I: confined to the vulva
- Stage II: show local spread
- Stage III: regional lymph node involvement
- Stage IV: extensive local spread and/or distant metastases

Management

Treatment is individualised to take account of the patient's wishes and fitness for surgery.

Surgery

The mainstay of treatment for vulval cancer is surgery. Tumours are excised with a 1 cm disease-free margin to reduce the risk of recurrence. This may require vulval skin flaps to close the wound (**Figure 12.10**). If the depth of invasion is > 1 mm, groin lymphadenectomy is needed to identify and remove lymph node metastases. Sentinel lymph node dissection reduces the morbidity of full groin lymphadenectomy.

> **Ipsilateral groin lymphadenectomy,** i.e. removal of groin nodes on the same side as the lesion, is appropriate for lateral vulval tumours that are 1 cm away from midline structures. If tumours impinge on the midline, bilateral groin lymphadenectomy is needed because the lymphatic drainage of midline structures can be to either groin, and there can be considerable crossover.

The morbidity of groin lymphadenectomy includes wound infection and breakdown

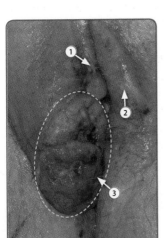

Figure 12.9 Malignant vulval cancer. ①, clitoris; ②, left labium majus; ③, vulval tumour. Courtesy of Richard Slade.

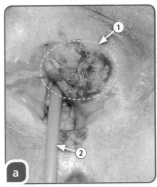

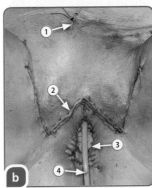

Figure 12.10 Surgery for vulval cancer. (a) Malignant vulval tumour ①. ②, urethral catheter. (b) The same patient after excision and flap reconstruction. ①, surgical drain; ②, vulval wounds; ③, vagina; ④, urethral catheter. Courtesy of Richard Slade.

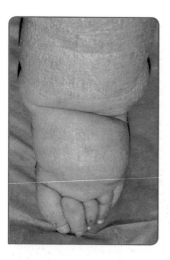

Figure 12.11 Chronic lymphoedema.

(20–40% of cases), and lymphocyst and lymphoedema (30–70%) (**Figure 12.11**).

- A lymphocyst is a localised swelling of accumulated lymph fluid after removal of the underlying lymph glands
- Lymphoedema is chronic lower limb swelling as a result of disrupted lymphatic drainage; it is treated with massage, the use of compression stockings and leg elevation

> The sentinel lymph node is the first node to receive lymphatic drainage from a tumour. If the sentinel node is negative, the rest of the lymph nodes are negative too. This allows full lymphadenectomy to be restricted to those who need it, i.e. those with lymph node metastases. For midline tumours, bilateral sentinel lymph nodes are assessed. The sentinel node is identified using blue dye and radioactive tracer injected into the tumour and subsequently detected in the groin(s).

Chemoradiotherapy

Adjuvant radiotherapy is used to reduce the risk of recurrence when surgical margins are involved or close, i.e. there is < 0.5 mm of healthy tissue, or when groin lymph node metastases are present.

Neoadjuvant chemoradiotherapy is used to treat extensive vulval tumours when primary surgery would compromise continence. The chemoradiotherapy may shrink the tumour completely so that surgery is no longer required, or shrink it sufficiently to allow sphincter-sparing surgery.

Prognosis

Early stage disease has an excellent prognosis. Overall 5-year survival rates vary according to stage as follows:

- 90% for stage I
- 50% for stage II
- 30% for stage III
- 15% for stage IV

Recurrent vulval tumours can be excised in most cases, but groin recurrences are usually fatal. For this reason, adequate groin node assessment and treatment at the time of primary surgery are critical.

Vaginal cancer

Vaginal cancer is rare, accounting for 1–2% of gynaecological malignancies. Metastatic spread from the cervix or endometrium is responsible for 80% of these tumours. Over 90% of vaginal tumours are squamous cell carcinomas (**Table 12.11**). Peak incidence is at 60–70 years of age.

Aetiology

Human papillomavirus, especially type 16, is found in 60% of tumours. Risk factors for vaginal cancer are:

- previous cervical intraepithelial neoplasia

Vaginal tumours: classification	
Type	**Features**
Primary	
■ Squamous cell carcinoma	Associated with human papillomavirus infection
■ Sarcoma botryoides	Embryonal rhabdomyosarcoma affecting young children (mean age 2 years)
■ Clear cell adenocarcinoma	Affects young women whose mothers were exposed to diethylstilbestrol in pregnancy
■ Malignant melanoma	Rare
Secondary	
■ Metastatic	Usually from cervix or endometrium, and much more common than primary vaginal cancer

Table 12.11 Classification of vaginal tumours

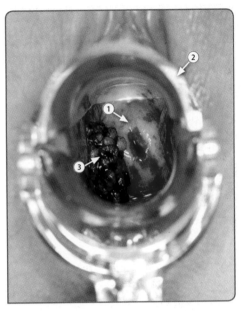

Figure 12.12 Malignant tumour in the right upper vagina. ①, cervix; ②, speculum; ③, vaginal tumour.

- vaginal intraepithelial neoplasia, a premalignant condition with a 10% risk of progression to invasive disease
- previous radiotherapy

Clinical features

Common presenting symptoms include vaginal bleeding or discharge. Late disease presents with haematuria, urinary retention, constipation or tenesmus. Vaginal examination finds a mass or ulcer, usually at the top of the vagina (**Figure 12.12**).

Investigations

Investigations are necessary for diagnosis and to guide treatment. Examination under anaesthetic and biopsy establish the diagnosis.

An MRI scan, cystoscopy and sigmoidoscopy are carried out to stage the disease. Vaginal cancer is surgically staged according to the FIGO system:

- Stage I: confined to vagina
- Stage II: extends to adjacent pelvic structures, but not to pelvic sidewall
- Stage III: invades pelvic sidewall and/or involves regional lymph nodes

- Stage IV: involves bladder or bowel, or distant metastases

Management

Most vaginal cancers are treated with radiotherapy. Radical surgery is an option for localised, stage I disease.

Prognosis

This depends on stage, with 5-year survival rates in the region of:

- 75% for stage I
- 40% for stage II
- 30% for stage III
- 0–20% for stage IV

Advanced cancer of all types is incurable, therefore palliative care is given to relieve symptoms and improve quality of life. Support from palliative care specialists is needed. For example, advanced cancer causes pain but effective analgesia causes nausea, vomiting and constipation, which themselves need treatment.

Answers to starter questions

1. Ovarian cancer is known as the 'silent killer' because it only becomes symptomatic in its late stages. As a result, ovarian cancer has a poor prognosis compared to other common cancers.

2. Mounting evidence supports the concept that some ovarian cancers actually arise in the fallopian tube. Studies have detected fallopian tubal intraepithelial lesions in the fimbriae of BRCA mutation carriers undergoing risk reducing surgery. These lesions are believed to represent precursor lesions for high-grade serous ovarian cancers.

3. The main reason for endometrial cancer becoming more common is the increase in obesity rates. Every 5 kg/m^2 increase in BMI confers a 60% increase in the risk of developing endometrial cancer. Increases in life expectancy and fewer women undergoing hysterectomy for benign gynaecological diseases also contribute to the increased rate.

4. Cervical screening reduces cervical cancer rates by identifying and treating precancerous cervical disease (cervical intraepithelial neoplasia, CIN). It therefore prevents the cancer from progressing into invasive, malignant disease.

Chapter 13
Urinary incontinence and genital prolapse

Starter questions

Answers to the following questions are on page 345.

1. Why does pregnancy cause genital prolapse and urinary incontinence?
2. Why is stress urinary incontinence a confusing term?
3. Why are mesh repairs controversial?

Introduction

Urinary incontinence, the involuntary leakage of urine, is not life-threatening but can cause discomfort and distress. The condition affects up to 10% of women but more than half of cases go undetected and untreated, because many find it difficult to discuss with health care professionals.

Genital prolapse is also common. However, its exact prevalence is difficult to ascertain because some women have no symptoms and others fail to seek help.

Urinary incontinence and genital prolapse often coexist. They also share risk factors, including advanced age and parity. Both conditions can greatly reduce a woman's quality of life, leading to physical, functional and psychological morbidity. Gentle enquiry and an empathic approach encourage disclosure and subsequent referral for specialist help.

Case 16 Weak bladder

Presentation

A 55-year-old woman, Amanda Edwards, presents to the gynaecology clinic with a history of urinary incontinence.

Initial interpretation

Detailed enquiry is necessary to establish the extent of the problem, including its effects on Mrs Edwards' quality of life. Are there any provoking factors? Are there any features that suggest urinary infection as a possible cause? Could there be an underlying malignancy?

Further history

Mrs Edwards says that she leaks urine when she coughs, sneezes or laughs. It is usually just a dribble, but she can lose a large volume if her bladder is full. She worries about being in a public place when this happens. She wears a pad to prevent embarrassment, and avoids going out and meeting new people.

To keep her bladder as empty as possible, Mrs Edwards limits the amount of fluid she drinks, and she avoids tea and coffee. She has no associated urgency, dysuria or haematuria.

She has no other gynaecological symptoms. She had two children, now adults, by vaginal delivery. She has chronic obstructive pulmonary disease, type 2 diabetes mellitus and hypertension, and takes medications for these conditions. Mrs Edwards is a lifelong smoker and struggles to keep to a healthy weight; however, she drinks alcohol only occasionally. She is divorced, lives alone and works in a supermarket.

Managing stress incontinence

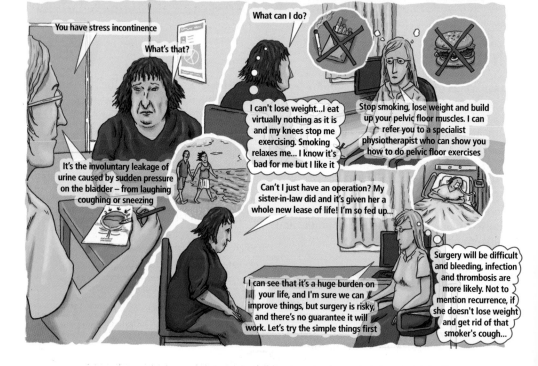

Examination

Mrs Edwards' body mass index is 38 kg/m². She coughs intermittently during the consultation, particularly after exertion. Her abdomen is soft and non-tender, with no palpable masses. Vulval inspection is normal, but Mrs Edwards leaks a few drops of urine when she is asked to bear down. The pelvic examination is otherwise unremarkable.

Interpretation of findings

Mrs Edward's description of leaking when she coughs, sneezes or laughs is characteristic of stress urinary incontinence. She was also able to demonstrate this by leaking when she bears down. The increased bladder pressure caused by these actions exceeds the urethral pressure, resulting in leakage of urine. This is particularly problematic if the bladder is full as the volume of urine leaked is greater; women limit the amount of fluid they drink to minimise this problem. Stress urinary incontinence is more common in women who have been pregnant and, particularly, had vaginal deliveries; damage to the pelvic floor muscles and nerves reduces their ability to contract the urethral sphincter.

The absence of urgency, dysuria or haematuria makes the differential diagnoses of urge incontinence, urinary tract infection and a bladder tumour, respectively, less likely. Similarly, the absence of a palpable mass on abdominal or pelvic examination excludes the pressure effect of an ovarian cyst or fibroid on the bladder as a cause of her symptoms.

The amount of tea and coffee consumed is important in urge incontinence as caffeine irritates the bladder muscle; it is less important when diagnosing stress incontinence.

The incontinence is substantially reducing her quality of life. The majority of women will have had symptoms for some time before they present to their doctor. Acknowledging the effect on their quality of life is essential; it reassures them that they are being taken seriously and that treatments are available.

In this case, obesity, smoking and chronic cough are modifiable precipitating factors. A bladder diary is needed to confirm the association between coughing, laughing etc. and the episodes of incontinence and to monitor fluid intake. A urine dipstick will exclude urinary tract infection as a cause of her symptoms.

Investigations

The results of dipstick urinalysis are normal, and a midstream specimen of urine is negative for infection. Mrs Edwards is asked to record her fluid intake, urine output and episodes of incontinence over 3 days in a bladder diary. This shows multiple provoked episodes of urinary leakage during the day, and one complete emptying of the bladder during a coughing fit.

Diagnosis

The description of urinary incontinence on coughing and following other provoking activities has confirmed the diagnosis of stress urinary incontinence. Unprovoked episodes of leakage are seen in urge incontinence, where the bladder muscle contracts involuntarily.

On the basis of this, Mrs Edwards is offered physiotherapy to strengthen her pelvic floor muscles. She is also advised to lose weight and stop smoking and is referred to the smoking cessation service for support and nicotine replacement therapy. A review appointment is arranged for 3 months' time. If Mrs Edwards' incontinence fails to improve with these simple measures, surgery may be considered.

Urinary incontinence

Urinary incontinence is the involuntary leakage of urine. The four main types of urinary incontinence are stress, urgency, overflow and functional incontinence (**Table 13.1**). Risk factors for urinary incontinence are shown in **Table 13.2**.

Types of urinary incontinence	
Type	Cause
Stress	Poor closure of the bladder
Urge	Overactive bladder
Overflow	Poor bladder contraction or blockage of urethra
Functional	Difficulty reaching the toilet because of medical comorbidities

Table 13.1 Types of urinary incontinence

Risk factors for urinary incontinence	
Risk factor	Comment
Obesity	Triples the risk of urinary incontinence
Parity	Risk increases with number of children born
Mode of delivery	Risk is higher with vaginal delivery than with caesarean section
Family history	Established genetic link for overactive bladder and urge incontinence
Age	Risk highest in elderly women
Medical history	Recurrent urinary tract infections and bladder symptoms in childhood, including enuresis, increase risk of urinary incontinence in adulthood
High-impact activities	High-impact activities such as running and jumping are associated with stress urinary incontinence
Others	High caffeine intake, diabetes, stroke, depression and vaginal atrophy are risk factors

Table 13.2 Risk factors for urinary incontinence

Stress urinary incontinence

Stress urinary incontinence is the involuntary loss of urine that occurs when bladder pressure exceeds urethral pressure, in the absence of activity of the detrusor (a muscle that forms a layer of the bladder wall). The condition is the most common cause of urinary incontinence in women, responsible for up to 50% of cases.

> **Urinary incontinence has a significant effect on women's lives.** It causes embarrassment, resulting in avoidance of leaving the house, drinking and socialising with friends. The cost of pads is also prohibitive for some.

Aetiology

Stress urinary incontinence is associated with pregnancy and childbirth, and is particularly common after prolonged labour and forceps deliveries. It commonly coexists with genital prolapse (see page 342). Obesity and chronic cough, for example in smokers and patients with chronic obstructive pulmonary disease, exacerbate symptoms.

Clinical features

The symptom of stress incontinence is urinary leakage provoked by coughing, laughing, sneezing or exercise. The observation of urinary leakage from the urethra with cough or Valsalva's manoeuvre is a sign of the condition. This sign is unlikely to be elicited if the patient has emptied her bladder immediately before examination.

Diagnostic approach

The diagnosis of stress incontinence is suspected on clinical grounds. The condition is only diagnosed formally with confirmation by urodynamic testing, in which case it is called urodynamic stress incontinence.

Investigations

Investigations are carried out to exclude other causes of urinary incontinence and establish the diagnosis.

Bladder diary

A record of fluid intake, urinary output and incontinent episodes over 3 days is essential to identify patterns and potential contributing factors.

The information in bladder diaries is rarely sufficient to determine the cause of the incontinence, but it does indicate the severity. The information is also used to assess fluid intake and the maximum time between voids, which is used to guide bladder training. Normal voiding frequency is less than eight times a day and once at night. The total volume passed is < 1800 mL/24 h.

Dipstick urinalysis and midstream urine specimen

Infection is excluded if the dipstick test results are negative for white blood cells, nitrites or both. If either are present, a midstream specimen of urine is sent for culture and sensitivities. Undiagnosed diabetes is excluded if dipstick testing is negative for glycosuria. Cases of haematuria (blood in the urine) in which menstruation has been eliminated as a cause are investigated to exclude bladder cancer.

Urodynamics

These tests are carried out to assess bladder and urethral function (**Figure 13.1**). They are used when empirical medical treatment fails, outflow obstruction is suspected or the woman has already had surgery for incontinence. Urodynamic testing is also recommended before surgery to identify women who are likely to have voiding difficulties postoperatively. Preoperative detection allows appropriate counselling and instruction in self-catheterisation to be provided.

> **Urodynamic testing is not offered at the first evaluation of women with stress urinary incontinence, because it is invasive and not necessary to initiate therapy.** It is also insufficiently sensitive to predict outcomes from non-surgical treatment.

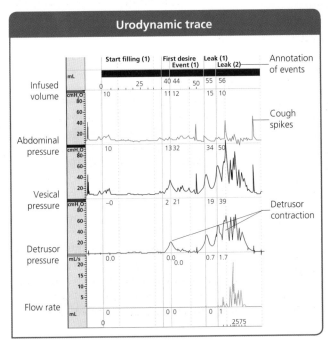

Figure 13.1 Urodynamic trace showing detrusor overactivity. The trace has five lines, which record infused volume, abdominal pressure, vesical pressure, detrusor pressure (vesical pressure minus abdominal pressure) and flow rate (i.e. leakage). Two detrusor contractions are labelled. The associated increases in pressure are shown on both the detrusor line and the vesical line but not on the abdominal line. During the second, greater detrusor contraction, leakage is shown by the increased flow rate, measured by urinary flow meter. Cough spikes are labelled. Patients are regularly asked to cough during urodynamic testing; coughing should consistently provoke similar changes in vesical and abdominal pressure and is used to ensure the measurements are valid. It is also an opportunity to monitor for stress incontinence provoked by coughing.

Management

Management focuses on improving symptoms and quality of life. It follows a stepwise approach. Conservative treatment is initially trialled; it is cheap, has no side effects and, if effective, avoids surgery.

Conservative treatment

This starts with lifestyle changes, including reducing caffeine and alcohol intake, and normalising body mass index through weight loss. Pelvic floor muscle exercises can be effective, particularly when performed with biofeedback and supervised by a specialist physiotherapist. Biofeedback is the process of gaining greater awareness of physiological processes, such as the strength of pelvic floor contractions. A specially designed device monitors the efficiency of pelvic floor muscle exercises and 'feeds back' to the woman, so that she can learn how to perform these exercises most effectively.

> **Pelvic floor muscle (Kegel) exercises improve the symptoms of urinary incontinence and genital prolapse.** Women are advised to repeatedly contract and relax the muscles of the pelvic floor 10 times 3 times a day over 12 weeks. Those who receive individualised treatment and supervision are more likely to achieve a benefit. Satisfaction rates of up to 70% are achieved; if no improvement after 12 weeks, surgical treatment is offered.

Surgery

In most developed countries the most common treatment for stress urinary incontinence is midurethral tape surgery. A midurethral sling is inserted through the retropubic approach (for transvaginal tape) or the transobturator approach (for transobturator tape). A synthetic tape is placed under the midurethra, which leads to scar formation and subsequent augmentation of the urethral angle. The procedure is effective in up to 90% of women. An equally effective alternative is the Burch colposuspension, which supports the bladder neck with a hammock of sutures attached to the pubic bone. This procedure can be done laparoscopically or through a pfannenstiel incision.

Injection therapy

Injectable periurethral bulking agents such as collagen are tried for women who are medically unfit for surgery or who wish to have another pregnancy. However, the benefits are usually short-lived: symptoms recur within 2 years in up to half of women.

Urge incontinence and overactive bladder

Urge incontinence is a sudden, urgent need to pass urine, accompanied by involuntary micturation.

Epidemiology and aetiology

Up to 35% of women have overactive bladder at some point in their life. The condition is caused by detrusor overactivity. It is usually idiopathic, although women who have had surgery for stress incontinence are predisposed to overactive bladder as a consequence of bladder neck obstruction. Central nervous system lesions or local irritants also cause overactive bladder.

Clinical features

Women with overactive bladder often drink an excessive amount of fluid and have high caffeine intake. History taking focuses on the effect of symptoms on quality of life (**Table 13.3**). Examination is normal.

Diagnostic approach

Overactive bladder is diagnosed when women complain of urgency with or without urge incontinence, urinary frequency or nocturia.

Investigations

A bladder diary shows frequent small-volume voids day and night.

Urinary incontinence and quality of life	
Domain	Effects
Quality of life	Anxiety, depression, social isolation, work impairment
Sexual function	Fear of incontinence during sexual activity impairs sexual function
Morbidity	Perineal infections, falls and fractures are more common
Increased caregiver burden	Increased likelihood of admission to a nursing home

Table 13.3 Effects of urinary incontinence on quality of life

Management

Both non-pharmacological and pharmacological methods are used. Conservative treatment is trialled first as it is non-invasive and has no side effects. Anti-muscarinic drugs are prescribed alongside bladder training if there is no improvement in symptoms.

Conservative treatment

Helpful lifestyle changes include caffeine reduction and restriction of fluid intake. Bladder retraining enables patients to regain some control of bladder function. This is done by delaying micturition by gradually increasing the time between visits to the toilet to empty the bladder.

Bladder training starts with timed voiding: the woman is instructed to empty her bladder by the clock at regular intervals. Urgency between voiding is controlled by distraction or relaxation techniques. When she can manage 2 days without leakage, the interval between scheduled voids is extended. Intervals are gradually increased until voiding is every 4 h without accidents. Successful bladder training requires patience and perseverance.

Medication

Long- and short-acting antimuscarinic anticholinergic drugs relax bladder smooth muscle and increase bladder capacity. Short-acting oxybutynin is the first-line therapy. Poor compliance is common, because of adverse effects, e.g. dry eyes and mouth.

After menopause, vaginal atrophy may coexist with overactive bladder; vaginal oestrogens improve symptoms in 60% of women.

Second-line treatments include injections of botulinum toxin type A into the bladder wall, sacral nerve stimulation or posterior tibial nerve stimulation. Botox treatment can cause difficulty voiding in up to 20% of women, necessitating short-term self-catheterisation until injection effects have worn off.

Surgery

Intractable symptoms may be improved by 'clam' augmentation ileocystoplasty, in which a loop of small bowel is used to increase bladder capacity. However, this procedure is generally the last resort, because of the risk of long-term complications including malignancy in the grafted bowel.

Most women with urinary incontinence use pads to keep their clothes dry. These should be incontinence pads: sanitary towels designed for use in menstruation are insufficiently absorbent. Pads must be changed regularly, because chronic exposure to urine-soaked pads causes contact dermatitis. This is a particular problem in nursing homes.

Overflow incontinence

Overflow incontinence is combined continuous urinary leakage and incomplete bladder emptying. The condition is caused by impaired detrusor contractility or bladder outlet obstruction. Bladder outlet obstruction may be the result of scarring from previous prolapse or incontinence surgery. It is rarer in women than in men.

Treatment focuses on the underlying cause, such as division of a previous tension-free tape, or alpha-blockers to relax the bladder and improve emptying. Intermittent self-catheterisation may be necessary in the short or long term.

Genital prolapse

Prolapse occurs when one or more pelvic organs descend through the pelvic floor into the vagina. The cervix, vaginal vault (after hysterectomy) and vaginal walls are most typically involved.

> **Prolapse can significantly impair a woman's quality of life.** Its presence can cause embarrassment, discomfort and avoidance of sexual intercourse.

Epidemiology

About half of all parous women have some degree of genital prolapse. However, only 10–20% of the women with genital prolapse seek medical help.

Aetiology

The pathophysiology of genital prolapse is multifactorial. Childbirth, ageing and family history are significant contributors. Pregnancy and childbirth damage the levator ani (muscle forming the pelvic floor), the pudendal nerve or both, thereby weakening the mechanical and neurological support of the pelvic floor. Postmenopausal oestrogen deficiency leads to atrophy of the pelvic architectural support and therefore exacerbates prolapse.

A further contributing factor is increased intra-abdominal pressure. Causes of this include obesity, chronic cough (e.g. from smoking, chronic obstructive pulmonary disease or gastro-oesophageal reflux), constipation and heavy weightlifting.

Clinical features

Women describe a sensation of dragging or 'a lump coming down', which worsens as the day progresses (**Table 13.4**). In severe prolapse (**Figure 13.2**), the tissues become ulcerated from friction against clothing, resulting in bleeding or discharge. There may be associated urinary incontinence or difficulty with defecation.

Symptoms of genital prolapse	
Type	Description
Bulge or pressure symptoms	Lump, bulge, something coming down, dragging sensation, backache, vaginal discharge, ulceration and bleeding
Urinary symptoms	Incomplete emptying, need to digitate to void, frequency, urgency, urinary incontinence, recurrent urinary tract infections
Bowel symptoms	Incomplete emptying, need to digitate to defecate, constipation, faecal incontinence
Sexual symptoms	Obstructed penetration, reduced sensation, reduced libido, altered body image, dyspareunia

Table 13.4 Symptoms of genital prolapse

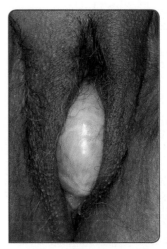

Figure 13.2 Vaginal vault prolapse following hysterectomy.

Diagnostic approach

Prolapse is diagnosed on clinical examination during Valsalva's manoeuvre or cough. Bimanual pelvic examination is required to exclude pelvic masses.

Careful examination with a Sims speculum (see page 95) enables the anterior and posterior vaginal walls to be examined separately. **Table 13.5** shows a classification system commonly used to describe prolapse. Prolapse can also be quantified by using the pelvic organ prolapse quantification system (**Figure 13.3**).

Classification of prolapse	
Classification	**Description**
Cystocele	Prolapse of bladder base or anterior vaginal wall
Enterocele	Hernia and prolapse of rectouterine pouch (pouch of Douglas)
Rectocele	Prolapse of rectum or posterior vaginal wall
Uterine prolapse	Descent of uterus
Vault prolapse	Descent of vault after hysterectomy
Procidentia	Complete prolapse of uterus and vaginal walls

Table 13.5 Classification of prolapse

Always examine the patient while she is standing up or squatting. This is necessary to assess the full extent of the prolapse.

Management

Management focuses on reducing symptoms and restoring pelvic floor support.

Conservative treatment

Symptoms of genital prolapse are improved by conservative measures such as weight loss and smoking cessation. Pelvic floor muscle

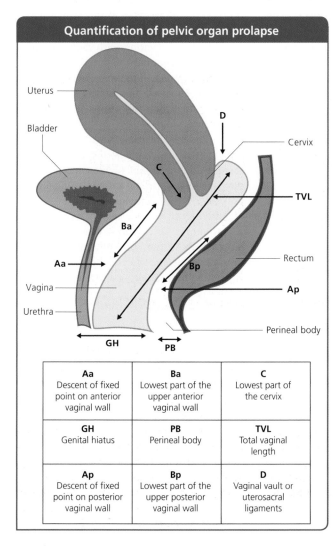

Figure 13.3 The pelvic organ prolapse quantification system is used to classify and assess the extent of genital prolapse.

Quantification of pelvic organ prolapse

Aa	Ba	C
Descent of fixed point on anterior vaginal wall	Lowest part of the upper anterior vaginal wall	Lowest part of the cervix
GH	**PB**	**TVL**
Genital hiatus	Perineal body	Total vaginal length
Ap	**Bp**	**D**
Descent of fixed point on posterior vaginal wall	Lowest part of the upper posterior vaginal wall	Vaginal vault or uterosacral ligaments

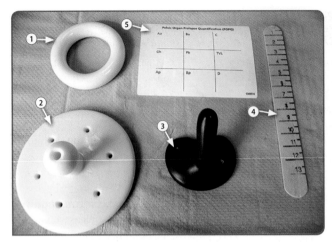

Figure 13.4 Different types of pessaries used to manage genital prolapse, and the pelvic organ prolapse quantification form. ① Ring pessary; ②, Gellhorn pessary; ③, shelf pessary; ⑤, POPQ chart used for assessing genital prolapse. The centimetre ruler ④ is used with the pelvic organ prolapse quantification form to measure the extent of the prolapse.

exercises (see page 109) help in cases of mild to moderate prolapse.

Pessaries are the first-line conservative treatment for prolapse. Several types are available, including the ring, shelf and Gellhorn pessary (**Figure 13.4**). The pessary is placed in the vagina and acts as a mechanical support. It does not treat the underlying prolapse but reduces the severity of symptoms associated with it. Drawbacks include the need to regularly remove, clean and replace it, possible trauma to the vagina from friction and the fact that it can fall out if incorrectly sized. Sexual intercourse is possible with ring pessaries, but not with shelf or Gelhorn ones. Low-dose oestrogen pessaries and cream are also useful for postmenopausal women with mild to moderate prolapse.

Surgery

Many types of surgery are used for prolapse repair. The choice of procedure depends on the anatomical location of the prolapse and whether the repair is primary or secondary.

Vaginal hysterectomy with vault support is the first-line treatment for uterine prolapse. An alternative first-line treatment if a woman wishes to conserve her uterus is sacrohysteropexy, in which the uterus is secured to the sacrum.

In post-hysterectomy vaginal vault prolapse repair, the vault is suspended to the sacrospinous ligament (sacrospinous colpopexy) or secured to the sacrum using a polypropylene mesh (sacrocolpopexy).

Anterior or posterior vaginal repair is used when anterior or posterior vaginal wall prolapse occurs without uterine prolapse. In this procedure, the endopelvic fascia is reinforced with either buttress sutures or a mesh.

Answers to starter questions

1. Fifty per cent of cases of urinary incontinence and 75% of cases of genital prolapse are caused by pregnancy and childbirth. The mechanisms are not fully understood, but compression, stretching or tearing of nerves, muscles and connective tissues of the pelvic floor are implicated. Childbirth, particularly prolonged labour and forceps delivery, is believed to be a more significant factor than pregnancy alone.

2. The term stress incontinence describes a symptom, a sign and a diagnosis, which causes confusion. The symptom of stress incontinence is urinary leakage on coughing, laughing, sneezing or exercising. The sign is the visualisation of urine at the urethral meatus during cough or Valsalva manoeuvre. A diagnosis is only made by a urodynamic investigation, when urinary leakage is witnessed following provocation and in the absence of detrusor activity.

3. Mesh is a mostly non-absorbable synthetic polypropylene used to treat genital prolapse. However, its long-term use has been shown to be associated with pain, infection, bleeding, dyspareunia, organ perforation, urinary problems, mesh erosion, recurrent prolapse, neuro-muscular problems and vaginal shrinkage in some patients. Lawsuits have been filed against mesh-producing companies by women who felt uninformed about the possible risks before they had a mesh repair, particularly in the USA. Mesh is now only used selectively in cases where the benefits outweigh the risks. This includes women who have had previous prolapse surgery without mesh that has failed and for the treatment of vault prolapse. The majority of women undergoing prolapse surgery do so without the use of mesh.

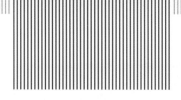

Chapter 14
Emergencies

Introduction

Emergencies occur at any time and in any setting. Previously healthy women are able to compensate for physiological stress for a long time before their condition deteriorates precipitously, so it is vital to heed subtle changes in vital signs, such as blood pressure, pulse, urine output, oxygen saturations, temperature, respiratory rate. Judicious and timely intervention can prevent or reduce the severity of emergency events.

Various systems are put in place to support the appropriate management of emergencies in gynaecology and maternity care. In the UK these include:

- early warning score alert systems
- induction of new healthcare professionals with team training and skills drills
- debriefing after an event, including the use of reflective practice and targeted supervision or training
- systematic reporting of near misses, critical incidents and maternal deaths, so as to learn from them and identify system errors and weaknesses

Case 17 Abdominal pain and unconsciousness

Presentation

Lucy Connor, aged 23 years, has been bought to hospital by a friend after she fainted at home. She is complaining of abdominal pain. On examination, she is pale and unable to lie flat because of the pain. She is clearly distressed. Her blood pressure is 85/50 mmHg, and her heart rate is 105 beats/min. A urinary pregnancy test gives a positive result.

Initial interpretation

This clinical presentation of collapse with a positive pregnancy test is consistent with a diagnosis of a ruptured ectopic pregnancy. The hypotension and tachycardia suggest hypovolaemic shock as a result of bleeding into the abdominal cavity.

> **Ruptured ectopic pregnancy is a life-threatening emergency that requires urgent surgical intervention.** It should always be considered and excluded in a woman of childbearing age who presents with collapse.

Further history and examination

Lucy's last period was 7 weeks ago. She did not know she was pregnant until now. She has had intermittent pain in her lower abdomen for the past 2 days. She now has constant severe pain in her left iliac fossa. She has had light vaginal bleeding today, similar to that at the start of a period. She felt dizzy at home and fainted when she got up from the sofa.

On examination, Lucy's abdomen is extremely tender, especially in the left iliac fossa, with rebound tenderness and involuntary guarding. Vaginal examination is poorly tolerated because of pain on movement of the cervix (cervical excitation) and an exquisitely tender mass in the left adnexa.

Working diagnosis

The working diagnosis is ruptured ectopic pregnancy resulting in intra-abdominal bleeding and hypovolaemic shock (**Figure 14.1**). The presence of iliac fossa pain and a positive pregnancy test are classical of an ectopic pregnancy. The tachycardia and hypotension indicate hypovolaemic shock. It is imperative to start fluid resuscitation immediately to start correcting the hypovolaemia and proceed to emergency surgery to stop the bleeding.

Immediate intervention

Help from senior colleagues is requested urgently. Two large bore intravenous cannulae are inserted, and blood is taken for a full blood count, coagulation tests, measurement of serum β-human chorionic gonadotrophin concentration and

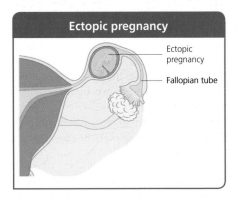

Ectopic pregnancy

Ectopic pregnancy

Fallopian tube

Figure 14.1 Ectopic pregnancies that implant and grow within the fallopian tube stretch the walls of the tube until its elastic limit is reached. Rupture occurs when the tube is stretched beyond this point; this causes bleeding into the peritoneal cavity. Tubal ectopic pregnancies usually become symptomatic between 6 and 8 weeks' gestation.

Case 17 *continued*

crossmatch. The cannulae allow intravenous access whilst the bloods confirm the pregnancy, anaemia and exclude any clotting abnormalities that may complicate management. A cross match ensures blood is available for transfusion. A blood gas shows a haemoglobin concentration of 68 g/dL, indicating significant intra-abdominal haemorrhage. Fluid resuscitation with intravenous crystalloid is continued while crossmatched blood is awaited. Lucy requires emergency surgery to remove the ectopic pregnancy and stop the bleeding.

Ectopic pregnancy

Haemorrhage from a ruptured ectopic pregnancy is the leading cause of pregnancy-related maternal death in the first trimester. Death usually occurs out of hospital or shortly after presentation to emergency services.

Modern ultrasound techniques mean that most ectopic pregnancies are diagnosed in women who have few symptoms or who are completely asymptomatic. Current guiding principles are to adopt a conservative approach to save the fallopian tube, if possible. Management is expectant, medical or surgical, depending on the stage at which the extrauterine pregnancy is detected, the health of the contralateral tube and the clinical condition of the patient (see page 179). Any patient presenting with an acute abdomen or haemodynamic compromise is managed surgically as an emergency. Expectant or medical management is never appropriate in these circumstances.

Case 18 Heavy vaginal bleeding and severe abdominal pain in pregnancy

Presentation

Sandra Jones, a 37-year-old homemaker, is 39 weeks into her third pregnancy. She attends the obstetric triage unit with a history of heavy vaginal bleeding and severe abdominal pain. She has not felt the baby move since the pain started 1 hour ago.

On admission, her blood pressure is 120/70 mmHg and her heart rate is 130 beats/min. The midwife is unable to auscultate the fetal heart.

Initial interpretation

Causes of antepartum haemorrhage are shown in **Table 14.1**. Severe abdominal pain accompanied by fresh vaginal bleeding is typical of placental abruption. The history and examination seek to quantify the amount of bleeding and the degree of maternal and fetal compromise. Sandra is haemodynamically compromised, and there is concern about fetal viability. If the fetus is still alive, expedited delivery by emergency caesarean section is required.

Further history and examination

Sandra's pregnancy has been uncomplicated until now, but she has not managed to give up smoking and admits to occasional cocaine use during the pregnancy,

Case 18 *continued*

			Antepartum haemorrhage: causes		
Diagnosis	Cause of bleeding	Source of bleeding	Clinical features		
			Abdominal pain	Maternal haemodynamic compromise	Fetal distress
Placental abruption (30% of cases)*	Premature separation of placenta from uterine wall	Maternal	Yes	Yes	Yes
Placenta praevia (20% of cases)*	Low-lying placenta	Maternal	No	Yes	No
Vasa praevia (rare)*	Rupture of fetal vessels	Fetal	No	No	Yes
Uterine rupture (rare)*	Uterine rupture	Maternal	Yes	Yes	Yes

*In the remaining 50% of cases, an exact cause is not found, so marginal placental separation is assumed to be the cause of bleeding.

Table 14.1 Key causes of antepartum haemorrhage

including today. Her previous pregnancies were normal and delivered vaginally at term.

Abdominal examination finds a very hard, 'woody' uterus (feels firm, like wood, and fetal parts cannot be distinguished), which is tender to palpation. It is not possible to establish fetal presentation. Speculum examination confirms heavy loss of fresh red blood, with large clots. Auscultation fails to detect any fetal heart activity.

Ultrasound confirms fetal death in utero, cephalic presentation and anterior placenta (not low lying). Digital cervical examination finds the cervix to be 3 cm dilated.

Working diagnosis

Antepartum haemorrhage accompanied by severe abdominal pain, haemodynamic compromise and fetal death in utero is likely to be caused by a large placental abruption. Bleeding from a placenta praevia is painless and rarely causes fetal compromise. Uterine rupture is rare unless following a previous casesarean section. Vasa praevia is extremely rare and does not cause maternal compromise. Therefore, placental abruption is the working diagnosis.

Immediate intervention

Resuscitation follows the ABCD approach. Supplemental oxygen is used, large bore intravenous access is obtained, and blood samples are taken for full blood count, coagulation tests and urgent crossmatch of 6 units of blood. Initial fluid resuscitation is with intravenous crystalloids. Once Sandra's condition has been stabilised, delivery is expedited by artificial rupture of the membranes and synthetic oxytocin (Syntocinon) augmentation.

Placental abruption

Placental abruption is separation of the placenta from the uterine wall before delivery of the fetus (**Figure 14.2**). The amount of bleeding is not a reliable indicator of the degree of placental separation, because blood loss is often concealed, being retained in the uterine cavity.

Few abruptions are visualised on ultrasound. The main indication for ultrasound is to exclude placenta praevia and establish fetal viability. Large placental abruptions cause disseminated intravascular coagulopathy, and it is essential to manage coagulation abnormalities aggressively.

Management is with maternal resuscitation, stabilisation and delivery. In prelabour abruptions, delivery is by caesarean section, particularly if there is acute fetal distress. In cases of fetal death, vaginal delivery is preferable to avoid the additional haemorrhagic complications of caesarean section and the resulting uterine scar.

Placenta praevia

Placenta praevia is when the placenta partially or completely covers the internal cervical os. Bleeding occurs when gradual changes in the lower uterine segment and cervix cause shearing forces and partial placental detachment.

Placenta praevia should be excluded in all women presenting with vaginal bleeding in the third trimester. An ultrasound scan to establish placental site must precede assessment by digital vaginal examination.

> **Never carry out a digital vaginal examination on a woman presenting with antepartum haemorrhage until placenta praevia has been excluded.** Injudicious vaginal examination can precipitate life-threatening haemorrhage.

Uterine rupture and vasa praevia

Uterine rupture is a rare and potentially catastrophic event for both mother and fetus. The uterine cavity is breached, usually along a scar from a previous caesarean section, after the onset of uterine contractions. In vasa praevia, fetal vessels lie in the

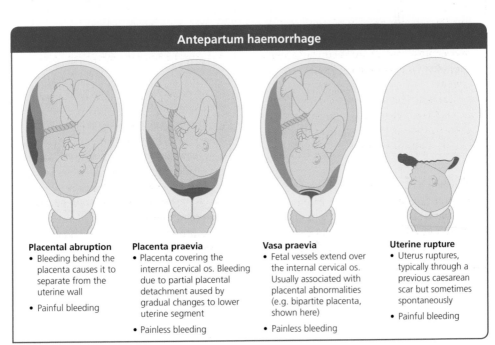

Antepartum haemorrhage

Placental abruption
- Bleeding behind the placenta causes it to separate from the uterine wall
- Painful bleeding

Placenta praevia
- Placenta covering the internal cervical os. Bleeding due to partial placental detachment aused by gradual changes to lower uterine segment
- Painless bleeding

Vasa praevia
- Fetal vessels extend over the internal cervical os. Usually associated with placental abnormalities (e.g. bipartite placenta, shown here)
- Painless bleeding

Uterine rupture
- Uterus ruptures, typically through a previous caesarean scar but sometimes spontaneously
- Painful bleeding

Figure 14.2 Aetiology of antepartum haemorrhage.

membranes covering the internal cervical os. If these fetal vessels rupture, for example at the time of rupture of the membranes, fetal exsanguination and death quickly follow. Acute management of uterine rupture or vasa praevia is emergency caesarean section.

Case 19 Headaches and visual disturbances in pregnancy

Presentation

Priya Dutta, a 38-year-old primigravida, has been brought to hospital after her husband found her collapsed on the floor of their kitchen. She had been drowsy and confused, and had urinated in her clothes and bitten her tongue.

When the ambulance crew arrived at her home, Priya's blood pressure was 190/110 mmHg. Her husband told them that she is 35 weeks pregnant and has been complaining of headaches and visual disturbances for the past few days.

Initial interpretation

Seizures in the third trimester of pregnancy are considered to be caused by eclampsia until proven otherwise (**Table 14.2**). The preceding headaches and visual disturbances, combined with severe hypertension at the time of the seizure, make eclampsia the most likely diagnosis. To confirm this a urine protein level should be checked. The combination of a seizure in the presence of proteinuria and hypertension is classical of eclampsia.

Further history and examination

Priya's repeat blood pressure measurement is 185/120 mmHg. She has clonus and brisk reflexes on examination. No focal neurological signs are present. Dipstick urinalysis gives a ++++ result for protein.

Seizures in pregnancy: causes		
Cause of seizure	Aetiology	History or clinical features
Eclampsia	Pre-eclampsia	Severe hypertension, proteinuria
Epilepsy	Idiopathic	History of epilepsy; check adherence to antiepileptic medication
Stroke	Intracerebral bleed or infarction	Headache, visual disturbances, focal neurological signs
Space-occupying lesion	Brain tumour, abscess	Headache, visual disturbances, focal neurological signs
Infection	Encephalitis, meningitis	Symptoms and signs of sepsis (high temperature, tachycardia, hypotension) clinically unwell
Electrolyte imbalance	Hypoglycaemia, uraemia, syndrome of inappropriate antidiuretic hormone secretion (SIADH)	Diabetes (electrolyte imbalance caused by excessive use of insulin), known renal impairment
Use of recreational drugs	Effects of cocaine, methamphetamine, alcohol withdrawal	History of recreational drug use or alcohol dependency

Table 14.2 Key causes of seizures in pregnancy

Case 19 *continued*

Working diagnosis

The working diagnosis is severe pre-eclampsia complicated by eclampsia. Pre-eclampsia is new onset hypertension and proteinuria after 20 weeks of pregnancy. Eclampsia refers to the development of grand mal seizures in a woman with pre-eclampsia, in the absence of other neurological conditions that cause seizures. Epilepsy rarely presents for the first time in pregnancy and Priya has no history of hypertension or renal disease. This is a life-threatening diagnosis that requires immediate intervention to prevent recurrent seizures and other sequelae of severe hypertension such as a cerebrovascular accident.

Immediate intervention

Priya is transferred to the obstetric high-dependency unit. Because she is post-ictal (has had a seizure), maintaining a clear airway is the primary concern. Supplemental oxygen is given via face mask. Large bore intravenous access is achieved, and blood samples are taken for full blood count (for platelet count), renal function tests (for urate levels), liver function tests, clotting tests and for identification of blood group. The results of these tests will confirm or refute the diagnosis of pre-eclampsia and determine the extent of organ damage.

An intravenous infusion of magnesium sulfate is administered to prevent further seizures. Intravenous labetalol is used to stabilise Priya's blood pressure, and blood pressure is measured every 15 min to check the effectiveness of this treatment. A urinary catheter is inserted and a sample sent for quantification of urinary protein. Strict restriction of total fluid intake (80–85 mL/h) is started and hourly urine output measured.

Once Priya's condition is stable, consideration is given to fetal well-being. External fetal monitoring via cardiotocography is started. Delivery needs to be expedited, so antenatal corticosteroids are given to promote maturation of the fetal lungs (see page 143), and the neonatal team are informed.

Severe pre-eclampsia and eclampsia

Severe pre-eclampsia is a progressive disorder associated with serious and potentially fatal maternal complications. Delivery reduces the risk of these complications. Expedited delivery is always in the best interests of the mother, but extreme prematurity can have catastrophic consequences for the infant (see page 221). It is sometimes appropriate to delay delivery, if the mother's condition allows, by 24–48 h to give time for antenatal corticosteroids to be administered to help mature the fetal lungs.

Severe pre-eclampsia has one or more of the features shown in **Figure 14.3**.

HELLP syndrome is a rare variant of pre-eclampsia complicated by haemolysis, elevated liver enzymes and low platelets (see Chapter 6, page 192).

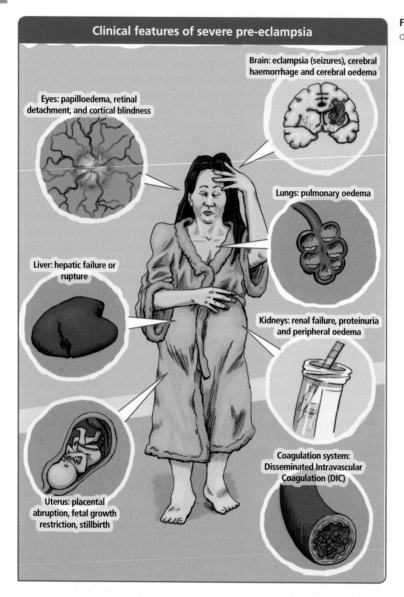

Clinical features of severe pre-eclampsia

Brain: eclampsia (seizures), cerebral haemorrhage and cerebral oedema

Eyes: papilloedema, retinal detachment, and cortical blindness

Lungs: pulmonary oedema

Liver: hepatic failure or rupture

Kidneys: renal failure, proteinuria and peripheral oedema

Uterus: placental abruption, fetal growth restriction, stillbirth

Coagulation system: Disseminated Intravascular Coagulation (DIC)

Figure 14.3 Features of severe pre-eclampsia.

Case 20 Spontaneous rupture of membranes

Presentation

Anita Nelson is 37 weeks into her fifth pregnancy. Her baby is in a breech position, and she attends the antenatal clinic to discuss mode of delivery. She has had a normal pregnancy and is keen to try a vaginal birth. As she is leaving the department, her membranes rupture spontaneously. The midwife helps her to a bed and starts external fetal monitoring and establishes that the fetal heart rate is only 60 beats/min.

Initial interpretation

Sudden fetal bradycardia after rupture of the membranes suggests cord prolapse, which is more common in multiparous

Case 20 *continued*

women with non-cephalic presentations. Anita should be examined vaginally to check for cervical dilatation accompanied by the umbilical cord below the fetal presenting part.

Further history and examination

On examination, clear liquor is draining from the vagina. The cervix is 4 cm dilated. The umbilical cord has prolapsed through the cervix and is palpable in the vagina. It is not pulsating. Pushing down on the cord from above are the fetal buttocks.

Immediate intervention

The presence of the cord below the presenting part of the fetus is diagnostic of cord prolapse. The midwife pushes the fetal buttocks up to relieve compression of the cord. She is careful to maintain elevation of the presenting part and avoid handling the cord (excessive handling causes the cord vessels to constrict and reduce blood flow to the fetus). She calls for help and a junior physician attends immediately.

The junior physician places a pillow under Anita's buttocks to help relieve the cord compression. He encourages the midwife to stay as she is while he covers Anita with a modesty sheet and pushes the bed to the operating theatre. Senior help arrives quickly, and the decision is made to proceed immediately to delivery by caesarean section.

Cord prolapse

Cord prolapse is a rare obstetric emergency that occurs when the umbilical cord descends through the open cervix before the presenting part of the fetus (**Figure 14.4**). It is suspected when there is a sudden decrease in fetal heart rate (bradycardia or decelerations) after rupture of the membranes. Cord compression compromises blood supply to the fetus, and thereby rapidly causes fetal hypoxia and death if prompt intervention is not forthcoming.

The immediate priority is to elevate the fetal presenting part to relieve compression of the cord. This can be achieved:

- digitally via vaginal examination
- by moving the patient into an all fours position with her head lower than her buttocks
- by using an indwelling catheter to fill her bladder with saline

It is essential to avoid handling the cord, because this can cause it to spasm, further restricting blood flow to the fetus. Prompt delivery via

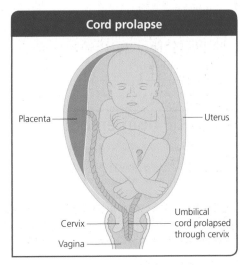

Figure 14.4 Cord prolapse. The fetus is in complete breech presentation, the placenta is on the lateral uterine wall, and the umbilical cord has prolapsed through the cervix into the vagina.

the quickest and safest route is the next step. This is usually caesarean section, unless the cervix is fully dilated and an instrumental delivery is feasible.

Case 21 Collapse and tachycardia after delivery

Presentation

Osma Omar had a vaginal delivery 30 min ago. Her partner calls for help because she has become unresponsive. On arrival, the midwife finds Osma collapsed and unresponsive on the bed. Her lips are blue and she is tachycardic, with a heart rate of 150 beats/min.

Initial interpretation

Collapse after delivery is a rare event. It is usually caused by post-partum haemorrhage, but amniotic fluid embolism must also be considered. In the absence of obvious bleeding, amniotic fluid embolism is the most likely cause.

Further history and examination

Osma has just had her fifth baby. She had a normal pregnancy and an uncomplicated delivery. Before this, she was fit and well.

She did not report chest pain or complain of breathlessness before she collapsed.

On examination, Osma has a high respiratory rate (26 breaths/min), an increased heart rate (155 beats/min) and low blood pressure (90/40 mmHg). There are no cardiovascular, respiratory or abdominal signs on examination.

Immediate intervention

Collapse following delivery in the absence of preceding symptoms or overt signs on clinical examination means that amniotic fluid embolism is the working diagnosis. The midwife pulls the emergency buzzer to summon help. Resuscitation follows the ABCD approach. Supplemental oxygen is used; large bore intravenous access is obtained; blood samples are taken for full blood count, urea and electrolytes, liver function and clotting tests; an arterial blood gas test is done to assess oxygenation levels; and a chest X-ray carried out to exclude chest pathology.

Amniotic fluid embolism

Amniotic fluid embolism occurs when amniotic fluid enters the maternal circulation and triggers a massive allergic reaction, which usually leads to cardiorespiratory failure and development of disseminated intravascular coagulopathy (**Figure 14.5**).

The clinical features of amniotic fluid embolism are consistent with those of cardiorespiratory failure: shortness of breath and hypoxia followed rapidly by maternal collapse. It is a rare event, occurring in about 1 in 20,000 births, but is responsible for around 10% of direct maternal deaths.

Management

In cases of amniotic fluid embolism, care is mostly supportive. Maternal mortality after amniotic fluid embolism is about 25%.

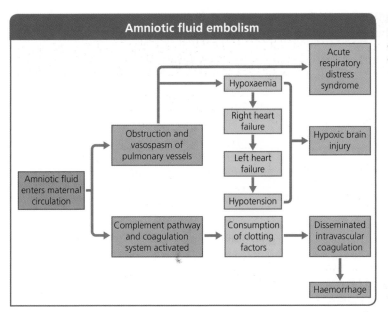

Figure 14.5
Pathophysiology of amniotic fluid embolism.

Case 22 Failure to deliver

Presentation

Maria Ramos is a 34-year-old primigravida whose labour has been induced with vaginal prostaglandins 2 weeks after her due date. After artificial rupture of her membranes and augmentation of her contractions with intravenous synthetic oxytocin (Syntocinon), she has finally reached full cervical dilation. After nearly 2 h of pushing, the head is delivered at 11:02. At 11:03, the emergency buzzer is pulled because the midwife cannot deliver the baby.

Initial interpretation

Shoulder dystocia is diagnosed when the shoulders fail to emerge shortly after the fetal head. It is an obstetric emergency, because the fetal blood supply is obstructed as a result of compression of the umbilical cord within the birth canal.

Further history and examination

Maria had a normal pregnancy. It took three prostaglandin pessaries to induce her labour, and progress was slow during both first and second stages. The fetal heart rate has been reassuring throughout. On examination, the fetal head is tight against the perineum, and firm axial traction with maternal contraction fails to deliver the baby.

Immediate intervention

Shoulder dystocia occurs when, after delivery of the fetal head, additional manoeuvres are required to deliver the fetal shoulders. Help from senior colleagues is summoned immediately. Maria's legs are hyperflexed on to her

Case 22 *continued*

chest to widen the pelvic outlet. An assistant applies suprapubic pressure to disimpact the fetal shoulder. This manoeuvre is successful, and the baby is delivered at 11:07.

The baby is floppy and makes no spontaneous respiratory effort at birth. He is towel dried and given oxygen via bag and mask. Within minutes the baby splutters and takes its first breath.

Shoulder dystocia

Shoulder dystocia is a rare event with potentially catastrophic consequences for the fetus. Shoulder dystocia is caused by impaction of the anterior fetal shoulder against the maternal symphysis pubis (**Figure 14.6**). The diagnosis is made when the fetal body fails to deliver with axial traction after delivery of the fetal head. Fetal hypoxia follows, and if delivery is not forthcoming, permanent hypoxic brain damage with severe neurodevelopmental consequences, including death, occur.

Risk factors include fetal macrosomia, instrumental delivery and maternal diabetes, but most cases of shoulder dystocia cannot be predicted. Poor management of shoulder dystocia can cause fetal brachial plexus injury as a result of injudicious pressure applied to the fetal neck.

Management

The HELPERR mnemonic is used to guide management of shoulder dystocia (**Table 14.3**). The stages involved are described below. They do not need to be carried out sequentially or in a particular order.

Help

In a hospital setting, help from an experienced midwife, obstetrician, neonatologist and paediatrician is summoned immediately.

Evaluate for an episiotomy

An episiotomy will not relieve the bony obstruction of shoulder dystocia but may be required to create more space for internal manoeuvres.

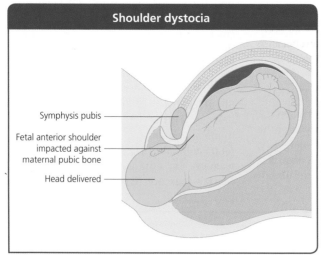

Shoulder dystocia

Symphysis pubis

Fetal anterior shoulder impacted against maternal pubic bone

Head delivered

Figure 14.6 Pathophysiology of shoulder dystocia.

Management of shoulder dystocia: HELPERR mnemonic	
Letter	Meaning
H	Call for help
E	Evaluate for episiotomy
L	Legs (the McRoberts manoeuvre)
P	Suprapubic pressure (Rubins 1)
E	Enter (internal manoeuvres)
R	Remove posterior arm
R	Rotate

Table 14.3 The HELPERR mnemonic for the management of shoulder dystocia

Legs (the McRoberts manoeuvre)

In this manoeuvre, the maternal position is changed to hyperflex the legs on to her chest. This will deliver 40% of babies in cases of shoulder dystocia. The position widens the anteroposterior diameter of the pelvic outlet.

Suprapubic pressure (Rubin's 1 manoeuvre)

Continuous pressure, applied over the posterior aspect of the anterior fetal shoulder can rotate it, thereby disimpacting it from the pelvic brim. If this manoeuvre is unsuccessful, then pulsatile pressure is tried.

Enter (internal manoeuvres)

If less invasive manoeuvres have failed, attempts are made to rotate the fetal shoulders vaginally using internal pressure, to allow them to pass under the pelvic brim.

Remove the posterior arm

Another internal manoeuvre is attempting to deliver the posterior fetal arm so that the lodged anterior arm can pass below the pelvic brim.

Rotate

Rotating the mother into an all fours position widens the anteroposterior diameter of the pelvic outlet to facilitate delivery.

Extreme cases

These have been managed successfully by breaking the fetal clavicle, or clavicles; symphysiotomy, i.e. cutting the cartilaginous connection between the maternal pubic bones; and Zavanelli's manoeuvre, in which the fetal head is pushed up into the uterus and a caesarean delivery carried out.

> **Maternity staff do not regularly encounter shoulder dystocia, so there is a risk of becoming deskilled in carrying out the appropriate manoeuvres.** To combat this, obstetric units engage in team training exercises using mannequins and skills drills, aided by the use of the mnemonic HELPERR, to ensure that staff are ready to manage real life scenarios when they arise.

Case 23 Excessive bleeding after delivery

Presentation

Judith McLennan had a normal delivery at 17:18, and the placenta was delivered at 17:28. Since then she has continued to bleed, and the midwife has estimated the blood loss so far to be 750 mL.

Initial interpretation

Excessive bleeding after delivery is post-partum haemorrhage.

The aim of examination is to identify the cause of bleeding. The main causes are uterine atony, perineal trauma, retained placental tissue and coagulation disorders (**Table 14.4**).

A definition of post-partum haemorrhage based on the volume of blood lost is problematic in clinical practice, because obstetricians and midwives usually underestimate this. A practical definition is excessive bleeding that makes the patient symptomatic, results in signs of hypovolaemia, or both.

Immediate intervention

Help is sought immediately. Resuscitation follows the ABCD approach, with supplemental oxygen delivered via face mask,

Management of post-partum haemorrhage

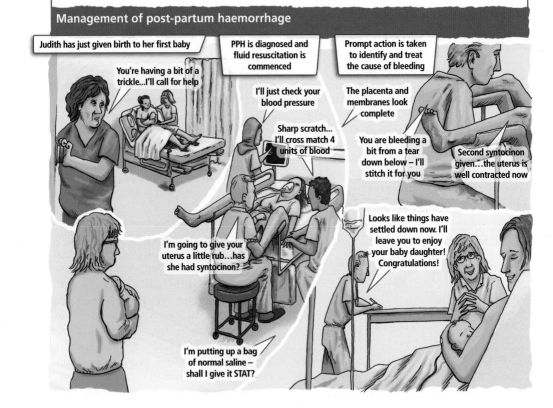

Judith has just given birth to her first baby

You're having a bit of a trickle...I'll call for help

PPH is diagnosed and fluid resuscitation is commenced

I'll just check your blood pressure

Sharp scratch... I'll cross match 4 units of blood

I'm going to give your uterus a little rub...has she had syntocinon?

I'm putting up a bag of normal saline – shall I give it STAT?

Prompt action is taken to identify and treat the cause of bleeding

The placenta and membranes look complete

You are bleeding a bit from a tear down below – I'll stitch it for you

Second syntocinon given...the uterus is well contracted now

Looks like things have settled down now. I'll leave you to enjoy your baby daughter! Congratulations!

		Post-partum haemorrhage: the four T's	
T	Cause of bleeding	Examination findings	Management
Tone	Uterine atony	The uterus fails to contract, and feels soft and floppy	'Rub up' a uterine contraction; give oxytocic drugs (e.g. synthetic oxytocin, Syntocinon; oxytocin–ergometrine, Syntometrine; or misoprostol)
Trauma	Lower genital tract trauma	Perineal, vaginal or cervical tears	Repair under local or regional anaesthesia
Tissue	Retained placental tissue	The placenta and membranes appear incomplete	Evacuate the contents of the uterus, usually in theatre under anaesthetic
Thrombin	Clotting problem	Non specific. A diagnosis of exclusion	Give blood products (e.g. fresh frozen plasma)

Table 14.4 The four T's of post-partum haemorrhage

large bore intravenous access is achieved and blood samples taken for full blood count, coagulation tests and crossmatch for 4 units of blood. Intravenous crystalloids are given to treat hypovolaemia while blood products are awaited.

Abdominal palpation to 'rub up' a uterine contraction is carried out while the placenta and membranes are checked for completeness and the perineum, vagina and cervix are inspected for lacerations. 'Rubbing up a contraction' is uterine massage either abdominally or bimanually, with one hand placed in the vagina. This stimulates myometrial contraction and reduces bleeding caused by uterine atony. The underlying cause of the bleeding is treated promptly while appropriate resuscitation with fluids and blood products is administered to prevent maternal deterioration as a result of hypovolaemic shock.

Post-partum haemorrhage

Post-partum haemorrhage is defined as blood loss of > 500 mL after delivery.

- If this occurs in the first 24 h after childbirth, this is is primary post-partum haemorrhage
- Bleeding more than 24 h after childbirth is secondary post-partum haemorrhage

Post-partum haemorrhage causes hypovolaemic shock, which is characterised by tachycardia, tachypnoea and hypotension. In severe cases, disseminated intravascular coagulation develops.

Management

The aim of management is to promptly treat the underlying cause while administering adequate resuscitation with fluids and blood products. Uterine atony contributes to 70% of cases of post-partum haemorrhage, so 'rubbing up' a uterine contraction or carrying out bimanual uterine compression is recommended while other causes are ruled out; the latter procedure is shown in **Figure 14.7**. Drugs that cause the uterus to contract, including synthetic oxytocin (Syntocinon), oxytocin-ergometrine (Syntometrine) and misoprostol, can also be given.

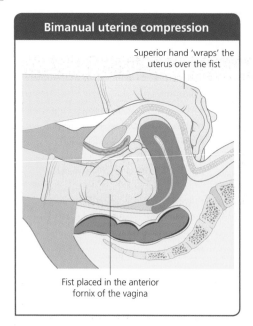

Bimanual uterine compression

Superior hand 'wraps' the uterus over the fist

Fist placed in the anterior fornix of the vagina

Figure 14.7 In bimanual uterine compression, the uterus is compressed between the upper hand on the abdomen, pushing down on the fundus, and the lower hand in the vagina.

Trauma is repaired. Retained tissue is removed, often in the operating theatre under regional or general anesthesia. If simple measures fail to stop the bleeding, urgent review by senior colleagues is required.

A haemostatic balloon (i.e. a Bakri balloon) in the uterine cavity has a tamponade effect, as does a uterine compression suture (i.e. a B Lynch suture). If bleeding persists despite all interventions, a hysterectomy is carried out.

Case 24 Vaginal bulge and heavy bleeding after delivery

Presentation

Elena Bianchi gave birth 5 min ago. While carrying out controlled cord traction, the midwife noticed a smooth bulge developing at the vaginal opening (introitus). Elena is bleeding heavily and has now become unresponsive.

Initial interpretation

The development of the vaginal bulge during cord traction suggests uterine inversion. Elena should be examined abdominally, where absence of a normally positioned uterine fundus is the key finding, and vaginally, where the presence of a smooth, round mass protruding from the cervix or vagina is diagnostic.

Further history and examination

Examination finds Elena to be tachycardic and hypotensive. At the introitus is an expanding mass and heavy ongoing bleeding. The placenta is still attached. Abdominal examination fails to find the uterine fundus above the pelvic brim.

Working diagnosis

An adherent placenta, a non palpable uterine fundus per abdomen and a smooth round vaginal mass is the classic presentation of uterine inversion (**Figure 14.8**). The bulge developing at the introitus is the uterus, inside out.

Case 24 *continued*

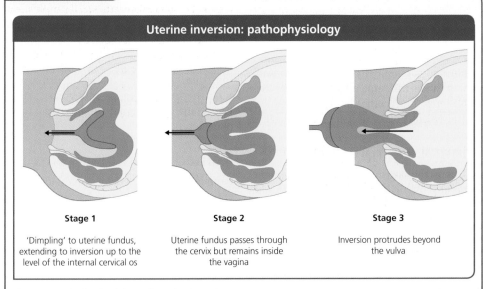

Uterine inversion: pathophysiology

Stage 1	Stage 2	Stage 3
'Dimpling' to uterine fundus, extending to inversion up to the level of the internal cervical os	Uterine fundus passes through the cervix but remains inside the vagina	Inversion protrudes beyond the vulva

Figure 14.8 Pathophysiology of uterine inversion

In most UK delivery suites there is an emergency buzzer in each room that sounds an alarm in the corridor and main delivery suite office. It triggers immediate response from all nearby staff members, including health support workers, midwifery and medical staff.

Immediate intervention

The midwife presses the emergency buzzer, and several members of staff arrive quickly. Resuscitation follows the ABCD approach, with supplemental oxygen given via face mask, venous access secured and intravenous crystalloid fluids administered. The senior obstetrician successfully replaces the uterus manually by pushing the uterine fundus along the long axis of the vagina towards the umbilicus. Elena is transferred to the operating theatre for careful manual removal of the placenta under anaesthesia.

Uterine inversion

Uterine inversion is the failure of the placenta to detach from the fundus, and the subsequent displacement of the uterine fundus to the level of the cervix, in incomplete inversion, or through the cervix, in complete inversion (see **Figure 14.7**).

This complication is more common when the placenta is in an abnormal location, for example in cases of placenta praevia or fundal placentation, and when vigorous attempts have been made to remove the placenta before it has separated from the uterine wall.

Uterine inversion is a rare but potentially life-threatening complication with an incidence of 1 in 2000–6500 deliveries. Immediate replacement of the uterus is recommended, because a uterine constriction ring (tight band of contracted myometrium) develops quickly and the prolapsed uterus becomes swollen and oedematous as a result, making replacement more challenging.

Case 25 Fever 2 days after delivery

Presentation

Lydia O'Reilly had her second uncomplicated vaginal delivery 2 days ago and went home the same day. She attends the obstetric unit with a high temperature and a history of feeling generally unwell.

Initial interpretation

This is the classic presentation of puerperal sepsis. History and examination is targeted towards identifying the source of sepsis, i.e. the presence of a cough, urinary symptoms and close contact with poorly family members.

Further history and examination

Lydia's eldest child has been unwell with a sore throat for the past week. Lydia is pale. Examination finds her heart and respiratory rates to be increased, and she has a temperature of 38.7°C.

Working diagnosis

The history and high temperature alongside a history of upper respiratory tract infection suggest a group A streptococcal infection. Other causes of upper respiratory tract infection, and sepsis originating from other sites, including urinary tract, perineum, uterus and breast are important differential diagnoses to consider.

Immediate intervention

Samples are obtained for microbiological testing from every possible site: swab samples from wounds, urine samples and blood culture samples. Early recourse to aggressive antibiotic therapy is required. Blood is sent for:

- full blood count and measurement of C-reactive protein concentration to monitor disease progression
- lactate concentration to determine the extent of compromise
- urea and electrolytes to check that renal function is normal

The choice of antibiotic depends on the working diagnosis. The selected antibiotic is usually given intravenously for the first 24 h.

Puerperal sepsis

Puerperal sepsis is systemic infection within the first 6 weeks after birth. Signs and symptoms vary with the source of sepsis. Endometritis, usually related to retained placental tissue, typically presents with lower abdominal pain and increased vaginal bleeding. Other sources of sepsis include:

- mastitis or breast abscess
- wound infection
- urinary tract infection
- pneumonia
- pharyngitis or group A *Streptococcus*
- gastroenteritis
- pyelonephritis
- endometritis or retained products (placental tissue)
- endocarditis

Over the past 10 years, the number of deaths related to group A streptococcal infection has increased.

Management

Severe sepsis mandates the immediate use of intravenous antibiotics alongside supplemental oxygen, fluid resuscitation, and appropriate monitoring of vital signs, urine output and the results of blood tests, including arterial blood gases to assess oxygenation and lactate concentration. In cases of suspected necrotising fasciitis, early surgical opinion is urgently required. If heart rate, respiratory rate, blood pressure, oxygenation levels and temperature indicate a worsening clinical picture, appropriate and early involvement of the critical care team is required. Ventilatory support, hemodialysis, and inotropes (drugs given to improve blood pressure) are necessary in some cases of severe life-threatening sepsis complicated by multiorgan failure.

Puerperal sepsis accounts for about 10 maternal deaths every year in countries like the UK. Previously healthy women can compensate for the physiological stress caused by sepsis for a long time before they finally succumb, so early warning signs must be heeded. The aim of management is to identify the source of infection and treat it aggressively with intravenous antibiotics, with the first dose given as soon as practicably possible and review after 24 hours to ensure that the patient is improving.

Chapter 15
Integrated care

Starter questions

Answers to the following questions are on page 387.

1. For how long after a sexual assault is DNA evidence retrievable?
2. Why isn't cervical screening performed during pregnancy?
3. What is the difference between audit and research?

Introduction

For care to be integrated, it must be co-ordinated and tailored to the needs and preferences of the individual. Good communication between primary care (community services, e.g. GPs, practice nurses, midwives) and secondary care (specialists based in hospitals, e.g. consultant obstetricians and gynaecologists) is vital (**Table 15.1** and **Figure 15.1**). The majority of patients in obstetrics and gynaecology are looked after in primary care, with referral to specialist services reserved for those at risk of complications, with worrying symptoms or where first line treatment has failed. Within secondary care,

patients are managed within multidisciplinary teams.

Integrated care in obstetrics and gynaecology looks after women 'from cradle to grave' and is frequently concerned with caring for healthy individuals. It becomes even more important, therefore, for clinicians to promote screening and good sexual health and be able to signpost services for women experiencing abuse as they may be the only health professionals they see.

This chapter covers the general principles of integrated care, but where specifics are unavoidable it refers to UK service structures.

Healthcare professionals and their roles

Area of care	Type	Role
Primary	General practitioner (GP)	First point of call for patient, initiate investigations and first line treatment, refer patients into secondary care as appropriate
	Health visitor	Work with families to promote child health
	Midwife	Look after pregnant woman and her baby before, during and after birth
	Practice nurse	Assess, screen and treat patients, with particular focus on cervical screening, contraception provision and reproductive health
Secondary care	Consultant obstetrician and gynaecologist	Provide specialist investigation and treatment, including management of complex health problems, complicated deliveries and surgical procedures
	Gynaecology clinical nurse specialist (CNS)	Patient advocate, provides holistic and flexible patient support
	Social worker	Supporting vulnerable individuals and families, including children, to live well
	Physiotherapist	Education and treatment of musculoskeletal and genitourinary problems

Table 15.1 Types of healthcare professionals and their roles within obstetrics and gynaecology

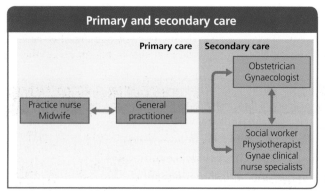

Figure 15.1 The structure of primary and secondary care.

Case 26 Late booking and abdominal bruising

Presentation

Amira attends her first midwife appointment at 22 weeks' gestation. She is accompanied by her husband, Samir, who answers all the questions on Amira's behalf. He explains that they moved to the UK from Egypt 6 months ago, and that his wife does not understand or speak English. Amira seems quiet and avoids eye contact with the midwife.

Initial interpretation

Amira is a late booker, because she is being seen for the first time after 14 weeks' gestation. This puts her at higher risk for maternal and fetal complications during the pregnancy, including maternal death. Her recent immigration status and the language barrier mean that her midwife needs to provide extra support to identify and manage any difficulties Amira is facing.

Case 26 *continued*

Further history

Samir tells the midwife that his wife is 19 years old and that this is her second pregnancy; they already have a 9-month-old son. She had a normal delivery last time and has no medical problems. They are living with relatives but are hoping to get their own home soon.

The midwife asks Amira for a urine sample and shows her to the toilet. It is essential that at the first booking visit every woman has a one-to-one conversation with their midwife about domestic abuse. When she is alone with Amira, the midwife locates a telephone interpreter and asks whether Amira is afraid of her husband and if he has ever hurt her. The midwife explains that all pregnant women are asked these questions, because abuse is common. Amira admits that Samir does not like her

leaving the house or talking to others. She also discloses that since she became pregnant again, he has started to hit her and punch her in the abdomen. She says that he has never hit their son.

> **Do not use family or friends to interpret when asking someone about potential domestic abuse.** Doing so breaches confidentiality and could put the woman at increased risk of violence. An independent interpreter, preferably with training in domestic abuse, is used instead.

Examination

Amira is thin and pale. She appears anxious. Her abdomen is distended, consistent with the reported number of weeks' gestation. She shows her midwife the

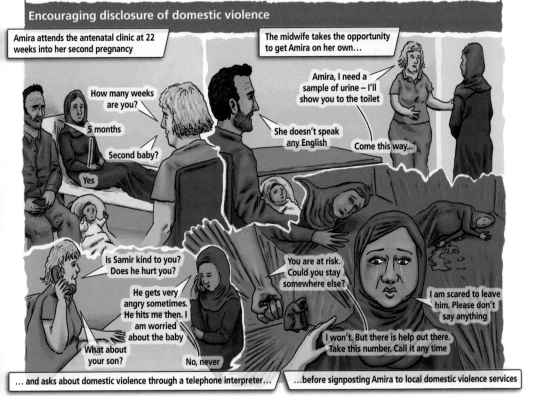

Encouraging disclosure of domestic violence

... and asks about domestic violence through a telephone interpreter... before signposting Amira to local domestic violence services

Case 26 *continued*

bruises on her abdomen, which are concealed by her clothing. No other physical injuries are found.

Interpretation of findings

Amira is describing domestic abuse, which has worsened since she became pregnant. Although her son is not being hurt physically, he is likely to be aware of or even witness the violence, with negative effects on his long-term emotional health. The unborn child is at risk of miscarriage, preterm birth and abruption from the attacks on Amira's abdomen, and infrequent attendance of antenatal visits means that opportunities to identify abnormalities of fetal growth and well-being are lost.

Investigations

Amira's midwife encourages her to talk about what is happening to her at home, reassuring her that she will not share this information with her husband or document it in her handheld notes.

An ultrasound scan is carried out to date Amira's pregnancy and to look for any fetal anomalies.

Blood and urine screening tests are done as per routine antenatal care at booking, and Amira's blood pressure is checked.

Diagnosis

Amira is asked whether she has considered leaving her husband and if she wants the police to be involved, because domestic violence is a criminal offence. The immediate safety of her and her son are discussed. Amira does not want the police to be contacted and wishes to return home, feeling able to do so with information about local domestic violence services. There is no perceived imminent threat of physical abuse so Amira's midwife is not legally required to report the domestic abuse to the police.

Amira is made aware via the interpreter that her midwife will discuss her disclosure with her supervisor and the safeguarding teams, and that social services will be notified to plan care for her and her children. Amira promises to try to attend antenatal clinic appointments, and she is given her midwife's telephone number in case of any problems with the pregnancy or further episodes of violence.

Domestic abuse and child protection

Domestic abuse is 'any incident of threatening behaviour, violence or abuse (psychological, physical, sexual, financial or emotional) between adults who are or have been intimate partners or family members, regardless of gender and sexuality'.

Domestic abuse is not pro-actively disclosed by the majority of victims. It is suspected on the basis of unexplained injuries, repeated attendances at general practitioners or hospital accident and emergency departments or failure to engage with medical and social services. Victims present to both primary and secondary care so all healthcare professionals need to be aware of domestic abuse and their responsibilities towards victims.

Epidemiology

Domestic abuse is common. One in four women in England and Wales experience domestic abuse in their lifetime, and 30% of cases begin or worsen when the woman is pregnant.

Risk factors

Risk factors include low income, young age (<25 years), mental health problems and alcohol and drug misuse, but domestic abuse can affect anyone. Domestic abuse is no more common in particular ethnic groups, but the types of abuse vary between communities, and religious and cultural differences, concerns about immigration status and language barriers reduce rates of disclosure. For example, women with insecure immigration status are warned by their abusers not to report domestic abuse for fear of deportation and are less likely to be aware of available services, such as domestic violence charities and women's refuges. In some communities, women face rejection and dishonour if they leave their husband, even because of domestic abuse.

Diagnostic approach

All women are asked routinely about domestic abuse. In the UK this is done at least three times during pregnancy: at the booking visit, in the second trimester and after the birth. This is done privately and with the expectation that they will be listened to and not judged by health care professionals.

> **Listen when someone discloses domestic abuse to you, and be supportive, non-judgemental and respectful.** It is extremely difficult for women to discuss domestic abuse. Your reaction to a woman's disclosure can increase her confidence or undermine it further.

Clinical features

Signs of abuse include:

- frequent visits with vague symptoms or regular non-attendance of appointments
- non-accidental injuries, including injuries to the genital tract
- poor past obstetric history, for example multiple miscarriages, stillbirth or growth restriction
- anxiety, panic attacks and self-harm
- presence of the woman's partner at every appointment, answering questions for her, or undermining or mocking her

- appearing frightened or evasive in the presence of a partner

The pregnant abdomen is commonly targeted during violent attacks, putting the fetus at risk of miscarriage, preterm birth and brain injury.

Other children in the household are also vulnerable; 50% of children whose mothers suffer will also be physically abused, and most will suffer long-term emotional problems as a result of being exposed to violence between their parents or between their mother and her partner.

Management

If domestic abuse is disclosed, the first concern is the safety of the woman and any children who are at risk.

- If there is an imminent threat of physical abuse, healthcare professionals should contact the police to ensure that the woman and her children are escorted to a place of safety. In the UK, this is a legal requirement. The police are contacted even if the woman does not want them to be involved.
- Lower levels of risk are managed by alerting women to local or national domestic abuse services like Women's Aid, a UK charity that offers help to women who experience domestic abuse

Independent domestic violence advisers are employed by health services, charities and local authorities and address the safety needs of women at high risk of harm. They create individualised plans to promote the safety of women and their children, which can include changing phone numbers and routes taken to children's schools, what to do if the abuser tries to enter the house and also provide mental health support and counselling. They participate in regular multiagency risk assessment conferences, at which information is shared between relevant organisations (e.g. housing associations, community mental health team, benefits agencies) so that these individualised support plans can be agreed and implemented jointly.

A referral is also made to the local children's safeguarding team, who liaise with social services and help plan care for children at risk. The mother's consent is not required for the team to be contacted, but it is good practice to inform her of the referral.

> **Confidentiality is not absolute in cases of domestic abuse, because others are likely to be at risk.** Women are reassured that their partner will not be informed of their disclosure of abuse and that no documentation will be placed in their handheld notes in case he looks through them. However, it is explained to them that information needs to be shared across agencies in cases in which the safety of others, particularly children, is compromised.

Victims of domestic abuse have many reasons for not wanting to leave their partner, including fear of retaliation, separation from their children, lack of money and having no place to go. The health care professional's role is not to encourage them to leave but to support them in finding ways to ensure their personal safety and the safety of other family members.

Female genital mutilation

Female genital mutilation (FGM) is any procedure in which the female external genitalia are partly or totally removed, or that causes any other injury to the female genital organs for non-medical reasons. It is divided into four types (**Figure 15.2** and **Table 15.2**). Type 4 FGM comprises all other non-medical procedures carried out on the female genitalia, including piercing, incising, stretching and cauterising.

The first time women with FGM present to health services is usually in pregnancy. All midwives should directly ask women from high-risk ethnic groups whether they have undergone FGM; UK midwives are legally required to do this. Women who have undergone FGM are referred to a designated obstetric consultant or midwife for individualised management.

Diagnosing FGM outside of pregnancy is unusual, unless a woman presents for cervical screening or with symptoms of obstructed urination and menstruation.

Epidemiology

Female genital mutilation is an international problem. It is most prevalent in north-eastern Africa, including Somalia, Sudan and Ethiopia. It is also practiced in migrant communities with cultural links to these areas.

The procedure is carried out on young girls, usually before the age of 5 years. In most cases it is done without anaesthesia and by untrained persons or family members using non-sterilised instruments.

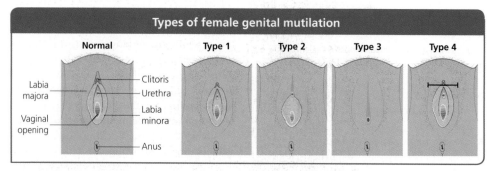

Figure 15.2 Types of genital mutilation

Female genital mutilation: types	
Type	Description
1a	Removal of clitoral prepuce only
1b	Removal of clitoral prepuce
	Partial or total removal of clitoris
2	Clitoris removed
	Partial or total removal of labia minora
3	Partial or total removal of labia minora
	Labia majora sewn together to cover the urethra and vagina, with only a small hole remaining for the passage of urine and menstrual blood
4	All other harmful non-medical procedures on the female genitalia, including tattoos and piercings

Table 15.2 Types of female genital mutilation

Complications

The short- and long-term complications of FGM are listed in **Table 15.3**.

It may be difficult for women who have undergone FGM to talk about its effects. They may be more at ease speaking with a female health care professional, or one from their own community. They may be unfamiliar with the terms 'female genital mutilation' and 'FGM', so it may be more helpful to use the words 'cut', 'closed' and 'open'. A trained interpreter is required if there is a language barrier.

Legality

FGM is illegal in a large number of countries including most of the countries where it is commonly practiced (e.g. Eritrea and Sudan). UK law is particularly exacting: FGM is illegal under the Female Genital Mutilation Act 2003 and the Female Genital Mutilation (Scotland) Act 2005. Under these Acts is also illegal to arrange or assist in arranging for a UK national or resident to be taken overseas to have the procedure carried out in another country. Furthermore, in the event of confirmation of FGM by examination or receiving a report of the procedure being carried out on a child (< 18 years old), they make it mandatory to record the presence of FGM in the clinical notes and to report this to the police within 1 month.

Female genital cosmetic surgery, for example labioplasty, is exempt from the UK's 2003 and 2005 Acts only if it is done to safeguard the woman's physical or mental well-being, and only if she is over 18 years old. Whilst performing genital piercings is illegal under the Act, there have been no prosecutions made and it is unlikely that women who have had the procedure performed voluntarily will be forced to remove their piercings.

Female genital mutilation: complications	
Short-term complications	Long-term complications
Haemorrhage	Genital scarring, causing pain, inclusion cysts (cyst resulting from implanation of epidermal elements into the dermis) and neuromas (a mass of nerve tissue)
Urinary retention	
Infection	Poor urinary flow, recurrent urinary tract infections, urinary obstruction, fistula
Swelling	Dyspareunia and impaired sexual function as a consequence of loss of the clitoris
Death	Psychological effects: flashbacks, anxiety, post-traumatic stress disorder
	Haematocolpos (accumulation of menstrual blood in the vagina) and dysmenorrhoea
	Genital infections, including bacterial vaginosis and genital herpes infection
	Infertility as a result of dyspareunia and associated decreased frequency or absence of sexual intercourse, pelvic infection and possibly primary infertility
	HIV and hepatitis B as a result of transmission via dirty equipment
	Adverse obstetric outcome: prolonged labour, post-partum haemorrhage, emergency caesarean section, perineal trauma, fear of childbirth

Table 15.3 Short- and long-term complications of female genital mutilation

A woman may be at risk of harm if her family become aware that she has disclosed information about FGM. If she wishes to be accompanied by someone she trusts, ensure that they understand the need for confidentiality.

Deinfibulation may need to be done quickly intrapartum, without prior assessment, especially if the baby shows signs of distress. It may not have been possible to carry out antenatal deinfibulation or plan the delivery. This is because women with FGM may not attend antenatal appointments, because of worries about how they may be treated because of it, and some have cultural reasons for being reluctant to undergo deinfibulation until the start of labour.

Management

In pregnancy

Women with FGM who become pregnant are referred by their midwives to a designated consultant or midwife for an individualised plan of care. This consists of:

- psychological assessment
- screening for hepatitis C in addition to routine antenatal tests
- assessment of the risk to the unborn child of also having FGM carried out
- a plan for delivery, which may include deinfibulation, a surgical procedure to open the vagina, done either antenatally or intrapartum

Reinfibulation, i.e. restitching of the vagina, is illegal in the UK.

In the UK, all baby girls born to women with FGM are referred to the safeguarding midwife so that the general practitioner (GP) and health visitor can be informed.

Outside of pregnancy

Women with FGM can self-refer or are referred by their general practitioner to a consultant gynaecologist with responsibility for looking after women and young girls with FGM. All recent cases are legally required to be reported to the police and social services to ensure safeguarding procedures are put in place to protect vulnerable individuals. As in pregnancy, psychological assessment and treatment and screening for HIV, hepatitis B and C and sexual health screening is offered. De-infibulation is performed if there is obstruction to normal urination and mictruition or the narrowed introitus prevents comfortable intercourse, vaginal examination or safe delivery. Referrals to infertility services are also made if necessary.

Forensic gynaecology

Forensic gynaecology concerns the care and management of girls and women who have been sexually assaulted.

The UK's Sexual Offences Act 2003 gives the definition that a male commits rape if he 'intentionally penetrates the vagina, mouth or anus of another person with his penis, in the absence of consent or reasonable belief that the person consents'. Assault by penetration is the intentional penetration with a body part, for example a finger, or an object of the vagina or anus of another person without their consent.

A person under the age of 13 years is unable to consent to sexual activity, so any type of sexual intercourse with a young child is considered rape. Assault by penetration and sexual assault are also non-consensual offences against children in this age group.

Epidemiology

More than 400,000 women are sexually assaulted annually in England and Wales. However, only 13% of sexual assaults are reported to the police.

Investigations and management

Severe physical injuries are managed by acute medical or trauma teams in hospitals. Once it is medically safe to do so, patients are transferred to a specialist sexual assault referral centre.

Swabs are used to collect samples from all applicable areas for DNA testing before wounds are cleaned and dressed. A chain-of-evidence form is used to provide accountability in the transportation of samples; properly completed chain-of-evidence forms and body diagrams increase the likelihood of achieving a successful prosecution. Injuries are documented by clear descriptions on body diagrams.

Urine and blood samples are taken for toxicology screens, including tests for alcohol and flunitrazepam (Rohypnol, a benzodiazepine sometimes used in drug-facilitated sexual assualt to cause amnesia). Forensic time frames (persistence of DNA) for different types of assault are shown in **Table 15.4**.

The risk of pregnancy is assessed and emergency contraception provided, if necessary.

Post-exposure prophylaxis is given to women at high risk of HIV infection, and hepatitis B vaccination is given immediately for all victims. Screening for other sexually transmitted infections is carried out 10–14 days after the

Forensic timeframes for sexual assault	
Type of assault	Forensic timeframe (persistence of DNA)
Penile penetration	
■ Oral	48 h
■ Vaginal	7 days
■ Anal	3 days
Digital (any orifice)	12 h
Skin swabs	2 days (up to 7 days if area not washed)

Table 15.4 Forensic timeframes (persistence of DNA) for different types of sexual assault

assault, allowing for the incubation period for these infections.

Emotional support is offered to all women. Emergency psychiatric referral is warranted for those identified as being at high risk of self-harm because of underlying mental health problems.

A forensic gynaecologist is required to attend court to present evidence for the prosecution.

Cervical screening and management of cervical intraepithelial neoplasia

Persistent human papillomavirus (HPV) infection causes cervical cancer. It leads to the development of precancerous cervical intraepithelial neoplasia and, over 10–20 years, to cervical cancer in a small proportion of untreated women. Cervical screening prevents 75% of cervical cancers by enabling early diagnosis and treatment of asymptomatic cervical intraepithelial neoplasia.

As an additional preventive measure, girls are offered vaccination against HPV to reduce the risk of becoming infected by the two strains that most commonly cause cervical cancer and two strains that commonly cause genital warts. HPV vaccination is discussed in more detail on pages 327–328.

Vaccinated women still need to attend for cervical screening when invited. They remain vulnerable to infections with types of HPV not covered by the vaccine, and long-term immunity has yet to be demonstrated. Furthermore, if they have beome infected with HPV prior to vaccination, the vaccine does not provide any protection.

Cervical screening

Cervical screening is carried out in general practice or hospital colposcopy departments. In England, Scotland and Wales, tests are offered to:

- women aged 25–49 years every 3 years
- women aged 50–64 years every 5 years

Cervical screening requires a sample of cells to be taken from the cervix; this is done by a cervical broom (cervical cytology sampling device). The cells are then examined in a laboratory using liquid-based cytology and a high-risk HPV test is carried out, if required. The results determine whether or not further investigation is required (**Figure 15.3**).

In 2012, 79% of eligible women in the UK had attended a cervical screening appointment within the previous 5 years; 5% of women had an abnormal result and < 1% of these had cervical cancer.

> **Cervical cytology is unnecessary for women in whom cervical cancer is suspected; these patients are referred directly to colposcopy.** Cervical screening is for detection of asymptomatic lesions only. It is of no value if the woman has an obvious cervical cancer.

Cervical screening is not offered to women under 25 years of age, because cervical cancer is rare in this group and the risks of harm from screening, such as psychological distress associated with abnormal results, unnecessary additional tests and risk of miscarriage or preterm labour if excisional treatments are performed, outweigh any benefits. Short-term HPV infections are common but usually resolve without treatment.

Older women who have had three tests with a negative result within the cervical screening programme are unlikely to develop new abnormalities over the age of 65 years.

Cervical cytology

Figure 15.4 shows the equipment used for obtaining a cervical cytology sample. A primary care nurse or doctor uses a cervical broom to obtain a sample of cells from the cervix. The tip of the broom is gently inserted into the external cervical os and rotated by 360° five times. The broom remains in contact with the cervix whilst it is rotated, so that the entire transformation zone is sampled. The transformation zone is a dynamic area of the cervix where columnar epithelium has or is being replaced by squamous epithelium. It

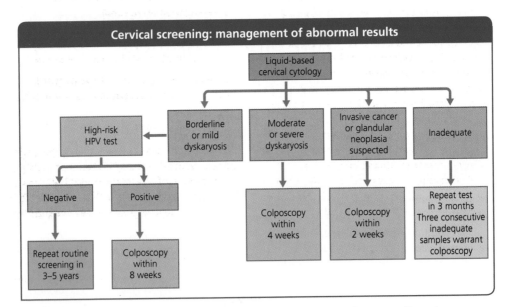

Figure 15.3 Cervical screening: management of abnormal test results. HPV, human papillomavirus.

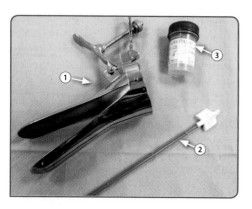

Figure 15.4 ① Cusco speculum, ② cervical broom and ③ vial containing fixative for liquid-based cervical cytology.

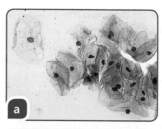

Figure 15.5 Liquid-based cytology results. (a) Normal cervical cytology. (b) Severe dyskaryosis.

changes location depending upon a woman's hormonal status and is the area in which cervical intraepithelial neoplasia develops.

The head of the broom is placed in a vial of preservative fluid and detached from the handle. This is then sent to be tested using liquid-based cytology.

Liquid-based cytology

The cervical cytology sample is examined under a microscope by a cytologist, who looks for signs of dyskaryosis. This may indicate the presence of cervical intraepithelial neoplasia, and the features observed include a range of nuclear abnormalities in which the chromatin pattern is abnormal (either coarse and clumped or pale and speckled) and the nuclear:cytoplasmic ratio is increased (i.e. the nucleus is proportionally larger than in a normal cell). See **Figure 15.5** for a comparison of normal and abnormal cytology.

Dyskaryosis is classified as mild, moderate or severe. Minor cytological abnormalities include mild dyskaryosis and borderline

nuclear change, in which the nuclei are abnormal but do not amount to dyskaryosis. The degree of dyskaryosis determines subsequent management (**Figure 15.3**).

Patients with a negative test result are invited to re-attend for screening in 3–5 years time, depending on their age.

- Patients with borderline change or mild dyskaryosis are referred for a high-risk HPV test to determine if further investigation is required
- Patients with moderate or severe dyskaryosis or with invasive cancer are referred for investigation by colposcopy

The results of liquid-based cytology investigation are usually available within 2 weeks.

High-risk HPV test

High-risk HPV tests involve the use of polymerase chain reaction (PCR) tests to identify the presence of the commonest HPV types that cause cervical cancer. They are required for all samples with borderline change or mild dyskaryosis to determine whether colposcopy referral is required. They are carried out by virologists on the cervical cytology sample currently being stored in the hospital laboratory.

Women who have a negative result from the high-risk HPV test have a repeat cervical screening test in 3–5 years, depending on their age, because they are extremely unlikely to develop cervical cancer in the meantime. Women who test positive for high-risk HPV are referred directly to colposcopy for further assessment.

An inadequate cervical cytology result is one which has not sampled the transformation zone. Patients with an inadequate result are retested within 3 months and referred for colposcopy if the inadequate result is repeated three times in a row. Referral to colposcopy can be made directly by the laboratory staff, without consulting the patient's GP.

> **Human papillomavirus primary screening is being trialled in England.** Under this new scheme, the high-risk HPV test is carried out first. A positive test result warrants referral for liquid-based cytology. The benefit of this system is that high-risk HPV testing detects more abnormalities than liquid-based cytology, so in future women with a negative HPV test result only need to be screened every 5–6 years, rather than every 3–5 years as at present.

Colposcopy

In colposcopy a specialised microscope (colposcope) is used to examine the cervix in detail. It is carried out in secondary care by specially trained nurses and doctors.

Colposcopy enables identification of areas of cervical intraepithelial neoplasia (CIN). Areas of CIN are identified with a 3–5% acetic acid solution and an iodine solution. CIN stains white with acetic acid due to the high nuclear protein content of the abnormal cells. It does not stain with iodine because the cells have a low glycogen content. The presence of CIN 3 or invasive disease is indicated by the presence of mosaics (cobblestone patterns) and punctation (dots) within areas of dense aceto-white staining; they are caused by capillaries becoming visible in abnormal epithelium on the surface of the cervix.

Figure 15.6 shows normal and abnormal results obtained by colposcopy.

Management of CIN

The approach depends on the amount of abnormal tissue that needs to be removed and the severity of tissue abnormalities. Cervical intraepithelial neoplasia is classified in order of increasing severity as CIN 1, 2 and 3 (**Figure 15.7**). Subsequent management is based on these classifications (**Table 15.5**).

Large loop excision of the transformation zone

The most common treatment of cervical intraepithelial neoplasia is large loop excision of the transformation zone (LLETZ). This is the removal of abnormal cells from the cervix, and is done at the same time as colposcopy. The procedure takes less than 5 minutes and is done preferably under local anaesthetic.

> **To reduce the risk of infection, women are advised to avoid sexual intercourse, the use of tampons and swimming for 4 weeks after treatment by LLETZ.** Heavy or offensive-smelling bleeding indicates infection, so antibiotic treatment is required.

Cone biopsy

This procedure is similar to a LLETZ. However, a cone biopsy involves removing a larger, cone shaped piece of tissue from the cervix with a knife or electric wire and the patient requires general rather than local anaesthesia. Compared with LLETZ, cone biopsy is used for large areas of CIN 3 and invasive cancers.

Cold coagulation

This is traditionally used for CIN 1, but recent years have seen a return in the popularity of cold coagulation for treatment of all severities of CIN, because LLETZ and cone biopsy are associated with obstetric sequelae. In cold coagulation, the abnormal cells are

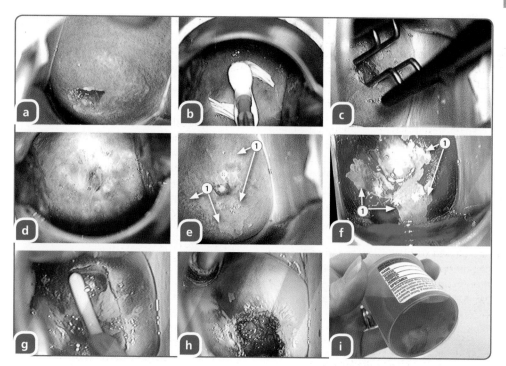

Figure 15.6 Colposcopic appearance of (a) a normal cervix; (b) a cervical broom sampling the transformation zone (TZ) for cervical cytology screening (smear test); and (c) the squamocolumnar junction (SCJ) within the endocervical canal, exposed with kogan forceps; (d) high grade CIN prior to application of acetic acid; (e) high grade CIN shown as a well-demarcated acetowhite area following application of acetic acid ①; (f) the same areas ① also fail to take up the brown iodine stain (Schiller's test negative); (g) large loop excision of the transformation zone (LLETZ); (h) post-treatment cervix showing area removed following diathermy for haemostasis; and (i) specimen removed for histopathological examination.

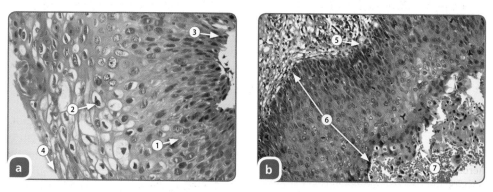

Figure 15.7 Histological appearance of (a) low grade cervical intraepithelial neoplasia (CIN 1) and (b) high grade CIN (CIN 2-3). There is increased mitotic activity in CIN and atypical mitotic figures are seen. (a) In CIN 1, atypical nuclei are most prominent in the basal third ①. Cytoplasmic maturation is present in the upper two-thirds of the epithelium, where koilocytosis ② is also visible. ③ Basement membrane. ④ Epithelial surface. (b) In CIN 2-3, nuclear atypia extends through the full epithelial thickness and is more marked than in CIN1 ⑥. Cytoplasmic maturation is only present in the upper third of the epithelium (CIN 2), or is not seen at all (CIN 3). ⑤ Basement membrane. ⑦ Epithelial surface.

Cervical intraepithelial neoplasia: classification and management		
Classi-fication	Fraction of epithelium occupied by abnormal cells	Management
CIN 1	One third	Resolves spontaneously Repeat colposcopy at 12 months to check that CIN has resolved Persistent CIN1 treated with LLETZ or cold coagulation
CIN 2	Two thirds	LLETZ
CIN 3	All	LLETZ Cone biopsy Hysterectomy

LLETZ, large loop excision of the transformation zone.

Table 15.5 Classification and management of precancerous cervical intraepithelial neoplasia

destroyed by a probe heated to 120 degrees. This is an ablative treatment, whilst LLETZ and cone biopsy are excisional treatments for CIN.

Follow-up

A 'test of cure' is carried out 6 months after treatment. This consists of repeat cervical cytology, with the sample sent for both cytological investigation and testing for the presence of high risk HPV.

■ If high risk HPV is absent, routine screening is required, with a repeat test in 3 years, even for women over 50 years old
■ If high risk HPV is present, or if moderate or severe dyskaryosis is detected, colposcopy is carried out to determine the need for further treatment

Women are advised that repeated LLETZ treatments and cone biopsies increase the risk of preterm birth. However, a single LLETZ procedure does not significantly increase the risk of delivery before 37 weeks' gestation.

Prognosis

CIN 1 resolves spontaneously in 70% of women within 1 year, and in 90% within 2 years. Without treatment, half of cases of CIN 2 regress within 2 years.

Left untreated, cervical intraepithelial neoplasia progresses to invasive cancer in 1% of CIN 1 cases, 5% of CIN 2 cases and ≥ 12% of CIN 3 cases. Ninety-five per cent of women are cured by a single LLETZ treatment. Women who have had an abnormal result with cervical screening have a fourfold increased risk of developing cervical cancer compared with those who have not. This means that continued surveillance for recurrent abnormalities is critical.

Management of gynaecological cancer

The incidence of gynaecological cancer is lower than that of breast cancer; on average, a GP in the UK would expect to come across one new case of ovarian cancer every 5 years and one of endometrial cancer every 3–4 years. To improve survival rates and patient quality of life, the management of gynaecological cancers needs an integrated approach. In the UK this based on coordination between health care professionals working at three levels of care; together, they form a cancer network (**Table 15.6**). This model of care ensures optimal investigation and assessment and specialist treatment by clinicians with large enough caseloads to maintain the key skills. It also improves continuity of care and patient satisfaction.

Multidisciplinary team meetings

All cases of gynaecological malignancy are discussed at weekly specialist multidisciplinary team meetings, at which treatment decisions are made. The core team compromises:

Gynaecological cancer care			
Level of care	Care provider	Site of care	Type of care
1	GP	GP surgery	Recognition of cancer symptoms
			Prompt referral to secondary care: the 2-week urgent referral pathway for suspected cancer
2	Local gynaecological cancer multidisciplinary team	Cancer unit at district general hospital	Rapid assessment of all types of gynaecological cancer
			Surgical treatment of microscopic stage 1 cervical cancer and low-risk endometrial cancer (grade 1 or 2, stage 1a)
3	Specialist gynaecological cancer multidisciplinary team	Cancer centre at university hospital	Management of all ovarian, vulval, vaginal, high-risk endometrial and cervical cancers not suitable for management in a cancer unit
			Provision of level 2 service to local population
			Management of all cases of recurrence of gynaecological cancer
GP, general practitioner.			

Table 15.6 Levels of care for gynaecological cancer

- two surgical gynaecological oncologists
- a medical oncologist (specialising in chemotherapy)
- a clinical oncologist (specialising in radiotherapy)
- a radiologist
- a histopathologist
- a cytopathologist
- a gynaecological clinical nurse specialist
- a multidisciplinary team coordinator

Gynaecological clinical nurse specialists

Gynaecological clinical nurse specialists have particular expertise in cancer and palliative care. They work in hospitals and in the community to assess the complex needs of cancer patients. They give advice and support to both health care professionals and patients. As well as reviewing pain and physical symptoms, they provide psychological, financial and practical support to patients during oncological treatment and follow-up. The UK's clinical nurse specialists are Macmillan nurses. They are funded by the Macmillan charity but work as part of the integrated health care team.

Management of terminal disease

Management of cancer in the last few weeks and months of life includes caring for the physical, emotional, psychological and spiritual needs of the patient to increase the likelihood of a peaceful and pain-free death. It requires multidisciplinary care from GPs, district and specialist nurses, oncologists, palliative care consultants, pastoral care workers and other allied health care professionals, such as physiotherapists and dieticians.

Guidance

In the UK, the Gold Standards Framework sets out an evidence-based approach to looking after patients at the end of life, with the aim of improving the seven C's:

- communication
- coordination of services
- control of symptoms
- continuity of care
- continued learning
- carer support
- care in the dying phase

Place of care

Most patients prefer to die at home rather than in hospital, and the proportion who do so is increasing with improved frameworks for integrating care by diverse professionals. Involvement of the palliative care team ensures adequate back-up 24 h a day and avoids unnecessary hospital admissions.

Hospice care is also available when a patient's needs are too great to be managed at home or when family carers need respite. Hospice care is not necessarily continuous or terminal: a patient may go home on improvement and return during a period of deterioration. Complementary therapy, rehabilitation and spiritual support facilities are available to provide holistic care.

Medication

The aim of medical treatment is to relieve symptoms rather than to treat chronic illness. Therefore drug therapy for the management of hypertension, hypercholesterolaemia and other long-term conditions is discontinued.

> Syringe drivers are frequently used for the continuous subcutaneous administration of drugs required to relieve severe pain in patients who are being cared for at home. Several drugs can be delivered simultaneously in this way, thereby avoiding the need for multiple injections.

The underlying cause of pain is assessed and appropriate analgesia given. Opioids of differing strengths are used to treat moderate to severe pain; they are given by mouth in tablet or liquid form; transdermally as skin patches; and subcutaneously, intramuscularly or intravenously. Antiemetics and laxatives are given at the same time to manage nausea and constipation, which are adverse effects of long-term opioid treatment.

Adjuvant drugs are used alongside opioids to treat other causes of pain:

- bisphosphonates strengthen bones and reduce bone pain
- steroids reduce pain and swelling caused by tumour compression
- antiepileptic and antidepressants, for example gabapentin and amitriptyline, reduce nerve pain
- muscle relaxants control muscle spasms

Cancer and its treatment cause loss of appetite, eating difficulties related to sore mouth, diarrhoea, fatigue and breathlessness. These are managed with steroids and mouthwashes (to treat sore mouths), loperamide (for diarrhoea) and anxiolytics, opiates and hyoscine (to treat breathlessness).

Do not attempt resuscitation orders

When cardiac or respiratory arrest is an expected part of the dying process and cardiopulmonary resuscitation is unlikely to be successful, an advance decision not to attempt resuscitation allows patients to die in a dignified and peaceful way.

A do not attempt resuscitation (DNAR) order is discussed with the patient or, if they find this too upsetting, with a relative or carer, with the patient's permission. If the patient lacks capacity, a physician can write a DNAR order in their best interests but must inform the patient's legal proxy or relative of the reasons for this decision.

> A signed DNAR form travels with the patient to inform health care professionals of the decision. Therefore, the order applies whether the individual is at home, in hospital or in an ambulance.

Contraception: special circumstances

Contraceptive services are provided by many different healthcare professionals in various locations, including the GP surgery, hospital, family planning clinic and pharmacy. The basis of a high-quality service is the provision, to individuals of all ages, of contraceptive choice and control over reproduction, thereby enabling them to avoid unwanted pregnancies and to plan their families. In the UK, contraception is provided free of charge.

When assessing whether a young person is in an abusive relationship, the partner's age is useful information. A large age gap increases suspicion of coercion into sexual activity. If sexual abuse is suspected, safe-guarding teams are alerted and referrals to the police and social services made as appropriate.

Under 16s

The law regarding the provision of contraceptive services to girls varies between countries. In the UK and in countries which draw on UK case law, for example Australia, the law for under 16s was established in the case of Gillick v West Norfolk and Wisbech Area Health Authority in 1985. Children are said to be Gillick competent if they are mature enough to understand the nature of the advice that is being given and what is involved. This was originally applied only to the provision of contraception, but it is now used more broadly when assessing whether a child is capable of making their own decisions regarding any medical treatment.

The Fraser guidelines arose out of the Gillick case and apply specifically to provision of contraceptive and sexual health services to under 16s without parental knowledge or consent. These are lawful if if the child satisfies all the Fraser guidelines:

- the child understands all aspects of the advice and its implications
- the child cannot be persuaded to tell their parents or allow them to be told
- the child is very likely to have sexual intercourse with or without treatment
- the child's physical or mental health is likely to suffer unless the advice or treatment is given
- it is in the best interests of the young person to receive the advice and treatment without parental knowledge or consent

Confidentiality is essential to build trust and encourage the use of contraceptive and sexual health services. It should be breeched only to prevent serious harm to the child or others, for example if the child is at risk of abuse, when the child does not have sufficient maturity or understanding to make a decision about disclosure or when the clinician is required to do so by law. In the UK, the last of these criteria is met in any case concerning children under the age of 13 years, with whom any sexual intercourse is illegal.

Patients who lack capacity

Legislation covers contraceptive decision making for people older than 16 years who lack capacity (lack ability to make their own decisions). In England and Wales, for example, this is the Mental Capacity Act 2005, which states that a person is assumed to be competent until proven otherwise and that demonstration of competence is situation specific. Accordingly a woman who lacks capacity for some decisions may nevertheless have capacity to make contraceptive decisions: such women are encouraged to make contraceptive choices themselves rather than have decisions made for them. This is facilitated by providing support, easily understood information and adequate time to consider options.

If a woman still lacks capacity to make contraceptive choices despite such support, most countries have legislation that allows decisions to be made in her best interests by a health care professional (HCP) taking into account the risk of falling pregnant. HCPs must consider the views of others involved in the woman's care and weigh up the least restrictive contraceptive option against the likelihood of adherence. For example, the combined oral contraceptive pill is reversible but remembering to take a pill daily is often difficult for women with learning difficulties; conversely, after sterilisation no additional precautions are required but the procedure is irreversible.

Sterilisation and abortion are considered differently. For example, the Mental Capacity Act 2005 classes these as 'serious medical treatment' and provides for them to be dealt with by a specialist court (Court of Protection): a family member or an independent advocate is appointed to make decisions in the best interests of the woman.

Neonatal resuscitation

Nearly half of all newborn deaths occur within the 24 hours of delivery and many are associated with a period of hypoxia. Effective resuscitation in the first few minutes of life dramatically improves long-term outcomes. All delivery staff are trained in neonatal resuscitation so they are able to respond to emergencies during delivery.

Ten per cent of neonates require some assistance breathing after birth and a further 1% require extensive resuscitation.

Fetal response to in utero hypoxia

Hypoxia is a lack of oxygen reaching the tissues . In babies it is the most common reason for needing resuscitation. Causes of hypoxia in utero include cord prolapse, uterine hyperstimulation and shoulder dystocia.

In utero, a fetus with hypoxia will attempt to breathe. If the insult is not removed, the fetus loses consciousness and brainstem centres involved in controlling breathing shut down, resulting in primary apnoea. The heart rate is initially unchanged, but decreases as the myocardium switches to anaerobic metabolism to maintain an energy supply. Perfusion of non-vital organs is reduced in an attempt to preserve circulation to the heart and brain.

If the hypoxia continues, primitive spinal centres initiate whole-body gasping or shuddering before the fetus enters terminal hypoxia. Cardiac function is impaired by el-evated lactic acid levels and eventually the heart stops. The whole process from the start of hypoxia to cardiac arrest and death takes 20 minutes in a healthy fetus.

Getting air to the lungs is therefore the key element of neonatal resuscitation: the circulation is usually sufficient to deliver oxygenated blood to the heart and brain if enough oxygen can be provided.

Resuscitation

Figure 15.8 shows the UK guidelines for resuscitating the neonate.

Dry and wrap

Babies are small and wet when they are born; a cold baby is more difficult to resuscitate than a warm one. A towel is used to dry and wrap the baby, who is kept under a radiant heater while the initial assessment is performed. Premature babies are placed in plastic bags without drying to reduce evaporation loss.

Assess

At birth, the need for resusciation is assessed in all babies. This is done using a scoring system called Apgar: activity (muscle tone), pulse, grimace (reflex irritability), appearance (skin colour) and respiration. Changes in Apgar score over time are used to monitor response to resuscitation. A healthy baby:

■ cries within a few seconds of delivery
■ has good tone

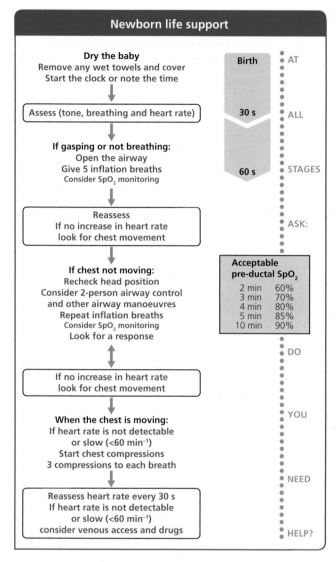

Newborn life support

Dry the baby
Remove any wet towels and cover
Start the clock or note the time

Assess (tone, breathing and heart rate)

If gasping or not breathing:
Open the airway
Give 5 inflation breaths
Consider SpO$_2$ monitoring

Reassess
If no increase in heart rate
look for chest movement

If chest not moving:
Recheck head position
Consider 2-person airway control
and other airway manoeuvres
Repeat inflation breaths
Consider SpO$_2$ monitoring
Look for a response

If no increase in heart rate
look for chest movement

When the chest is moving:
If heart rate is not detectable
or slow (<60 min⁻¹)
Start chest compressions
3 compressions to each breath

Reassess heart rate every 30 s
If heart rate is not detectable
or slow (<60 min⁻¹)
consider venous access and drugs

Birth — AT
30 s — ALL
60 s — STAGES
ASK:

Acceptable pre-ductal SpO$_2$
2 min	60%
3 min	70%
4 min	80%
5 min	85%
10 min	90%

DO
YOU
NEED
HELP?

Figure 15.8 Guidelines for neonatal resuscitation. Reproduced with the kind permission of the Resuscitation Council (UK).

- has a heart rate >100 bpm
- is often blue in colour initially, particularly at the peripheries

An ill baby:

- is pale
- is floppy
- is not breathing
- has a slow or non-existent heart rate

Airway

The neonate's airway is opened by placing it in the neutral position, i.e. with the neck neither flexed nor extended. The large occiput causes the neck to flex when the baby is on its back obstructing the airway. Airway suctioning is only used if there is a visible obstruction; meconium is not aspirated in an otherwise healthy, crying baby.

Breathing

Babies are born with lungs full of fluid, which must be forced into the circulation to aerate the lung tissue effectively. Sustained, high-pressure inflation breaths are delivered, looking for evidence of chest wall movement and an increase in fetal heart rate as signs of successful oxygenation.

Circulation

If there is no improvement in heart rate despite chest wall movement, chest compressions are commenced at a ratio of 3:1 ventilation breaths (shorter-lasting, lower-pressure breaths than inflation breaths).

Drugs

Drugs are rarely needed for resuscitation, but include adrenaline, sodium bicarbonate to correct acidosis, dextrose to treat hypoglycaemia and blood or intravenous fluid if there has been loss of circulating volume, for example in the case of a vasa praevia.

> **Cooling is used in term babies with evolving moderate to severe hypoxic brain injury within 6 hours of birth.** It is continued for 72 hours to improve outcomes.

Prognosis

The majority of neonates who require resuscitation are successfully resuscitated after birth with no long-term morbidity. Moderate to severe hypoxic ischaemic encephalopathy develops in 0.2–0.3% of babies, with a mortality rate of 6–30% and cerebral palsy and significant long-term disabilities in 20–30% of survivors.

Resuscitation is discontinued after 10 minutes without a heartbeat because the outlook is extremely poor.

Risk management

Risks are high in obstetrics and gynaecology as a specialty, because it involves the management of a large number of emergency situations. Risk management is the process of proactively identifying what could go wrong as well as retrospectively reviewing incidents to highlight areas for improvement and thereby prevent future adverse events. The main aim of risk management is to improve patient safety.

Risks are identified in various ways:

- by conducting a risk assessment in a specific clinical area, such as the delivery suite or theatre
- incident reporting of specific outcomes on a prespecified trigger list
- complaints and claims
- staff consultation, for example through workshops and interviews
- clinical audit (**Figure 15.9**)

> **Incident reporting is not punitive to the individual involved but an opportunity to improve patient care.** Risk management is a review of the whole system rather than a process to identify errors by specific individuals.

The maternity dashboard is software used to benchmark the performance of an individual maternity unit against nationally set standards. By providing contemporary information, it allows timely action in the case of deviation from agreed goals. A traffic light system is used to assess four broad categories:

- workforce
- clinical activity
- risk incidents and complaints
- clinical outcomes, such as the rate of third or fourth perineal tears and the number of cases of post-partum haemorrhage > 2500 mL

An investigation team is established to analyse each risk incident and determine its degree of severity and the likelihood of recurrence. The team is also charged with identifying contributory factors and problems with delivering care through root cause analyses, before devising an action plan to reduce future risk. The action plan may include the development of new guidelines, the provision of further training or an increase in staffing levels.

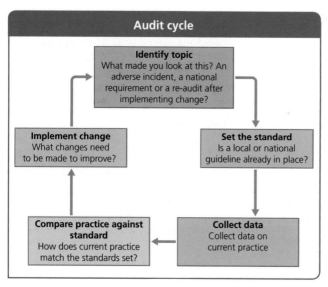

Figure 15.9 Audit cycle. Once a topic is identified, an appropriate standard is sought against which to measure local practice. Data are collected and compared with the standard and improvements identified. After implementing the necessary changes the cycle is repeated to ensure improvement in care.

Answers to starter questions

1. The retrieval of DNA depends upon the nature of the assault, whether the victim has washed themselves or their clothes, and the time that has elapsed since the assault. DNA can be retrieved up to 7 days after an assault involving vaginal penetration, but only for 2–3 days after an assault if oral or anal penetration was performed.

2. Cervical screening is not performed during pregnancy as the results are more difficult to interpret. Instead, routine screening is performed 3 months after delivery. The exception to this is if a follow-up to a previous abnormal result is required. Colposcopy can be performed safely in pregnancy and high-grade cervical intraepithelial neoplasia (CIN) is monitored with a repeat colposcopic examination at 28 weeks' gestation. Biopsies are only taken during pregnancy to exclude malignancy if absolutely necessary because the risk of bleeding is significantly increased. Definitive treatment of CIN 2/3 is performed postnatally.

3. A clinical audit is a quality improvement process in which patient care and outcomes are compared against specific criteria. Recommendations are based on the findings of the audit and implemented before the process is repeated. This is the 'audit cycle' (**Figure 15.9**). Research is a structured activity that provides new knowledge. Studies generate new hypotheses and test them, and can include comparing novel treatments or investigations with existing ones. Ethical approval is required to complete this work.

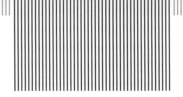

Chapter 16
Self-assessment

SBA questions

Normal pregnancy and delivery

1. A 29-year-old woman visits her midwife for the first time with a planned pregnancy. This is her first pregnancy. She missed her period 2 months ago, is a non-smoker and has no known medical conditions. Her mother and her sister required caesarean deliveries.
   What is the single most appropriate care schedule?
   A Consultant-led care, appointments and ultrasound scans every 4 weeks from 20 weeks
   B Consultant-led care, appointments every 4 weeks from 20 weeks
   C Midwifery-led care, appointments at first antenatal visit, 16, 20, 25, 28, 31, 34, 36, 38 and 40 weeks
   D Midwifery-led care, appointments at first antenatal visit, 16, 20, 28, 34, 36, 38 and 41 weeks
   E Shared care, alternate appointments at the hospital and in the community

2. A 26-year-old woman returns to her midwife after routine screening. Her test results are: A Rhesus positive, hepatitis B surface antibody-positive, hepatitis B surface antigen and core antibody negative, rubella IgG positive, urine culture positive.
   What is the single most appropriate course of action?
   A Anti-D at 28 weeks
   B Hepatitis B immunisation for infant
   C Hepatitis B immunisation for mother
   D Postnatal rubella immunisation

   E Repeat urine test and treat if result remains positive

3. A 40-year-old woman is pregnant for the first time. She attends her dating scan at 13 weeks. She opts for Down's syndrome screening. Her nuchal translucency scan and blood test results establish the likelihood of Down's syndrome is 1:50.
   What is the single most appropriate next step?
   A Chorionic villus sampling or amniocentesis
   B Quadruple test
   C Reassurance alone
   D Repeat combined test
   E Termination of pregnancy

4. A 33-year-old woman is booked for midwife-led antenatal care and is now 40 weeks pregnant. All her antenatal checks have been normal. She is worried that has not yet gone into labour. She has not experienced any change in her baby's movements.
   Which is the single most appropriate course of action?
   A Admit to labour ward for observation
   B Immediate caesarean section
   C Immediate induction of labour
   D Membrane sweep
   E Ultrasound

5. A 23-year-old woman is 40 weeks pregnant when she suddenly experiences a gush of clear fluid from the vagina. About 2 h later, she starts having contractions. When she calls the birth suite, her contractions are every 2–3 min. She attends the birth suite for assessment. Which single finding would require review by an obstetrician?

A Cervix fully effaced and 2 cm dilated
B Fetal heart rate 130–140 bpm
C Maternal pulse rate 88 bpm
D No further loss of liquor
E Temperature 38.5°C

6. A 39-year-old woman had a vaginal delivery 2 days ago. She went home the day after giving birth.
Which single symptom would prompt a midwife to refer her back to the hospital?

A Calf tenderness
B Mucousy red vaginal discharge
C Period-like pains
D Swollen, engorged breasts
E Tiredness

Complications in early pregnancy

1. A 19-year-old woman is 8 weeks pregnant when she attends the early pregnancy unit for light vaginal bleeding. She has a transvaginal ultrasound, which reveals a missed miscarriage.
Which single combination of ultrasound features is consistent with this diagnosis?

A Bright echogenic endometrial stripe. Normal ovaries
B Single intrauterine pregnancy. Crown–rump length, 5 mm. Fetal heartbeat not present
C Single intrauterine pregnancy. Crown–rump length, 7 mm. Fetal heartbeat present
D Single intrauterine pregnancy. Crown–rump length, 11 mm. Fetal heartbeat not present
E Thickened endometrium. Right ovary contains a corpus luteal cyst of 3 cm

2. A 24-year-old woman is 6 weeks pregnant when she is admitted to the emergency room with right iliac fossa pain and spotting. Her blood pressure is 80/63 mmHg, and her pulse rate is 125 bpm.
Which is the single most appropriate next step?

A Offer methotrexate
B Offer misoprostol
C Schedule for emergency surgery
D Serial measurements of β-human chorionic gonadotrophin (hCG)
E Refer for suspected appendicitis

3. A 22-year-old woman is 6 weeks pregnant when she returns to the early pregnancy unit for blood tests after mild right iliac fossa pain and spotting 2 days ago. At her first visit, her serum hCG concentration was 150 IU/L. Today, her serum hCG is 80 IU/L. She is haemodynamically stable.
Which is the single most appropriate step?

A Offer expectant management
B Offer methotrexate
C Offer misoprostol
D Schedule for urgent surgery
E Transvaginal ultrasound

4. A 21-year-old woman is 7 weeks pregnant and presents to her general practitioner (GP) having vomited constantly for the past 3 days. She is unable to keep food or fluids down. Her urine dipstick shows ketones 4+.
What is the single most appropriate next step?

A Admit for an insulin sliding scale
B Offer an ultrasound
C Offer oral antiemetics
D Reassure and give dietary advice
E Refer to the early pregnancy unit for intravenous rehydration

5. A 38-year-old woman is 8 weeks pregnant and has spotting, abdominal cramps and vomiting. Her ultrasound reveals an echogenic intrauterine mass with multiple cystic spaces giving it a 'snow storm' appearance. This is her second pregnancy.
Which is the single most appropriate management option?

A Offer methotrexate
B Offer misoprostol
C Offer surgical evacuation of the uterus
D Repeat ultrasound in 10–14 days
E Serial hCG measurements

Complications in mid to late pregnancy

1. A 32-year-old woman has a fasting blood glucose concentration of 6.7 mmol/L and a blood glucose concentration of 9.1 mmol/L after an oral glucose test at 28 weeks gestation. She is told she has gestational diabetes.
What is the single most appropriate next step?

A Dietary modification and home glucose monitoring
B Reassure and return to midwife-led care
C Repeat the glucose tolerance test postnatally
D Start insulin
E Start metformin

2. A 40-year-old woman attends her routine midwife appointment at 32 weeks. This is her first pregnancy. She has developed a headache, blurred vision and ankle oedema.

Her midwife finds her blood pressure to be 150/100 mmHg. Her urine dipstick analysis shows 3+ of protein.
What is the single most appropriate next step?

A Admit to the maternity unit for review
B Measure urinary catecholamines
C Reassure and advise simple analgesics
D Request an MRI and refer to neurology
E Send a urine specimen for culture

3. A 32-year-old woman attends her routine 34-week midwife appointment complaining of itching. She has noticed that her baby's movements have reduced.
Which is the single most appropriate course of action?

A Offer induction of labour
B Offer ursodeoxycholic acid
C Reassure and offer antihistamines
D Refer to the antenatal day assessment unit for fetal monitoring
E Take blood samples for LFTs and see in 2 weeks

4. A 35-year-old woman attends her antenatal appointment at 36 weeks. Her BMI was 50 at her first antenatal visit. She now measures large for dates. Her ultrasound confirms polyhydramnios.
What is the single most likely diagnosis?

A Pre-eclampsia
B Pre-labour rupture of membranes
C Gestational diabetes
D Intrauterine growth restriction
E Placental abruption

5. A 26-year-old woman is 32 weeks into her third pregnancy. She has steadily gained weight with each pregnancy. Her body mass index (BMI) at her first antenatal visit in this pregnancy was 48 kg/m^2.
What is the single most appropriate next step?

A Assess fetal growth using fundal height
B Avoid epidural anaesthesia in labour
C Encourage breastfeeding
D Recommend elective caesarean delivery
E Restrict calorie intake to aim to lose 10% of bodyweight before delivery

6. A 28-year-old woman is in her first pregnancy. She has had epilepsy since childhood. This is managed with lamotrigine.
What is the single most appropriate recommendation?

A Avoid breastfeeding
B Consider early epidural
C Consider induction of labour at 37 weeks
D Stop antiepileptics
E Take folic acid 400 µg daily

7. A 28-year-old woman is brought into the labour ward with fresh vaginal bleeding at 37 weeks. The blood has soaked through her clothing. She is Rhesus-negative.
What is the single most appropriate next step?

A Antenatal corticosteroids
B Anti-D
C Caesarean delivery
D Digital vaginal examination
E Intravenous access and taking of blood samples for full blood count and cross-match

Complications in delivery and the postnatal period

1. A 20-year-old woman is 29 weeks pregnant in her first pregnancy. While at work, she started to experience backache. Over the course of the day, she started to get painful contractions. She attends maternity triage, where she is found to have a positive fibronectin test and is 1 cm dilated.
What is the single most appropriate intervention?

A Antibiotics
B Caesarean delivery
C Corticosteroids
D Intravaginal prostaglandins
E Reassure and send home

2. A 25-year-old woman goes into spontaneous labour at 39 weeks. She has no antenatal risk factors and is admitted to the midwife-led birth suite. She is found to be 5 cm dilated at her first examination. At her next examination, 4 hours later, she is still 5 cm dilated.
What is the single most appropriate action?

A Amniotomy
B Epidural
C Give nifedipine
D Intravenous synthetic oxytocin (Syntocinon)
E Reassurance: she is still in early labour

3. A 26-year-old woman is 38 weeks pregnant when her waters break. Initially the liquor was clear, but it is now stained green. She is assessed by the obstetrician, who recommends that her labour be augmented by using synthetic oxytocin (Syntocinon).
Which is the single best setting for this intervention?

A Antenatal ward
B At home
C Consultant-led delivery suite
D Maternity theatre
E Midwife-led unit

4. A 34-year-old woman went into spontaneous labour at 39 weeks. Because of concerns regarding decelerations heard by her midwife during intermittent auscultation, she has been placed on continuous fetal monitoring. Her cardiotocography is pathological and fetal blood sampling confirms acidosis (pH 7.13). She is 9 cm dilated. The baby's head is two fifths palpable per abdomen.
What is the single best next step?

   A Caesarean delivery
   B Forceps delivery
   C Reassess in 1 hour
   D Recommend starting voluntary pushing
   E Ventouse delivery

5. A 36-year-old woman goes into spontaneous labour. She has had rapid deliveries with all six of her children. She delivers in the car on the way to the hospital. As she is transferred from her car to the maternity unit, she starts to bleed heavily, passing large clots. On examination, her uterus is soft and is three fingers' breadth above her umbilicus. Her perineum is intact and her placenta appears complete.
Which single cause is the most likely explanation for her bleeding?

   A Clotting disorder
   B Endometritis
   C Perineal trauma
   D Uterine atony
   E Retained placental tissue

6. A 32-year-old woman had her baby by caesarean section 3 days ago because of failure to progress in labour. She had been induced after failing to labour despite her membranes rupturing 2 days before. You are asked to review her urgently. She has a pulse rate of 120 bpm, and her blood pressure is 100/60 mmHg. Her respiratory rate is 18 breaths/min, and her oxygen saturation is 98% on room air. She has a temperature of 38.5°C.
What is the single most appropriate intervention?

   A Intravenous antibiotics and paracetamol
   B Magnesium sulphate
   C Oxygen and intravenous furosemide
   D Oxygen and low-molecular-weight heparin
   E Transfusion with cross-matched blood

Reproductive endocrinology

1. A 16-year-old girl has never had a period. She is in the national training squad for gymnastics and hopes to compete in the next Olympic Games. She presents with her mother to the gynaecology outpatient department. The gynaecologist suspects that her training regimen is the cause.
Which single finding would be in keeping with this diagnosis?

   A Breast development and no uterus seen on pelvic ultrasound
   B Breast development, polycystic ovaries and hirsutism
   C Breast development and uterus seen on pelvic ultrasound
   D High follicle-stimulating hormone (FSH) concentration and absent breast development
   E Low FSH and absent breast development

2. A 30-year-old woman has been trying to conceive for the past 2 years. She has always had irregular periods and since her early twenties has had to shave her excess facial hair on a daily basis. Her BMI is 35 kg/m².
Which single medication is most likely to help her conceive?

   A Clomifene
   B Co-cyprindiol (Dianette)
   C Desogestrel (Cerazette)
   D Eflornithine
   E GnRH analogues

3. A 6-year-old girl is brought to the clinic by her mother, who is concerned that her daughter is going through puberty early. She is the tallest in her class at school, and she has started developing breasts and pubic hair.
Which single statement is true regarding the management of this condition?

   A A pelvic examination is necessary to rule out an ovarian tumour
   B Bone radiographs are necessary to rule out McCune–Albright syndrome as a cause
   C Gonadotrophin-releasing hormone (GnRH) analogues may be of benefit
   D The mother can be reassured that this is a normal variation and requires no treatment
   E Most children with this condition have a hormone-secreting tumour and will require surgery

4. A 28-year-old woman is concerned because her periods have become irregular. She has noticed a milky discharge from her nipples, headache and blurred vision. She has always had regular periods until recently, and she is not on medication.
What single investigation is the most appropriate, given the above symptoms?

A Breast ultrasound
B Mammography
C MRI of the head
D Skull radiography
E Tonometry

5. A 28-year-old woman visits her GP because she has found it increasingly difficult to cope with her cyclical mood changes. Around the time of her period, she is tearful and feels low. She has been threatened with disciplinary action at work because she taken a lot of time off.
   What is the single most appropriate next step?

   A Evening primrose oil
   B Luteal phase selective serotonin reuptake inhibitors (SSRIs)
   C Progesterone-only pill
   D Reassure her that this is normal and requires no treatment
   E Refer to occupational health

6. A 39-year-old woman had a hysterectomy and bilateral salpingo-oophrectomy at the age of 38 years after trying a number of medical and surgical treatments for her endometriosis. Although this has helped her with her pain, she has had problems with severe hot flushes and mood changes. She is considering hormone replacement therapy (HRT) but is worried about the risks.
   Which single statement is true regarding her risks when using HRT?

   A Increased risk of colorectal cancer
   B Increased risk of dementia
   C Increased risk of endometrial cancer
   D Increased risk of osteoporosis
   E Increased risk of venous thromboembolism

Fertility and contraception

1. A 37-year-old woman smokes 20 cigarettes a day and has a BMI of 37 kg/m². She has two children; one is 5 years old and the other is 10 years old. She is in a new relationship and wishes to discuss contraception.
   Which single option is contraindicated?

   A Barrier contraception
   B Combined oral contraceptive pill
   C Contraceptive implant (Nexplanon)
   D Levonorgestrel-releasing intrauterine system (Mirena coil)
   E Progesterone-only pill

2. A 23-year-old non-smoker has had a copper intrauterine device for contraception since the birth of her son 2 years ago. She likes the reassurance of having a monthly bleed but finds this heavy and painful.

Which single option would reduce the bleeding while giving her a regular period?

   A Combined oral contraceptive pill
   B Contraceptive implant (Nexplanon)
   C Contraceptive injection (Depo-Provera)
   D Levonorgestrel-releasing intrauterine system (Mirena coil)
   E Progesterone-only pill

3. A 14-year-old girl visits her GP to request emergency contraception. She is alone. Four days ago, she has had consensual unprotected sexual intercourse with her boyfriend, who is in her year at school.
   She is deemed Fraser competent.
   Which single option would be the most effective to prevent pregnancy?

   A Barrier contraception
   B Contraceptive implant (Nexplanon)
   C Levonorgestrel (Levonelle)
   D Nothing can be prescribed without parental consent
   E Ulipristal acetate (EllaOne)

4. A 42-year-old woman has had four children. She and her husband feel that they have completed their family and are looking for the most reliable form of permanent contraception.
   Which single option is the most appropriate for their needs?

   A Barrier contraception
   B Hysteroscopic tubal sterilisation
   C Laparoscopic tubal sterilisation
   D Levonorgestrel-releasing interuterine system (Mirena coil)
   E Vasectomy

5. A 40-year-old woman and her partner have been trying to conceive for 2 years. She has never been pregnant, but her partner has a child from another relationship. The patient has irregular periods. Her day 2 FSH is 28 IU/L and her antimüllerian hormone (AMH) is very low (<5 pmol/L).
   Which single option would offer the best chance of a live birth?

   A Clomifene
   B Intracytoplasmic sperm injection (ICSI)
   C Intrauterine insemination (IUI)
   D In vitro fertilisation (IVF) using a donor egg
   E Metformin

6. A 35-year-old woman and her partner have tried to conceive for over 3 years. She has regular periods. Her partner's semen analysis results indicate azoospermia.
   Which single next best series of investigations will determine the cause of their subfertility?

A Day 21 progesterone, day 2 luteinising hormone (LH) and FSH

B Hysterosalpingo-contrast sonography

C Hysterosalpingogram

D Karyotype, FSH and LH, and screening for cystic fibrosis

E No further investigations, because the cause is likely to be idiopathic

7. A 29-year-old woman visits the emergency room with abdominal pain, nausea and shortness of breath. Her abdomen is distended. She has a history of polycystic ovary syndrome and has been undergoing IVF. She had egg retrieval 3 days ago, and 18 oocytes were retrieved.
   Which single course of management is most appropriate?

   A Antibiotics

   B Diuretics

   C Supportive management

   D Therapeutic dose low-molecular-weight heparin

   E Urgent surgery

Abnormal uterine bleeding

1. A 30-year-old woman has not had a period since her surgical evacuation of a miscarriage 6 months ago. She experienced abdominal pain and a foul-smelling discharge a few days after her surgery. This settled with oral antibiotics. She has taken a number of home pregnancy tests, which have all been negative.
   Which is the single most useful next investigation?

   A Hysteroscopy

   B Karyotyping

   C MRI head

   D Serum hCG

   E Triple swabs

2. A 47-year-old woman has heavy periods. Her cycles are regular and are 27 days long. She bleeds for 8–10 days of these. Over the past year, her bleeding has become heavier. Her pads are regularly flooded and she is embarrassed to leave her home in case she bleeds through.
   Which single term best describes her symptoms?

   A Amenorrhea

   B Dysmenorrhea

   C Menorrhagia

   D Polymenorrhea

   E Oligomenorrhea

3. A 39-year-old woman has had a levonorgesterol-releasing intrauterine system (Mirena coil) inserted 12 months ago to try to improve her heavy menstrual bleeding, but she continues to experience heavy irregular bleeding. She has completed her family.
   Which is the single most appropriate next stage of management?

   A Copper intrauterine device

   B Hysterectomy

   C Endometrial ablation

   D GnRH analogues

   E Ferrous sulphate

4. A 25-year-old woman has had heavy, painful periods and deep dyspareunia for the past 6 months. On pelvic examination, she has a tender nodule in her posterior fornix and a fixed uterus. She would like to try for a baby as soon as possible.
   Which is the single most appropriate treatment option?

   A Antibiotics

   B Endometrial ablation

   C Hysterectomy

   D Levonorgestrel-releasing intrauterine system (Mirena coil)

   E Operative laparoscopy

5. A 19-year-old girl has bleeding between her periods and after sex. She has had a copper coil for contraception for the past 3 months. On examination, her GP notes the coil threads, a reddened cervix and cervical excitation.
   What is the single most appropriate investigation to perform?

   A Cervical biopsy

   B Colposcopy

   C Genital tract swabs

   D Pelvic ultrasound

   E Smear test

6. A 62-year-old woman had her last period 5 years ago, but in the past 2 months she has experienced several episodes of light vaginal bleeding.
   What is the single most appropriate next step?

   A Oral HRT

   B Measurement of serum LH and FSH concentration

   C Urgent referral for colposcopy

   D Urgent referral for transvaginal ultrasound and biopsy

   E Vaginal oestrogen cream or pessaries

Inflammatory and infective disorders

1. A 26-year-old woman has severe cyclical pelvic pain, which is worse during sex. A pelvic MRI demonstrates bilateral endometrioma. She is trying for a baby and wants to conceive as soon as possible.
What is the single most appropriate treatment to give?

A Combined oral contraceptive pill
B GnRH analogues
C Hysterectomy
D Levonogestrel-releasing intrauterine system (Mirena coil)
E Operative laparoscopy

2. A 41-year-old woman complains of a white itchy vaginal discharge. On examination, the vaginal walls are erythematous and coated in a white cottage cheese-like discharge.
What is the single most appropriate treatment to give?

A Aciclovir
B Azithromycin
C Ceftriaxone
D Clotrimazole
E Metronidazole

3. A 20-year-old woman complains of increased vaginal discharge. She has a regular partner, but she admits that they occasionally forget to use condoms. She has swabs taken and is recalled a week later, because her swabs suggest she has gonorrhoea.
What is the single most appropriate next step?

A Emergency contraception
B Intramuscular penicillin
C Oral metronidazole
D Refer to genitourinary medicine
E Test of cure

4. A 21-year-old woman has severe abdominal pain and painful ulcers over her labia. She has been unable to pass urine for nearly 24 h.
What is the single most likely cause?

A Human papillomavirus (HPV)
B Herpes simplex virus
C *Klebsiella* granulomatosis
D Syphilis
E Varicella-zoster virus

5. A 25-year-old woman was diagnosed with HIV after routine screening at a sexual health clinic 3 years ago. She is now in a new relationship. Her partner is HIV negative. They wish to try for a baby.

What is the single most appropriate advice to give?

A Avoid pregnancy as the risk of vertical transmission is too high
B Breastfeeding is encouraged
C Caesarean delivery is required
D Consider intrauterine insemination
E Regular unprotected intercourse; there is no risk of transmission to her partner or child

6. A 33-year-old woman has a fever, abdominal pain and a mucopurulent vaginal discharge. Transvaginal ultrasound reveals a 6 cm right-sided tubo-ovarian mass. Her pregnancy test is negative.
What is the single most likely cause?

A *Candida albicans*
B Chlamydia
C Group B *Streptococcus*
D Human papillomavirus (HPV)
E *Treponema pallidum*

Gynaecological tumours

1. A 45-year-old woman has noticed her periods have become heavier and less regular. Her haemoglobin concentration is 89 g/L. She frequently has problems with constipation and after passing urine she often feels like she has not completely emptied her bladder. An ultrasound shows several large fibroids; the largest measures 15 cm.
What is the single most appropriate management to give?

A Blood transfusion
B Co-codamol
C Hysteroscopy
D Referral for fibroid embolisation
E Tranexamic acid

2. A 28-year-old woman has had left-sided pelvic pain for 6 months. A pelvic ultrasound scan reveals a 4-cm unilocular cyst on her right ovary. The cyst has no septation, no solid components and no vascularity. She is taking the oral contraceptive pill.
Which single blood test will confirm the diagnosis?

A α-Fetoprotein
B CA 125
C hCG
D Lactate dehydrogenase
E None of the above

3. A 40-year-old woman has been told her sister, who had breast cancer at the age of 38, carries the BRCA2 gene.

Which single statement is true regarding the patient's risks?

A If she has inherited the BRCA2 gene, her risk of ovarian cancer is 50–85%
B Prophylactic hysterectomy will reduce her risk of ovarian cancer by 90%
C Prophylactic surgery eliminates the risk of peritoneal cancer
D She has a 50% chance of carrying the BRCA2 gene
E Taking the oral contraceptive pill has increased her risk of ovarian cancer

4. A 28-year-old woman has a strong family history of bowel cancer. She is found to have a germline mutation of the DNA mismatch repair gene MLH1.
What is the single most appropriate recommendation?

A Bilateral mastectomy
B Prophylactic oophorectomy once her family is complete
C Regular colonoscopy and advise of the risk of endometrial cancer
D Screen any men in the family for cancer
E Screening for ovarian cancer

5. A 70-year-old woman has received a diagnosis of high-grade serous ovarian cancer. Her CT scan showed a large pelvic mass but no metastases to her lungs. Histological examination demonstrates cancer cells in both of her ovaries and into her omentum. All tumour deposits were completely resected at surgery.
Which single statement applies to her case?

A Her 5-year survival rate is 80–90%
B She has stage 1 cancer
C She has stage 4 cancer
D She will require adjuvant chemotherapy
E She will require adjuvant radiotherapy

6. A 73-year-old woman has had bilateral, painless leg swelling for a month since undergoing a wide local excision and bilateral lymph node dissection for vulval cancer.
What is the single most appropriate course of action?

A Admit to hospital for IV antibiotics
B Refer to rapid access clinic to rule out deep vein thrombosis
C Manual lymphatic drainage, compression stockings and exercise
D Offer diuretics
E Offer pelvic MRI to check for recurrence

Genital prolapse and incontinence

1. A 53-year-old woman requires further treatment because, despite physiotherapy, she still has problems with urinary leakage. She is unable to pick up her 2-year-old granddaughter without severe leakage, which also happens when she laughs, coughs or sneezes.
Which is the single next best course of action?

A Bladder retraining
B Oxybutynin
C Trimethoprim
D Tension-free vaginal tape
E Urodynamics

2. A 61-year-old woman has urine leakage. She finds that she frequently needs to pass urine but only passes small amounts. Occasionally she leaks before she is able to reach the toilet.
Which single additional feature of the patient's history would be consistent with a diagnosis of an overactive bladder?

A Digitating to void
B Dysuria
C Haematuria
D Nocturia
E Slow stream

3. A 73-year-old woman has noticed a lump in her vagina. She has osteoarthritis and is often constipated as a result of her pain medication. When she is constipated, her lump becomes more prominent and sometimes she needs to push it back to pass stool. She wants to avoid surgery as she is the main carer for her disabled husband.
What is the single most appropriate management option?

A Antimuscarinics
B Gelhorn pessary
C Posterior repair
D Sacrohysteropexy
E Transobturator tape

4. A 65-year-old woman underwent a mesh repair for a recurrent posterior wall prolapse 6 months ago and returns to see her surgeon with problems. Since her operation she has experienced dyspareunia and an offensive vaginal discharge. She says it feels like 'there is something sharp poking into her vagina'.
What is the single most likely cause?

A Atrophic vaginitis
B Bacterial vaginosis

C *Candida* infection
D Mesh erosion
E Vaginal cancer

Emergencies

1. A 23-year-old woman has abdominal pain
   and appears pale and clammy. She has
   irregular periods, her last being 7 weeks ago,
   and her pregnancy test is positive. Her pulse
   rate is 110 bpm, and her blood pressure is
   100/65 mmHg. She has guarding over her right
   iliac fossa on palpation.
   What is the single most appropriate next step?

   A Ask the patient to return in 48 h for a
      repeat hCG test
   B Book her into the early pregnancy unit next
      morning
   C Intravenous access, fluids and admission to
      the gynaecology ward
   D Pain relief and discharge
   E Referral to the surgical assessment unit

2. A 36-year-old woman has severe abdominal
   pain. This is her second pregnancy. In her first
   pregnancy, she was induced at 35 weeks for
   pre-eclampsia. Despite smoking cessation
   advice, she has continued to smoke heavily
   in this pregnancy. Her pulse rate is 110 bpm
   and her blood pressure is 100/65 mmHg. Her
   uterus is rigid and the cardiotocography results
   are pathological.
   What is the single most likely diagnosis?

   A Amniotic fluid embolism
   B Cord prolapse
   C Placental abruption
   D Pre-eclampsia
   E Sepsis

3. The same woman is given a general
   anaesthetic and her baby is delivered by
   caesarean section. Suddenly her oxygen
   saturations decrease, her heart rate increases
   to 140 bpm and her lips start to turn blue. Her
   chest is rising equally and there is air entry
   bilaterally.
   What is the single most likely cause?

   A Amniotic fluid embolism
   B Anaphylaxis
   C Disseminated intravascular coagulation
   D Hypovolaemia
   E Pneumothorax

4. A 22-year-old woman is 36 weeks pregnant
   when she complains of blurred vision
   and headache. Her blood pressure is
   180/110 mmHg and her urine dipstick shows
   protein +++. As she is being assessed, she has

a tonic clonic seizure.
Which single treatment will increase the risk of
complications due to her condition?

A Induction of labour
B Intramuscular bethamethasone
C Intravenous bolus of 1 L of Hartmann's
   solution
D Intravenous labetalol
E Intravenous magnesium sulphate

5. A 34-year-old woman who was induced
   for severe pre-eclampsia has a vaginal
   delivery but starts to bleed briskly after the
   placenta is delivered. Her blood pressure is
   160/100 mmHg and her pulse rate is 105 bpm.
   Which single treatment is contraindicated in
   the management of bleeding in this case?

   A Blood products
   B Ergometrine
   C Synthetic oxytocin (Syntocinon)
   D Tranexamic acid
   E Uterine massage

6. A 27-year-old woman has gestational diabetes
   and is being induced at 37 weeks. Her
   baby's growth was above the 90th centile at
   36 weeks. She has been fully dilated for over 2 h
   and has been pushing for the past hour and is
   exhausted. The obstetrician decides to perform
   a ventouse delivery. The head is delivered after
   three pulls, but the shoulders fail to deliver.
   Which single measure is the most likely to aid
   delivery?

   A Caesarean delivery
   B Catheterisation
   C Elevating the legs into McRoberts position
   D Episiotomy
   E Symphisiotomy

7. A 37-year-old woman has been progressing
   slowly in labour. A decision has been made
   to assist by rupturing her membranes. The
   midwife performing the procedure manages
   to break the waters but feels the umbilical cord
   descend into the vagina.
   What is the single best next step?

   A Call for help and transfer urgently to
      theatre for delivery
   B Check the fetal heart rate
   C Empty the bladder
   D Encourage the mother to push
   E Start synthetic oxytocin (Syntocinon)

8. A 29-year-old woman returned home 6 h
   after a normal delivery. Two days later, she
   started to experience fevers and rigors. Her
   temperature is 38.6°C. She also complains of
   a sore throat, a cough and arthralgia. A week
   ago, her toddler had been sent home from

nursery with a fever and a sore throat. What is the single most likely causative organism?

A *Escherichia coli*

B Group A *Streptococcus*

C Group B *Streptococcus*

D Methicillin-resistant *Staphylococcus aureus*

E *Streptococcus viridans*

Integrated care

1. A 17-year-old is 32 weeks pregnant and a regular attender at maternity triage. She has complained of a number of vague problems over the past few weeks. On this occasion, there is quite clearly bruising to her abdomen and her arms. When questioned, she admits that her partner has been hitting her. What is the single most appropriate course of action?

A Confront her partner

B Document your discussion in her handheld notes

C Encourage her to leave her partner

D Inform the safeguarding midwife and consider initiating a multiagency risk assessment conference

E Maintain her confidentiality and promise that you will tell no one else

2. A 21-year-old woman presents with contractions at 38 weeks gestation. She underwent female genital mutilation (FGM) at the age of 7 years in Somalia, and she came to the UK at the age of 12. On examination, her clitoris has been removed and the labia are fused, leaving a narrow opening that admits two fingers. Which single intervention is appropriate regarding her subsequent care?

A Caesarean delivery to prevent failure to progress

B Continuous fetal monitoring via a fetal scalp electrode

C Delivery at a standalone midwifery unit

D Offer defibulation postnatally if not performed in labour

E Reinfibulation at patient's request after delivery

3. A 28-year-old woman attends the emergency room with cuts and bruises to her face and abdomen. She reports she has been sexually assaulted by her ex-partner, who had come to her house to talk about the custody of their children. The forensic medical examiner is on their way. What is the single most appropriate intervention to offer?

A Assess the need for emergency contraception

B Assess the need for post-exposure prophylaxis

C Assess the risk of harm to her children

D Clean and dress the wounds

E Review her medically and ensure her injuries do not require further medical attention

4. A 25-year-old woman has her first cervical screening test. She is subsequently informed that her sample is inadequate. What is the single most appropriate next step?

A Colposcopy

B HPV test

C Repeat test in 3 months

D Repeat test in 1 year

E Repeat test in 3 years

5. A 55-year-old woman has started her treatment for stage 4 cervical cancer 2 years ago. Following diagnosis, she was treated with chemoradiation and recently had to have a nephrostomy to relieve pressure on her left kidney. Over the past few months, she has been losing weight and having more difficulty managing her pain. After discussion with her medical team, she decides that she wants no further active treatment. What single medication can be appropriately discontinued?

A Atorvastatin

B Diazepam

C Metoclopramide

D Morphine

E Paracetamol (acetominophen)

6. A 17-year-old woman has a spontaneous delivery at 38 weeks. The baby is born with its cord loosely around its neck. The midwife removes this, but the baby remains pale and floppy and is making no respiratory effort. What is the single next best step?

A Chest compressions

B Deliver inflation breaths

C Dry and stimulate the baby

D Place baby's head in the neutral position

E Suction the baby's airway

SBA answers

Normal pregnancy and delivery

1. C

A woman should receive regular antenatal appointments to monitor ongoing maternal and fetal wellbeing. If there are no risk factors for complications during pregnancy or delivery, midwifery-led care is appropriate. In their first pregnancy, mothers are offered 9 routine appointments. Low-risk, parous women are offered 7 routine appointments.

2. E

A positive urine culture at the first antenatal visit suggests possible asymptomatic bacteruria. Treating asymptomatic bacteruria reduces the risk of premature delivery and pyelonephritis. The culture should be repeated and antibiotics offered if the second urine culture is also positive. Anti-D is only required in women who are rhesus negative to prevent rhesus isoimmunisation. Being hepatitis B surface antibody positive, but surface antigen and core antibody negative is consistent with previous immunisation against hepatitis B and requires no further action.

3. A

The women should be referred to a specialist screening midwife or obstetrician to discuss the risks and benefits of having a diagnostic test such as chorionic villus sampling (performed between 11 and 14 weeks' gestation) or to wait until after the 14th week of pregnancy to perform an amniocentesis. Diagnostic testing provides a definitive result on which to base the decision whether or not to continue a pregnancy for which there is a higher risk of Down's syndrome, as in this case. A definitive result guides antenatal and postnatal management in cases where parents chose to continue a pregnancy when a chromosomal disorder has been confirmed.

4. D

Most women go into labour spontaneously before 42 weeks. Membrane sweeps and the use of prostaglandins to induce labour increase the likelihood of a vaginal delivery. The risk of stillbirth increases beyond 41 completed weeks. Induction of labour is therefore offered from 41 weeks. Caesarean delivery is not offered in the first instance to minimise the risk of complications in subsequent pregnancies. Women who choose to continue beyond 42 weeks are offered further tests of fetal wellbeing (ultrasound and cardiotocography).

5. E

A temperature of 38.5°C is a sign of possible infection. Sepsis is a leading cause of maternal death, so all signs of infections are acted on quickly to reduce the risk to mother and baby.

6. A

Calf tenderness and unilateral calf swelling may be symptoms of deep vein thrombosis. Venous thromboembolism is a leading cause of direct maternal death. Suggestive symptoms warrant urgent investigation and treatment.

Complications in early pregnancy

1. D

A missed miscarriage is when an early pregnancy stops developing but is not expelled. A fetal heartbeat should be visible from about 5 weeks, when the crown–rump length is 4–5 mm. If the crown–rump length is < 7 mm, the absence of a fetal heart beat cannot be definitively diagnosed so the woman is asked to return for a second scan 7–14 days later. A missed miscarriage is diagnosed at the second scan only if the embryo has not grown in size and a heartbeat is still not visible. At a crown–rump length of 11 mm, the expected value at about 7 weeks gestation, an absent fetal heart is diagnostic.

2. C

Women in early pregnancy and with localised pain and bleeding are presumed to have an ectopic pregnancy until proven otherwise. This patient is tachycardic and hypotensive, so she is likely to have a ruptured ectopic pregnancy and to have bled significantly. An emergency laparoscopy should be carried out to confirm the diagnosis and stop the bleeding. This procedure should not be delayed to await the result of other investigations or the outcome of methotrexate treatment.

3. A

Decreasing levels of hCG are consistent with a failing pregnancy. hCG levels in this patient are too low to determine the location of this pregnancy using ultrasound. All pregnancies of unknown location are presumed ectopic until proven otherwise. As with failing intrauterine pregnancies, ectopic pregnancies occasionally resolve with expectant management. Women with failing ectopic pregnancies are managed as outpatients if they are pain-free and haemodynamically stable. They are advised to return to the emergency room if they become unwell or develop any signs, such as dizziness or worsening pain, that may indicate a ruptured ectopic pregnancy.

4. **E**
This patient has severe ketonuria as a result of hyperemesis. The accompanying dehydration is unlikely to resolve without intravenous rehydration and parenteral antiemetics. Dietary advice, reassurance and oral antiemetics should be offered on discharge.

5. **C**
The ultrasound findings are consistent with a molar pregnancy. Molar pregnancies are managed by surgical evacuation. To confirm the diagnosis, the products of conception are sent for histology. In the UK, women with confirmed molar pregnancies are followed up by regional centres in London, Sheffield and Dundee, because there is a small risk of malignant change.

Complications in mid to late pregnancy

1. **A**
Management of gestational diabetes starts with home glucose monitoring and dietary modification; 80–90% of women are able to manage their blood glucose levels with these alone. Women who continue to have persistently high blood glucose levels despite these changes may be offered metformin and in rare instances insulin. A glucose tolerance test is offered 6 weeks postnatally to differentiate between those women with underlying type 2 diabetes from those with gestational diabetes.

2. **A**
This woman has signs and symptoms consistent with severe pre-eclampsia. She requires immediate admission to hospital and urgent review by a senior obstetrician. She should be offered one-to one-care in a critical care setting, medication to prevent an eclamptic seizure and have her blood pressure stabilised. Delivery should be considered once she is stable.

3. **D**
Itching is a common complaint and may be caused by obstetric cholestasis. Liver transaminases and bile acids should be measured. Of more concern is the history of reduced fetal movements, which must be investigated as a priority with fetal monitoring. Induction before 37 weeks is only considered if there is evidence of fetal compromise.

4. **C**
Polyhydramnios is often seen in women with gestational and pre-existing diabetes and is associated with an increased risk of preterm labour, placental abruption, post-partum haemorrhage and unstable lie. Pre-eclampsia, prelabour rupture of membranes and intrauterine growth restriction are causes of oligohydramnios.

5. **C**
Because this woman is obese, fetal growth monitoring by abdominal palpation and measurement of symphysis–fundal height is unlikely to be accurate. Women are advised to avoid actively trying to lose weight by dieting, but very overweight women may find that by adopting a healthy diet and lifestyle they lose a small amount of weight during pregnancy. Breastfeeding can help weight loss postnatally. Obese women are less likely to breastfeed and therefore should be offered opportunities to discuss its benefits and offered support whilst breastfeeding. Obesity in itself is not an indication for elective caesarean delivery, nor a contraindication to epidural anaesthesia.

6. **B**
Women with epilepsy should be encouraged to attend for preconception counselling to optimise epilepsy management before becoming pregnant. Most women with epilepsy present when already pregnant. These women should remain on the medication on which their condition has been stable before the pregnancy and take a higher daily dose of folic acid (5 mg). Women with epilepsy have the highest risk of seizures when tired and in pain, so early epidural is recommended to reduce the risk of a seizure intrapartum. Epilepsy is not an indication for early induction because it does not increase the risk of stillbirth. Lamotrigine is considered safe in breastfeeding and therefore breastfeeding is encouraged.

7. **E**
Antepartum haemorrhage is an obstetric emergency and is managed by an ABC approach. Obtaining intravenous access and taking blood samples allow intravenous fluids and blood products to be given, if needed. Resuscitation and stabilisation of the mother take priority over assessment of fetal well-being.

Complications in delivery and the postnatal period

1. **C**
Admission for observation and antenatal corticosteroids is offered to women with symptoms of threatened preterm labour who have a positive fibronectin test. Corticosteroids stimulate the production of fetal surfactant, reducing the risk of neonatal respiratory distress. Threatened preterm labour is not an indication for delivery unless there is evidence of fetal distress. Antibiotics are not indicated unless there is clinical evidence of infection.

2. **A**
During the established first stage of labour (4–10 cm dilated), dilation should progress at a rate of at least 0.5 cm/h. Progress should be plotted on a partogram. When progress does not occur as expected, action is required. In the first instance, if the membranes remain intact, amniotomy is carried out; this often increases the frequency and strength of contractions.

3. **C**
Augmentation of labour with intravenous synthetic oxytocin (Syntocinon) requires one-to-one care, close maternal and fetal observation and easy access to obstetric care if the fetus becomes distressed. This level of care is best provided by a consultant-led delivery suite.

4. **A**
The cardiotocography and fetal blood sampling show evidence of fetal compromise. Emergency delivery is advised to prevent neonatal morbidity and intrapartum stillbirth. As the woman is not fully dilated, assisted vaginal delivery is contraindicated. Spontaneous vaginal delivery is unlikely to occur within 30 minutes. Caesarean delivery is therefore recommended to expedite delivery.

5. **D**
Grand multiparity (having delivered 5 or more infants previously) and precipitous (rapid) delivery are risk factors for uterine atony (a failure of the uterus to contract). If the uterus does not contract sufficiently following delivery to compress the uterine blood vessels, excessive blood loss occurs. Uterine atony is the most common reason for post-partum haemorrhage. Atony should be suspected if the uterus feels soft and the fundus is still felt above the umbilicus following delivery.

6. **A**
Maternal sepsis is a leading cause of maternal mortality. Signs of sepsis, such as pyrexia and tachycardia, must be acted on quickly to prevent the mother's condition from deteriorating.

Reproductive endocrinology

1. **E**
Excessive exercise can cause a state of hypothalamic hypogonadotropic hypogonadism. A finding of low FSH and absent breast development is consistent with this diagnosis.

2. **A**
Women with polycystic ovary syndrome commonly have anovulatory cycles leading to subfertility. Clomifene is used to stimulate ovulation by inhibiting the negative feedback of oestrogen on the hypothalamus. When taken at the beginning of a menstrual cycle, it causes increased amounts of FSH and LH to be released. This results in a larger number of follicles to mature and rupture resulting in ovulation.

3. **C**
This patient's advanced growth and sexual development suggest precocious puberty, which can be delayed with the use of GnRH analogues. This allows time for the child's growth potential to be achieved, otherwise early fusion of the growth plates reduces the child's final height. Precocious puberty is usually idiopathic; rare causes include pituitary and ovarian tumours and genetic conditions such as McCune–Albright syndrome. Pelvic examination is not carried out in children. Bone radiographs are used principally to establish the child's bone age and the condition of the growth plates.

4. **C**
Galactorrhoea can be caused by a number of factors. Bilateral discharge suggests a central cause. Given the blurred vision and headaches,

an MRI of the head, along with measurement of serum prolactin concentration, should be performed to exclude a pituitary tumour.

5. **B**
Premenstrual dysphoric disorder can affect up to 2% of women. It can significantly reduce a woman's self-esteem and social functioning. Cognitive behavioural therapy, selective serotonin reuptake inhibitors and the combined oral contraceptive pill are all first-line treatments. Progesterone-only pills can worsen symptoms and are not advised.

6. **E**
There is a small increased risk of venous thromboembolism in women taking HRT; however, this is still less than the risk for women using the oral contraceptive pill or during pregnancy and the puerperium. The risks associated with HRT increase with age and duration of HRT, but it reduces the risk of osteoporosis and should be offered to women whose menopause is induced by surgery until the 'normal' age of menopause (about 50 years).

Fertility and contraception

1. **B**
Smokers >35 years old and women with BMI >35 kg/m² are at higher risk of venous thromboembolism on the combined oral contraceptive pill. Therefore the risks outweigh the benefits of this method of contraception. Other methods of contraception, such as the progestogen-only pill or non-hormonal methods, should be considered.

2. **A**
Use of the combined oral contraceptive pill results in a regular, lighter withdrawal bleed. Copper intrauterine devices are associated with heavier menstrual bleeding, which some women find troublesome. Progestogen-based contraceptives are associated with lighter bleeding, but this can be irregular. Some users of progestogen-based contraceptives become amenorrhoeic.

3. **E**
EllaOne (ulipristal acetate) is a selective progesterone receptor modulator that prevents pregnancy up to 5 days after unprotected intercourse in 95% of cases. It works by preventing ovulation and making the endometrium less receptive to implantation. Contraceptive services may be offered to under 16's without parental knowledge, provided that the Fraser guidelines are satisfied.

4. **E**
Vasectomy is 30 times less likely to fail and has a 20 times lower rate of complications than female sterilisation. Sterilisation should be regarded as a permanent procedure and cannot reliably be reversed. With the advent of long-acting reversible contraceptives with failure rates similar to those for surgical procedures, fewer women are choosing to undergo surgical sterilisation.

5. **D**
The combination of high FSH concentration and very low AMH concentration is a sign of low ovarian reserve. This does not preclude conceiving naturally or after induction of ovulation, but the chances of pregnancy are low. The best chance for a live birth is to consider IVF using a donor egg.

6. **D**
An estimated 1% of men have azoospermia (no sperm in their ejaculate). Azoospermia accounts for 10–15% of cases of male factor infertility. It can be caused by inadequate production of sperm or an obstruction of sperm transport. Investigating the cause of azoospermia by offering karyotyping, measurement of serum LH and FSH concentration and screening for cystic fibrosis may identify a genetic or treatable cause.

7. **C**
This patient has ovarian hyperstimulation syndrome. Women undergoing IVF treatment take gonadotrophins and hCG; a side effect of this is the overproduction of cytokines that promote vascular permeability. This causes a shift of fluid from the vascular space to the abdominal and pleural cavities. In severe cases, this results in ascites and pleural effusion that require hospital admission and supportive management in the form of pain management, thromboprophylaxis and, rarely, drainage of excess fluid.

Abnormal uterine bleeding

1. **A**
Secondary amenorrhea is the absence of menstruation for greater than 6 months which occurs after menarche and is unexplained by pregnancy, lactation, hysterectomy or the menopause. Intrauterine adhesions (Asherman's syndrome) resulting from surgical evacuation of the uterus are a cause of secondary amenorrhea. Hysteroscopy

is offered if intrauterine adhesions are suspected.

2. **C**
    The medical term for heavy menstrual bleeding is menorrhagia. Polymenorrhoea is the term for frequent menstrual cycles, i.e. cycles of less than 21 days.

3. **C**
    Endometrial ablation is a procedure that destroys the endometrial lining, thereby reducing menstrual bleeding. It can be carried out as a day case and in some cases while the patient is awake. It is less radical than hysterectomy and causes fewer surgical complications. Gonadotrophin-releasing hormone analogues are rarely used to treat excessive menstrual bleeding, because they cause menopausal adverse effects and bleeding returns to pretreatment levels on discontinuation of treatment.

4. **E**
    Laparoscopy is used to confirm the diagnosis of endometriosis and to simultaneously diathermy or resect endometriotic lesions that are causing pain. Hormonal therapy such as the combined oral contraceptive pill, progestogen-based contraceptives and GnRH analogues are effective treatments of endometriosis-related pain. Their contraceptive effect limits their use in women trying to conceive.

5. **C**
    Cervicitis and cervical excitation are signs of genital tract infection. Swabs should be taken for nucleic acid amplification testing for chlamydia and gonorrhoea, as well as for culture. Women with intrauterine devices are at the highest risk of pelvic infection in the first month after insertion. Thereafter, they have the same risk of infection as women without an intrauterine device.

6. **D**
    Women who present with post-menopausal bleeding, i.e. bleeding over a year since their last menses, require urgent referral for transvaginal ultrasound and biopsy. One in 10 women with these symptoms have an underlying malignancy. Treatment should not be instigated until after investigation.

Inflammatory and infective disorders

1. **E**
    Women with secondary dysmenorrhoea often have endometriosis. This can be managed medically with hormonal therapies and non-steroidal anti-inflammatories, or surgically with resection or ablation of deposits of endometriosis. Rarely, women may require a hysterectomy to manage their pain. Therefore it is necessary to discuss a woman's fertility intentions when devising a management plan. Hormonal therapies have a contraceptive effect and are not be suitable for women wishing to conceive immediately.

2. **D**
    A diagnosis of *Candida* infection (thrush) is based on clinical history and examination. *Candida* is a normal vaginal commensal, so genital swabs are usually unhelpful. Cultures may help guide treatment in cases of recurrent or resistant thrush. Antifungals such as topical clotrimazole in conjunction with oral fluconazole are first-line treatments.

3. **D**
    Gonorrhoeal infection is treated in conjunction with genitourinary medicine specialists because of multi-drug resistance. The first-line treatment for gonorrhoea is intramuscular ceftriaxone and oral azithromycin. Test of cure and partner notification is offered to ensure that the infection has been treated and the risk of transmission of resistant strains is mitigated. These are best provided by specialist services.

4. **B**
    Primary herpes simplex infection can cause florid painful ulcers and in severe cases urinary retention. Some patients require hospital admission for pain relief and catheterisation. Subsequent episodes tend to be less acute. Treatment with aciclovir early after development of symptoms can shorten the length of an episode.

5. **D**
    Preconceptual counselling in HIV-positive women with HIV-negative partners limits the risk of transmission of the virus to her partner and unborn child. These couples are offered

intrauterine insemination to reduce the risk of infection to the partner. Women with HIV with an undetectable viral load are offered vaginal delivery. In high-income countries, HIV-positive mothers are advised not to breastfeed.

6. **B**

Chlamydia is the most common cause of pelvic inflammatory disease leding to the development of tubo-ovarian abcesses. Gonorrhoea, *Gardenerella* and *Mycoplasma* are less common causes. *Candida* and group B *Streptococcus* are commensals commonly present on vaginal swabs and do not cause systemic disease.

Gynaecological tumours

1. **D**

Fibroids are benign tumours of the myometrium; they are present in nearly 50% of women. Most women have no problems related to their fibroids. The two main reasons for seeking help are heavy menstrual bleeding or pressure effects, such as constipation, urinary frequency and incomplete bladder voiding, related to the fibroids. Fibroid embolisation reduces blood flow to fibroids and shrinks them. This reduces bleeding and pressure symptoms, and is useful when dealing with multiple, large fibroids. Hysteroscopic resection of fibroids is more suited to single submucosal fibroids (fibroids protruding into the uterine cavity).

2. **E**

It is often not possible to determine the cause of chronic pelvic pain. Cysts are common findings on pelvic ultrasound in premenopausal women, but they may be incidental and unrelated to the pain. The finding of a unilocular cyst of < 5 cm with no solid elements or abnormal bloodflow is consistent with a functional cyst. These rarely cause pain, settle without treatment in premenopausal women and require no further investigation.

3. **D**

Women with a BRCA2 mutation have a 45% chance of developing breast cancer by the age of 70 and a 15% chance of developing ovarian cancer. This predisposition is inherited in an autosomal dominant manner. Women with a first degree relative who has a BRCA2 mutation have a 50% chance of carrying the gene. They are offered genetic testing and if positive are offered screening or prophylactic

surgery to reduce their risk of breast and ovarian cancer. Removal of tubes and ovaries reduces the risk of premenopausal breast cancer by 50% and the risk of ovarian cancer by 95%.

4. **C**

Mutations of DNA mismatch repair genes cause Lynch syndrome, a genetic predisposition to cancers; especially bowel and endometrial cancer. People with Lynch syndrome will be offered surveillance for colorectal cancers. Evidence of a link between Lynch syndrome and breast and ovarian cancer is much weaker; therefore screening and prophylactic surgery to prevent these cancers in people with Lynch syndrome is not recommended.

5. **D**

Surgical staging and histological findings guide discussions about prognosis and further management. In this case, the patient has stage 3 disease and requires adjuvant chemotherapy. Radiotherapy is not used as first-line treatment for ovarian cancer because the disease is often widespread rather than localised. To be effective large areas of the abdomen and pelvis would need to be treated, leading to an unacceptable level of gastrointestinal toxicity.

6. **C**

Bilateral painless leg swelling following lymphadenectomy (lymphoedema) affects over a third of patients who receive treatment for vulval cancer. The swelling is a consequence of impaired flow of lymph fluid back into the lymphatic system. Treatments include massage techniques such as manual lymphatic drainage, increased physical activity, leg elevation and compression stockings. Unlike in peripheral oedema, diuretics are unhelpful. Deep vein thromboses and cellulitis present acutely with unilateral, painful leg swelling. Nodal recurrence is unlikely a month after surgery.

Genital prolapse and incontinence

1. **E**

Stress incontinence can usually be diagnosed by history alone. Before surgery for stress incontinence is offered, urodynamics should be carried out to check for signs of outflow obstruction and detrusor overactivity. These signs may predict how effective a midurethral tape procedure will be in preventing urinary leakage, as well as the likelihood of needing to self-catheterise because of resultant outflow obstruction.

2. D
Frequency and nocturia are the most common symptoms of overactive bladder. Dysuria and haematuria suggest underlying infection, inflammation and in rare cases malignancy. Hesitancy and slow flow are usually associated with outflow obstruction.

3. B
This patient has symptoms of a posterior wall prolapse, which is associated with chronic constipation. Management includes physiotherapy, stool softeners and laxatives, vaginal pessaries or surgery. Decision-making regarding the most appropriate option is shared between the patient and the clinician. In this case, the woman has specified she wishes to avoid surgery and therefore a Gelhorn pessary would be best suited.

4. D
Mesh repair of pelvic organ prolapse is associated with a 2–15% risk of complications, including mesh erosion, dyspareunia and chronic pain. Women with mesh erosion can present with increased vaginal discharge, vaginal bleeding and dyspareunia. In postmenopausal patients, atrophic vaginitis, candida infection and bacterial vaginosis cause similar symptoms, but are likely to predate surgery. Mesh seen protruding through the vaginal wall at examination is diagnostic of mesh erosion.

Emergencies

1. C
Women attending with pain in early pregnancy are presumed to have an ectopic pregnancy until proven otherwise. The patient is tachycardic, so it would be unsafe to send her home; the tachycardia may be a sign of bleeding from a ruptured ectopic pregnancy. Admission to the ward for observation allows further assessment. In the event of deterioration overnight, she may require emergency surgery. However, if her condition improves, the location of the pregnancy can be determined by transvaginal ultrasound.

2. C
Constant abdominal pain and a rigid uterus suggest placental abruption. Women with

concealed abruptions may not have any vaginal bleeding. Shearing of the placenta away from the uterine wall can lead to fetal compromise. The baby should be delivered via the fastest mode of delivery. This allows haemostasis to be achieved as well as preventing further fetal injury. Risk factors for placental abruption include pre-eclampsia, smoking, hypertension, multiparity, maternal trauma and substance abuse.

3. A
Amniotic fluid embolism is a rare obstetric emergency caused by the passage of amniotic fluid or fetal cells into the maternal circulation via the placental bed. It presents with hypotension, cyanosis and altered mental state, and rapidly leads to cardiorespiratory collapse and coagulopathy. Amniotic fluid emboli are more likely to occur after a placental abruption.

4. C
Pre-eclampsia is a condition characterised by hypertension and proteinuria towards the end of pregnancy. The typical symptoms are headache, blurred vision and swelling. It is a systemic disease that affects multiple organ systems. Increased vascular permeability predisposes women with pre-eclampsia to pulmonary oedema, so large intravenous boluses of fluid must be avoided.

5. B
Blood pressure should be kept below 160/100 mmHg to reduce the risk of intracerebral bleeding. Ergometrine is a drug commonly used in conjunction with synthetic oxytocin (Syntocinon) to facilitate post-partum haemostasis. It can exacerbate hypertension, so is avoided in women with pre-eclampsia.

6. C
Shoulder dystocia occurs when the body of the fetus fails to deliver after delivery of the head, because the anterior shoulder of the fetus becomes impacted behind the maternal symphysis pubis. It is associated with neonatal morbidity and mortality, even when managed appropriately. Flexion and abduction of the mother's hips, positioning her thighs on to her abdomen, is known as the McRoberts manoeuvre. This simple non-invasive manoeuvre flattens the lumbrosacral angle and increases the anterior posterior diameter and has a success rate of up to 90%.

7. A
Cord prolapse occurs when the cord descends through the cervix past the

presenting part. Compression of the cord and reflex vasospasm restrict blood flow to and from the fetus, thereby causing asphyxia. Perinatal mortality of up to 9% has been recorded in births complicated by cord prolapse. Delivery must occur by the fastest means possible to minimise the risk of fetal hypoxia. In most cases this is a caesarean delivery. Synthetic oxytocin and voluntary pushing are avoided because they exacerbate cord compression.

8. B
There has been a dramatic increase in the number of women dying because of group A streptococcal infections; this was the cause of nearly 50% of deaths from maternal sepsis in the UK between 2006 and 2008. The most common site of post-partum infection is the genital tract. A history of a sore throat or cough is often associated with group A streptococcal sepsis. Handwashing before and after using the toilet reduces the transmission of this bacterium from the pharynx to the genital tract. Group B *Streptococcus* causes severe neonatal infections but rarely causes severe illness in adults.

Integrated care

1. D
Domestic violence affects one in four women and often increases in frequency during pregnancy. Ensuring the safety of the woman and her children is the first consideration. The advice of specialist advisers in safeguarding should be sought. They will facilitate the involvement of multiple agencies in preparing individualised plans to support women and children at high risk. Information sharing is therefore essential. Confidentiality cannot be absolute.

2. D
Women who have had female genital mutilation are identified as early as possible in pregnancy. This facilitates assessment and discussion regarding whether a defibulation would be required prior to or during labour to facilitate examination, allow application of a fetal scalp electrode where necessary and accommodate vaginal delivery. Women with FGM are managed in consultant-led units where medical assistance is more readily available. FGM is not an indication in itself for caesarean delivery. Where caesarean

delivery occurs before a defibulation can be performed, defibulation should be offered postnatally to reduce the risks of maternal and neonatal morbidity in subsequent deliveries. It is illegal to perform FGM or re-infibulate women in Europe, North America, Australasia and much of Africa.

3. E
The primary duty of the emergency room physician is to attend the medical needs of the patient. If it is safe to do so, the cleaning of wounds should be avoided to ensure that DNA evidence that may help in the prosecution of an offender is not disrupted. Gathering of such evidence is part of the remit of professionals trained in the assessment of the needs of victims of sexual assault.

4. E
Cervical cytology is inadequate if there are insufficient cells within the sample to assess. This can occur due to poor sampling technique, a lack of oestrogen or, rarely, in the presence of a necrotic tumour. In women with a normal-looking cervix, repeat cytology is offered 3 months after the initial test. Women who have had 3 inadequate cervical cytology results are referred to colposcopy.

5. A
Medications for chronic conditions such as hypercholesterolaemia should be discontinued. This reduces the burden of unnecessary medications and their potential adverse effects. End-of-life care focuses on providing relief from disease-associated symptoms that cause distress, and providing emotional support for the individual and their family.

6. C
Drying and warming a baby is usually enough to trigger respiratory effort in infants; it also prevents hypothermia. Cold babies have increased oxygen consumption and are more likely to become acidotic. During this time, the baby's colour, tone, respiration and heart rate are assessed. If there is no improvement, the baby's airway is then opened by placing its head in the neutral position and inflation breaths are given. Chest compressions are carried out only if the chest is moving adequately with the ventilation and the heart rate is fewer than 60 bpm. Suction should only be used on the rare occasion when material can be seen blocking the airway.

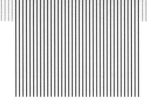

Index